GROUP

FITNESS

INSTRUCTOR

MANUAL

ACE's Guide

for Fitness

Professionals

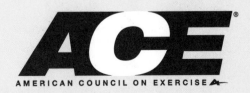

ACE
AMERICAN COUNCIL ON EXERCISE

Library of Congress Catalog Card Number: 99-069516

First edition
ISBN 1-890720-01-1
Copyright © 2000 American Council on Exercise® (ACE®)
Printed in the United States of America.

B C D E F

Distributed by:
American Council on Exercise
P. O. Box 910449
San Diego, CA 92191-0449
(858) 279-8227
(858) 279-8064 (FAX)
www.ACEfitness.org

Managing Editor: Daniel Green
Technical Editor: Richard T. Cotton, M.A.
Design: Karen McGuire
Production: Glenn Valentine
Publications Director: Christine J. Ekeroth
Associate Editor: Joy Keller
Index: Bonny McLaughlin
Copy Editor: Peter McCurdy
Proofreader: Mariapaz Ramos Englis

Acknowledgements:
Thanks to the entire American Council on Exercise staff for their
support and guidance through the process of creating this manual.

NOTICE

The fitness industry is ever-changing. As new research and clinical experience broaden
our knowledge, changes in programming and standards are required. The authors and
the publisher of this work have checked with sources believed to be reliable in their
efforts to provide information that is complete and generally in accord with the
standards accepted at the time of publication. However, in view of the possibility of
human error or changes in industry standards, neither the authors nor the publisher nor
any other party who has been involved in the preparation or publication of this work
warrants that the information contained herein is in every respect accurate or complete,
and they are not responsible for any errors or omissions or the results obtained from
the use of such information. Readers are encouraged to confirm the information
contained herein with other sources.

Reviewers

Stephen A. Black, M.Ed., P.T., A.T.C., C.P.T., opened Sports Performance in 1991, a company providing testing, coaching, educational, and consulting services to multisport and endurance athletes, corporations, clubs, and organizations, with offices located in Boulder, Colo., Orlando, Fla., and Austin, Texas. With close to 25 years experience in the sports medicine field as a physical therapist, athletic trainer, and certified personal trainer, Black assists with research and development of new products, and conducts ongoing research and educational programs.

Sabra Bonelli, M.S., is the head of the Fitness Programs Department for the Mission Valley YMCA in San Diego, Calif. Bonelli received her master's degree in exercise physiology from San Diego State University. She has authored several ACE *Fit Facts*, articles in *ACE Certified News* and, most recently, ACE's *Step Aerobics* specialty book.

Karen J. Calfas, Ph.D., is the director of Health Promotion at Student Health Services, San Diego State University. Dr. Calfas is assistant clinical professor in the Department of Family and Preventive Medicine of the School of Medicine at the University of California, San Diego.

Ann Cowlin, M.A., C.S.M., C.C.E., is assistant clinical professor at the Yale University School of Nursing and the movement specialist for the Yale University Athletic Department. Cowlin is the founder of Dancing Thru Pregnancy, Inc. and the author of the *U.S. Army Pregnancy Fitness Train-the-Trainer Program*.

Denise Fandel, M.S., A.T.C., has served as executive director of the NATA Board of Certification (NATABOC) since 1997. Prior to becoming executive director she served on the NATABOC Board for seven years and as president for four years. Previously, Fandel was the head athletic trainer at the University of Nebraska at Omaha as well as an instructor in the School of Health, Physical Education, and Recreation. She authored a chapter in the ACE *Personal Trainer Manual* and has been published in the *Journal of Athletic Training*.

Scott D. Flinn, M.D., is the director of the Sports Medicine Clinic at Marine Corps Recruit Depot, Parris Island, South Carolina. During his military career he worked with the U.S. Navy Seals for three years and in Italy as a family practice physician. He completed his Primary Care Sports Medicine Fellowship at San Diego Family and Sports Medicine Center affiliated with Stanford University. Dr. Flinn is board certified in family practice and has a Certificate of Added Qualification in Sports Medicine.

David L. Herbert, J.D., is senior partner of Herbert & Benson, Attorneys at Law, Canton, Ohio. He is the co-editor of the *Exercise Standards and Malpractice Reporter*, published by PRC Publishing, Inc. of Canton, Ohio. Herbert is a past presenter, consultant, or reviewer for ACSM, AFAA, ACE, NSCA, and a number of other organizations. He is the author or co-author of 10 books, a dozen book chapters, and more than 500 articles on a variety of topics dealing with the legal aspects of sport, sports medicine, negligence, exercise, and risk management.

Dale Huff, R.D., C.S.C.S., is co-owner of NutriFormance, a personal training and nutrition consulting company based in St. Louis, Missouri. Huff is a member of the *ACE FitnessMatters* Editorial Advisory Board and a frequent speaker and writer for IDEA and other professional organizations.

Irene Lewis McCormick, M.S., is an ACE, ACSM, and AFAA-certified group fitness instructor and personal trainer with more than 16 years experience She is a master trainer, ACE faculty member, national fitness lecturer, presenter, and educator, and has contributed to *ACE Certified News*, *Better Homes & Gardens*, *ACE Fitness-Matters*, and several specialty and instructional manuals. She is also the host of her own local cable fitness show. Lewis McCormick currently acts as the fitness program director at Ames Racquet & Fitness Center in Ames, Iowa and is the spokesperson for the Better Homes & Gardens fitness website "The Personal Trainer" available on-line at www.bhglive.com.

John P. Porcari, Ph.D., is a professor in the Department of Exercise and Sports Science and executive director of the La Crosse Exercise and Health Program at the University of Wisconsin – La Crosse. He is a fellow of the American College of Sports Medicine and the American Association of Cardiovascular and Pulmonary Rehabilitation (AACVPR) and is a vice president on the Executive Board of AACVPR. Dr. Porcari's research interests have focused on the acute and training responses to exercising on a variety of exercise modalities, particularly new products on the market. He has more than 30 peer-reviewed publications and 60 national presentations.

Brad A. Roy, Ph.D., F.A.C.S.M., is the director of The Summit, Kalispell Regional Medical Center's facility for health promotion and fitness. He has more than 20 years experience in the field of clinical exercise physiology and serves as a reviewer for a number of journals.

Steve Sanchez, M.S.P.T., is the director of Physical Therapy at the Head, Neck, & Spine Center of San Diego in La Jolla, California. He is also a physical therapist at the University of California, San Diego Medical Center.

Larry S. Verity, Ph.D., F.A.C.S.M., is a professor of exercise physiology in the Department of Exercise and Nutritional Sciences at San Diego State University. He is a fellow of the American College of Sports Medicine and is a certified Exercise Specialist. He has served as an editorial consultant for ACE and has published refereed manuscripts and chapters on fitness assessment and screening.

Table of Contents

Foreword

Today we find ourselves at a crossroads in the fitness revolution that began more than a quarter of a century ago.

Despite increasing data to support the importance and value of exercise, and ongoing coordinated efforts of organizations such as the Centers for Disease Control and Prevention, ACE, and others, a mere 20% of the U.S. population exercise regularly. The task of motivating millions of people to exercise is proving increasingly difficult as labor-saving devices and sedentary entertainments become more ubiquitous.

However, of all the variables that can affect exercise compliance, perhaps the most important is the fitness professional. Research bears out that qualified, enthusiastic group fitness instructors can influence exercise compliance among participants more than any other factor. How is this best accomplished? Through education and certification that ensure instructors are qualified to teach safe and effective exercise. Teaching a group exercise class is not just a matter of leading others through a series of choreographed or prescribed movements. It's about recommending progressive exercise to minimize injury, designing a variety of routines that are fun and challenging, establishing realistic goals, providing periodic evaluations, keeping adequate records, and recognizing accomplishments through rewards and recognition.

It is the drive and desire to motivate millions of people to exercise that continues to spur the growth of the fitness industry. The American Council on Exercise has demonstrated its commitment to this growth through the development of new products and the formation of key strategic alliances, such as the one forged with the International Health and Racquet Sports Association (IHRSA), which will serve to increase both the number of health-club members to 100 million by 2010 as well as the demand for ACE certification.

By the year 2005, the U.S. Department of Labor predicts a 14% to 24% increase in the number of people employed as fitness professionals. With this growth come innumerable opportunities for those who choose to be a part of a profession dedicated to the health and well-being of others. I urge you to stay in touch with the American Council on Exercise. You are our eyes and ears in the trenches. And to quote Helen Keller, "We can do so much alone, but so much more together."

*Ken Germano
Executive Director
American Council on Exercise*

Introduction

The Group Fitness Instructor Manual: ACE's Guide for Fitness Professionals was created, in part, in response to the rapid growth of today's fitness industry. Being a group fitness instructor is no longer just about teaching aerobics. The modern group fitness instructor may be expected to teach a variety of specialties, such as step, indoor cycling, yoga or cardiokickboxing. And yet the need for a basic understanding of exercise science and principles remains the same.

This new manual offers the most current, complete picture of the foundational knowledge, instructional techniques, and professional responsibilities group fitness instructors need to teach safe and effective exercise. Designed to serve as a study aid for the newly revised Group Fitness Instructor Certification Exam, it is also a comprehensive resource for new and veteran group fitness instructors.

It is important to note, however, that the scope of information presented in this manual will not exactly match the scope of information tested in the ACE certification exam. Exam candidates should refer to the Exam Content Outline in Appendix B for a detailed syllabus of information covered in the certification exam. In addition, ACE acknowledges various experience and skill levels among group fitness instructor exam candidates. As such, we encourage candidates lacking the practical skills and experience related to teaching group fitness classes to take advantage of ACE-approved training programs to prepare for the ACE examination.

The 11 chapters that comprise the *Group Fitness Instructor Manual: ACE's Guide for Fitness Professionals* represent a comprehensive review of the knowledge group fitness instructors need to perform their jobs with a basic level of competency. The first two chapters, Exercise Physiology and Fundamentals of Anatomy and Applied Kinesiology, feature the basics of cardiorespiratory, metabolic, neuromuscular, and environmental exercise physiology, as well as a detailed review of the cardiorespiratory and nervous systems and musculoskeletal anatomy. In addition, a thorough overview of basic nutrition as it applies to both health maintenance and weight control is presented in Chapter 3.

Chapters 4, 5, and 6 offer the "nuts and bolts" of the group fitness instructor profession. Chapter 4, Health Screening, presents the most up-to-date information related to the preexercise screening of fitness clients. In Chapters 5 and 6, class format, teaching strategies, and music selection are discussed and then implemented in a detailed review of the critical components of designing and leading a group fitness class.

Catering to individual needs of exercisers is, and will continue to be, a challenging task for group fitness instructors. Chapter 8, Disabilities and Health Limitations, and Chapter 9, Exercise and Pregnancy, each examine a wide range of issues related to the varied needs of these special populations.

The final two chapters provide information on the prevention, detection, and treatment of musculoskeletal injuries, basic emergency procedures, and the legal and professional responsibilities of group fitness instructors. While group fitness instructors may not need to draw upon this information on a daily basis, sound knowledge, judgment, and application of these principles are essential to your future success in this dynamic field.

The American Council on Exercise

Chapter 1

Christine L. Wells, Ph.D., professor emeritus of exercise science and physical education at Arizona State University, is a widely recognized authority on women and sports. She has been president of the Research Consortium of the American Alliance for Health, Physical Education, Recreation, and Dance (AAHPERD), a member of the Board of Trustees and vice-president of Education of the American College of Sports Medicine (ACSM), president of the Southwest Chapter of the ACSM, and a member of the IDEA Board of Advisors. Dr. Wells is the author of *Women, Sport, and Performance: A Physiological Perspective*.

John P. Porcari, Ph.D., is a professor in the Department of Exercise and Sports Science and executive director of the La Crosse Exercise and Health Program at the University of Wisconsin – La Crosse. He is a fellow of the American College of Sports Medicine and the American Association of Cardiovascular and Pulmonary Rehabilitation (AACVPR) and is a vice president on the Executive Board of AACVPR. Dr. Porcari's research interests have focused on the acute and training responses to exercising on a variety of exercise modalities, particularly new products on the market. He has more than 30 peer-reviewed publications and 60 national presentations.

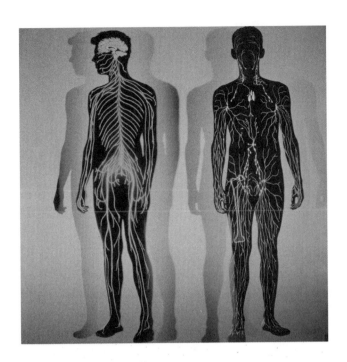

Exercise
Physiology

By Christine L. Wells and John P. Porcari

The structure and function of the human body allow an extraordinarily wide range of possible movements requiring very complex interactions of neuromuscular coordination and metabolism. For example, a pole vaulter needs to be able to couple the coordination and agility to maneuver over the crossbar with the explosive burst of energy needed to sprint down the runway. At the other extreme, an ultramarathoner needs to be able to generate low levels of energy repetitively for prolonged periods of time.

The study of **exercise physiology** allows us to understand how the body responds to the varied demands placed on it by exercise. It is essential for the group fitness instructor to understand the basics of exercise physiology so he or she can design safe and effective exercise programs.

Physical Fitness

Before we begin discussing the specific effects of exercise on the body, it is important to realize there are several areas that contribute to overall "**physical fitness**" and, hence, different body systems that need to be trained appropriately. Physical fitness is a complex concept that has different meanings to different people. In this manual, physical fitness refers to the **capacity** of the heart, blood vessels, lungs, and muscles to function at a high level of efficiency. The person who is physically fit has an enhanced functional capacity that allows for a high quality of life. Although a somewhat vague phrase, quality of life generally implies an overall positive feeling and enthusiasm for life and the ability to do enriching and enjoyable activities without fatigue or exhaustion from routine and required activities. A high level of physical fitness enables people to perform their required daily tasks without fatigue, thus enabling them to participate in additional pleasurable activities for personal enjoyment. As physiological or functional capacity increases, one's capacity for physical activity or exercise also increases. In other words, a person can lift heavier weights or run farther or faster — in short, can participate in more strenuous activities. Being physically fit makes possible a lifestyle that the sedentary cannot enjoy. Increased physical fitness is often reflected by physiological adaptations, such as a lowered heart rate during a standardized exercise test or an improved ability to mobilize and use body fuels. A high level of physical fitness implies optimal physical performance and good health.

There are five major components of physical fitness. It should be noted that the components are health-related as opposed to skill-related. The development of a high degree of **motor skill** is sometimes confused with physical fitness, but these two attributes are not necessarily related to each other. A highly skilled person may have a low level of physical fitness, and the reverse may also be true. Motor skill (sometimes referred to as motor performance or motor fitness) is thought to be related to such attributes as agility, balance, and coordination — terms that defy precise definition and do not necessarily affect a person's overall health or quality of life.

The five components of physical fitness are as follows:

1. **Muscular strength**. The maximal force a muscle or muscle group can exert during contraction. Muscular strength is essential for normal everyday functioning, as we all are required to lift and carry objects (e.g., groceries, suitcases) in our daily lives. Adequate muscular strength may even become more important as we age. In many cases, for instance, the elderly are not able to walk up stairs or even get up out of a chair due to inadequate strength in the lower extremities.

2. **Muscular endurance**. The ability of a muscle or muscle group to exert force against a resistance over a sustained period of time. Muscular endurance is assessed by measuring the length of time (duration) a muscle can exert force without fatigue or by measuring the number of times (**repetitions**) that a given task can be performed without fatigue. Many everyday activities require a significant amount of muscular endurance (e.g., walking up stairs, shoveling snow).

3. **Cardiovascular** or **cardiorespiratory endurance** (sometimes referred to as

aerobic power or **aerobic fitness**). The capacity of the heart, blood vessels, and lungs to deliver oxygen and nutrients to the working muscles and tissues during sustained exercise and to remove the metabolic waste products that would result in fatigue. Efficient functioning of the cardiorespiratory system is essential for optimal enjoyment of such physical activities as walking, running, swimming, and cycling. The performance of regular, moderately intense aerobic exercise is the key to developing and maintaining an efficient cardiorespiratory system.

4. **Flexibility**. The ability to move joints through their normal full **range of motion (ROM)**. An adequate degree of flexibility is important to prevent musculoskeletal injuries and to maintain correct body posture.

5. **Body composition**. Body composition refers to the makeup of the body considered as a two-component model: **lean body mass** and **body fat**. The lean body mass consists of the muscles, bones, nervous tissue, skin, blood, and organs. These tissues have a high metabolic rate and make a direct and positive contribution to energy production during exercise. Body fat, or **adipose tissue**, represents that component of the body whose primary role is to store energy for later use. Body fat does not contribute in a direct sense to exercise performance. Body fat is further classified into **essential body fat** and storage body fat. Essential body fat is that amount of fat thought to be necessary for maintenance of life and reproductive function; 3% to 5% body fat is generally thought to be essential for men, and 8% to 12% for women. (Percent body fat refers to the percentage of the total body weight that is fat.) Storage fat is contained in the fatty deposits or fat pads found under the skin (**subcutaneous fat**) and deep inside the body (**internal fat**). A large amount of storage fat is considered excess fat and results in the condition referred to as **obesity**.

Bioenergetics of Exercise

Our body's cells require a continuous supply of energy in order to function. Ultimately, the food we eat supplies this energy. However, our cells do not directly use the energy contained in the food we eat rather, they need a chemical compound called **adenosine triphosphate**, or **ATP**. ATP is the immediately usable form of chemical energy needed for all cellular function, including muscular contraction.

The foods we eat are made up of carbohydrates, fats, and proteins. The process of digestion breaks these nutrients down to their simplest components (**glucose**, **fatty acids**, and **amino acids**), which are absorbed into the blood and transported to metabolically active cells, such as muscle, nerve, or liver cells. These components either immediately enter a metabolic pathway to produce ATP or are stored in body tissues for later use.

For example, excess glucose will be stored as **glycogen** in muscle or liver cells. Fatty acids that are not immediately used for ATP production will be stored as adipose tissue (body fat). In contrast, relatively little of the protein (amino acids) one eats is used for energy production. Instead, it is used for the growth or repair of cellular structures or is excreted in our waste products. Figure 1.1 summarizes the fate of the carbohydrates, fats, and protein that we eat.

Figure 1.1

Foods consumed ultimately produce the chemical energy required for cellular function.

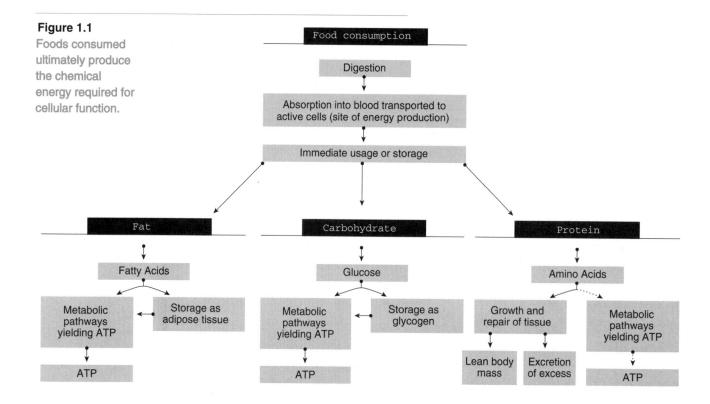

Stored ATP — The Immediate Energy Source

ATP is a complicated chemical structure made up of a substance called adenosine and three simpler groups of atoms called phosphate groups (P). Special high-energy bonds ($\frown$) exist between two of the phosphate groups (Figure 1.2a). Breaking the terminal phosphate bond releases energy (E) that the cell uses directly to perform its cellular function (Figure 1.2b). The specific cellular function performed depends on the cell type. In a muscle cell, the breakdown of ATP results in the mechanical work known as muscular contraction.

While ATP can be stored within the cells, the amount stored and immediately available for muscle contraction is extremely limited, sufficient for only a few seconds of muscular work. Therefore, ATP must be continuously resynthesized. ATP can be resynthesized in several ways — immediately with the phosphagen system, somewhat more slowly with the anaerobic production of ATP from carbohydrate, or still more slowly with the aerobic production of ATP from either carbohydrate or fat.

The Phosphagen System

Creatine phosphate (CP) is another high-energy phosphate compound found within muscle cells. Together, ATP and CP are referred to as the **phosphagens**. When

Figure 1.2

Breakdown of the ATP molecule

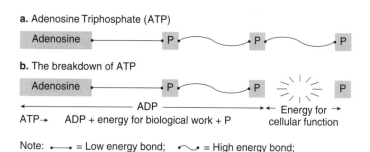

a. Adenosine Triphosphate (ATP)

| Adenosine | P | P | P |

b. The breakdown of ATP

| Adenosine | P | P | P |

← ——————— ADP ——————— → ← Energy for → cellular function

ATP→   ADP + energy for biological work + P

Note: •—— = Low energy bond; $\frown$ = High energy bond;
P = Phosphate group; ADP = Adenosine Diphosphate

ATP is broken down for muscular contraction, it can be resynthesized very quickly from the breakdown of CP. The energy released from breaking the high-energy phosphate bond in CP is used to reform ATP from **adenosine diphosphate** (**ADP**) and P (the phosphate group broken off from ATP), by-products of the initial reaction. This process is shown in Figure 1.3.

The total amount of ATP and CP stored in muscle is very small, and thus the amount of energy available for muscular contraction is extremely limited. In fact, there is probably enough energy available from the phosphagens for only about 10 seconds of all-out exertion. However, this energy is instantaneously available for muscular contraction, and therefore is essential at the onset of physical activity and during short-term, high-intensity activities such as sprinting 50 yards, performing a weight-lifting movement, or leaping across a stage.

Anaerobic Production of ATP from Carbohydrate

The anaerobic production of ATP from carbohydrate sources is known as **anaerobic glycolysis**. **Anaerobic** literally means "without the presence of oxygen," and **glycolysis** refers to the breakdown of glucose or its storage form, glycogen. Thus, anaerobic glycolysis is a metabolic pathway that does not require oxygen whose purpose is to transfer the bond energy contained in glucose (or glycogen) to the formation of ATP.

Anaerobic glycolysis is capable of producing ATP quite rapidly and thus is required when energy (ATP) is needed to perform activities requiring large bursts of energy over somewhat longer periods of time than the phosphagen system will allow. This metabolic pathway occurs within the cyto-

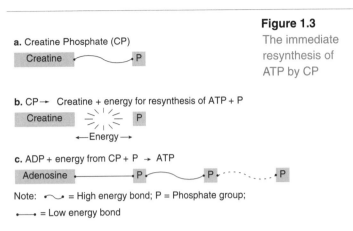

Figure 1.3
The immediate resynthesis of ATP by CP

plasm of the cell and involves the incomplete breakdown of glucose (or glycogen) to a simpler substance called pyruvic acid. If exercise intensity is very high and adequate amounts of oxygen are not available, pyruvic acid is converted into **lactic acid** (**LA**), as indicated in Figure 1.4a.

The formation of LA poses a significant problem because when it accumulates in

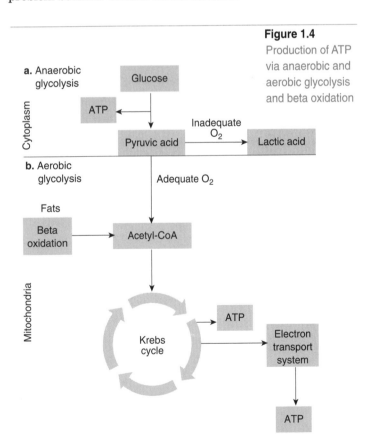

Figure 1.4
Production of ATP via anaerobic and aerobic glycolysis and beta oxidation

large amounts it is associated with changes in muscle pH and eventual muscle fatigue. If the removal of lactic acid by the circulatory system cannot keep pace with its production in the active muscles, temporary muscle fatigue occurs with painful symptoms usually referred to as "the burn." Thus, anaerobic glycolysis can only be used to a limited extent during sustained activity and provides the main source of ATP for high-intensity exercise lasting up to a maximum of approximately 3 minutes.

Aerobic Production of ATP from Carbohydrate or Fat

The aerobic production of ATP is used for activities requiring sustained energy production. Since **aerobic** literally means "in the presence of oxygen," aerobic metabolic pathways require a continuous supply of oxygen delivered by the circulatory system. Without oxygen, these pathways fail to produce ATP.

This metabolic pathway, called **aerobic glycolysis** or **oxidative glycolysis**, occurs within highly specialized cell structures called the mitochondria. **Mitochondria**, often called the powerhouses of the cell, contain specific enzymes (**oxidative enzymes**) needed by the cell to utilize oxygen. This highly efficient metabolic process is limited mainly by the capacity of the cardiorespiratory system to deliver oxygen to the active cells. When sufficient oxygen is available, pyruvic acid is converted into acetyl-CoA, which enters the Krebs cycle and the electron transport system, producing substantial amounts of ATP (Figure 1.4b).

Aerobic pathways are also available to break down fatty acids (the digested component of dietary fat) for the production of ATP. This metabolic pathway, called fatty acid, or **beta oxidation** (Figure 1.4b), also occurs within the mitochondria and requires a continuous supply of oxygen (as does aerobic glycolysis) as it proceeds through the Krebs cycle and electron transport system. The aerobic metabolism of fat yields a very large amount of ATP; therefore, fat is said to have a high caloric density. A calorie is a unit of energy. Fat yields 9 kilocalories of energy per gram compared to 4 kilocalories of energy per gram from glucose. That is why body fat is such an excellent source of stored energy.

At rest, the body uses both glucose and fatty acids for energy production via aerobic pathways. The cardiorespiratory system can easily supply the oxygen necessary for this low rate of energy metabolism. With exercise, however, supplying the required amount of oxygen rapidly enough becomes more difficult. Because glucose metabolism requires less oxygen than fatty acid metabolism, the body will use more glucose for energy production and less fat as exercise intensity increases. Table 1.1 provides a summary and comparison of the aerobic and anaerobic systems of ATP production.

Muscles and Metabolism

Our muscles are composed of several kinds of fibers that differ in their ability to utilize the metabolic pathways outlined above. **Fast twitch (FT) fibers** are rather poorly equipped in terms of the oxygen delivery system, but have an outstanding capacity for the phosphagen system and a very high capacity for anaerobic glycolysis. Therefore, fast twitch fibers are specialized for anaerobic metabolism. They are recruited by the nervous system predominantly for rapid, powerful movements such as jumping, throwing, and sprinting.

Table 1.1
Comparison of Anaerobic and Aerobic Systems of ATP Production

Anaerobic System	Rate of ATP Production	Substrate(s)	Capacity of System	Major Limitation(s)	Major Use
Phosphagens (stored ATP & CP)	Very rapid rate	Creatine phosphate (CP)	Very limited ATP production	Very limited supply of CP	Very high-intensity, short-duration sprint activities. Predominates during activities of 1–10 seconds.
Anaerobic glycolysis (GLU → ATP + LA)	Rapid metabolic rate	Blood glucose Glycogen	Limited ATP production	Lactic acid by-product causes rapid fatigue	High-intensity, short duration activities. Predominates during activities of 1–3 minutes.

Aerobic System	Rate of ATP Production	Substrate(s)	Capacity of System	Major Limitation(s)	Major Use
Aerobic glycolysis	Slow metabolic rate	Blood glucose Glycogen	Unlimited ATP production	Relatively slow rate of oxygen delivery to cells Glycogen storage	Lower intensity, longer duration, endurance activities. Predominates during activities longer than 3 minutes.
Fatty acid oxidation	Slow metabolic rate	Fatty acids	Unlimited ATP production	Relatively slow rate of oxygen delivery to cells Large amount of O_2 needed	Lower intensity, longer duration, endurance activities. Fatty acid oxidation predominates after about 20 minutes of continuous activity.

Note: GLU = Glucose; LA = Lactic acid; CP = Creatine Phosphate

Slow twitch (ST) fibers, on the other hand, are exceptionally well equipped for oxygen delivery and have a high quantity of aerobic, or oxidative, enzymes. Although they do not have a highly developed mechanism for use of the phosphagens or anaerobic glycolysis, ST fibers have a large number of mitochondria and, consequently, are particularly well designed for use of aerobic glycolysis and **fatty acid oxidation**. Thus, ST fibers are recruited primarily for low-intensity, longer-duration activities such as walking, jogging, and swimming.

Persons who excel in activities characterized by sudden bursts of energy, but who tire relatively rapidly, probably have a high percentage of fast twitch fibers. Persons who are best at lower-intensity, endurance activities probably have a large percentage of slow twitch fibers. Most people have roughly equal percentages of both fiber types. There are also a number of "intermediate" muscle fibers that have a fairly high capacity for both fast anaerobic and slow aerobic movements.

Muscle fiber distribution (fast twitch, intermediate, or slow twitch) is determined to a large extent by genetic makeup. This is not to say, however, that metabolic capacity is unresponsive to activity lifestyle. All three types of muscle fiber are highly trainable; that is, they are capable of adapting to the specific metabolic demands placed on them. If a person regularly engages in low-intensity endurance activities, improvement is seen in aerobic capacity. Although all three types of muscle fiber will show some improvement in aerobic ability, the ST fibers will be most responsive to this kind of training and will show the largest improvement in aerobic capacity. If, on the other hand, short-duration, high-intensity exercise such as interval training is pursued, other metabolic pathways will be emphasized, and the capabilities of the FT fibers to perform anaerobically will be enhanced. ST fibers will be less responsive to this kind of training.

It is important for group fitness instructors to have a thorough understanding of the different metabolic systems in order to prescribe specific exercise programs that will enable participants to achieve desired results. As discussed, exercise intensity and duration is directly related to the continuum of metabolic pathways and movement patterns. For example, prescribing quick, explosive movements specific to the use of the phosphagens and anaerobic glycolysis will be ineffective if the goal of the exercise program is to develop cardiorespiratory endurance. This concept, known as **exercise specificity**, is probably the single most important principle of exercise physiology.

The Neuromuscular System

Group fitness instructors need to understand how a motor skill is executed. To do so requires a basic appreciation of the neuromuscular system, which includes both the nervous and musculoskeletal systems. The nervous system is responsible for coordinating movement, while the musculoskeletal system is responsible for carrying out the movement.

Basic Organization of the Nervous System

The basic anatomical unit of the nervous system is the **neuron,** or nerve cell. There are two kinds of neurons, sensory and motor. **Sensory neurons** convey electrical impulses from sensory organs in the periphery (such as the skin) to the spinal cord and the brain (called the **central nervous system**, or **CNS**). **Motor neurons** conduct impulses from the CNS to the periphery. Because the motor neurons carry electrical impulses from the CNS to the muscle cells, they signal the muscles to contract or to relax and, therefore, they regulate muscular movement. The endings of the motor neuron connect, or synapse, with muscle cells in the periphery of the body. This motor neuron–muscle cell synapse is called the neuromuscular junc-

Figure 1.5

Basic anatomical structure of a neuron (or nerve cell) and motor end plate

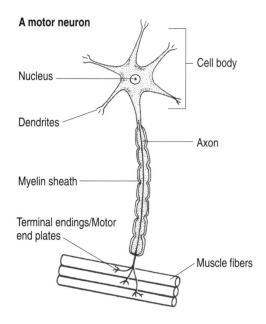

A motor neuron

Nucleus

Dendrites

Myelin sheath

Terminal endings/Motor end plates

Cell body

Axon

Muscle fibers

tion, or **motor end plate**. (Figure 1.5 shows a motor neuron and motor end plate.) The basic functional unit of the neuromuscular system is the **motor unit**, which consists of one motor neuron and the muscle cells that it innervates. Motor units are arranged according to muscle fiber type. A neuron capable of conducting nervous impulses very rapidly synapses with the cells of fast twitch muscle fibers. The cells of slow twitch muscle fibers are controlled by somewhat slower-conducting neurons.

Basic Organization of the Muscular System

The skeletal muscle is a complex tissue and is described only briefly here. Basically, muscle is entirely surrounded by a layer of connective tissue called the **epimysium**. At the ends of a muscle the epimysium thickens into a **tendon** that connects the muscle to the bone. Sublayers of connective tissue further divide each muscle into bundles of individual muscle cells, and finally each in-

dividual muscle fiber is covered by the **endomysium** (Figure 1.6).

An individual muscle cell is composed of many thread-like protein strands, called **myofibrils**, that contain the **contractile proteins**. The basic functional unit of the myofibril is the **sarcomere.** Within the sarcomere are two protein **myofilaments**: the thick myofilament is **myosin**, and the thinner myofilament is **actin** (see Figure 1.6). The myosin and actin myofilaments are arranged to interdigitate in a prescribed, regular way, revealing a pattern of alternating light and dark bands, or striations, within the sarcomere. Tiny projections called cross-bridges extend from the myosin myofilaments toward the actin myofilaments.

According to the **sliding filament theory**, muscular contraction occurs when the cross-bridges extending from the myosin myofilaments attach (or couple) to the actin myofilaments and pull them over the myosin myofilaments. As the cross-bridges produce tension, the muscle shortens. The actual

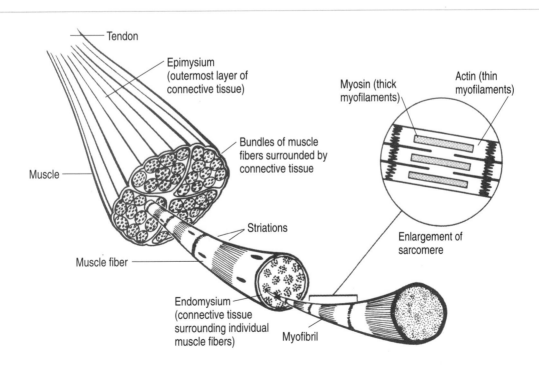

Figure 1.6
Organization of muscle

Tendon

Epimysium (outermost layer of connective tissue)

Muscle

Bundles of muscle fibers surrounded by connective tissue

Striations

Muscle fiber

Endomysium (connective tissue surrounding individual muscle fibers)

Myofibril

Myosin (thick myofilaments)

Actin (thin myofilaments)

Enlargement of sarcomere

Figure 1.7
The sliding filament theory

a. Myofibril at rest.

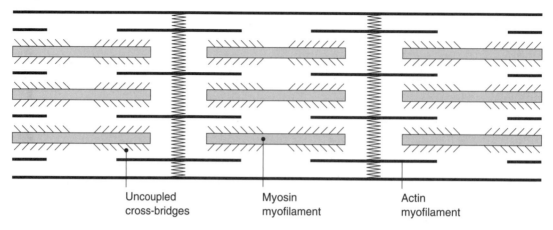

Uncoupled cross-bridges

Myosin myofilament

Actin myofilament

b. Contracted myofibril.

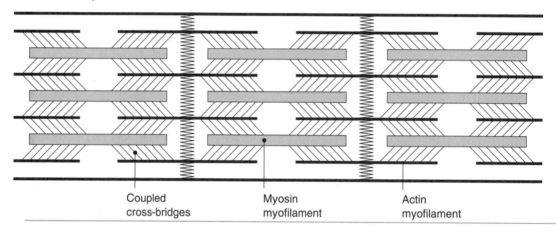

Coupled cross-bridges

Myosin myofilament

Actin myofilament

muscle shortening occurs as the actin myofilaments are pulled toward the center of the sarcomere, and the sarcomere shortens (Figure 1.7). The coupling of myosin and actin and the shortening process are dependent upon the breakdown of ATP for energy.

Types of Muscular Contraction

What has been described above is a form of **isotonic** muscular contraction, in that there is joint movement when the muscle is stimulated. Tension (or force) develops throughout the muscle as it contracts, but the tension changes with the total length of the muscle and the angle of the joint. The greatest force is generated at the muscle's optimal length, where the actin and myosin myofilaments are aligned so that the largest number of cross-bridges between the myofilaments is activated simultaneously. At all other lengths, fewer cross-bridges are simultaneously coupled to actin myofilaments and, therefore, less force can be developed. The relationship of muscle tension (force) to muscle length is illustrated in Figure 1.8a.

There are two types of isotonic contraction: **concentric** and **eccentric**. A concentric contraction occurs when the muscle shortens when it is stimulated. An eccentric contraction is the opposite of concentric contraction in that the muscle develops tension as it *lengthens* against a resistance (rather than as it *shortens* against a resistance). This is sometimes called "negative work." If we consider walking up and down a flight of stairs as an example, going up the stairs requires the quadricep muscle group to contract concentrically (shortening and lifting the weight of the body *against* gravity), while going down the stairs requires the quadriceps to contract eccentrically (slowly lengthening and lowering the weight of the body *with* gravity). In typical weight-lifting movements, eccentric contractions usually follow concentric contractions.

Isometric muscular contractions occur when actual muscle shortening does not take place. Since no joint movement occurs, this type of contraction is sometimes referred to as a *static* contraction. An example of an isometric muscle contraction is holding a weight at arm's length or attempting to move an immovable object (e.g., exerting force outward against a door frame). Isometric exercises are often used during physical rehabilitation and physical therapy when a joint has been injured. By contracting the muscles isometrically, an individual can maintain or increase muscular strength without aggravating the injured joint. It should be remembered, however, that, since no joint movement is taking place, increases in strength are very specific to the joint angle at which the contractions are carried out and that contractions should be carried out at several joint angles.

Isokinetic contractions, in outward appearance, look much like isotonic contractions (Figure 1.8b). In this kind of contraction, however, tension within the muscle changes throughout the range of motion. To accomplish an isokinetic contraction, special equipment is required to alter the resistance offered the muscle as it contracts at a constant velocity. This approach is sometimes referred to as "accommodating-resistance" or "variable-resistance" exercise. Isokinetic

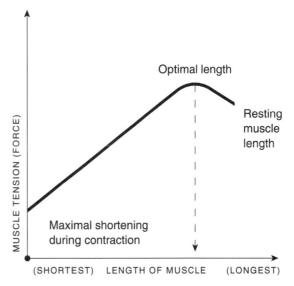

a. Isotonic contraction

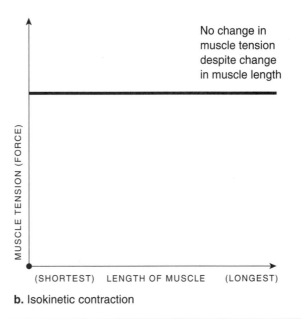

b. Isokinetic contraction

Figure 1.8
The muscle length-tension curve during two forms of contraction

exercise enables maximal tension to develop in a muscle throughout its entire range of motion; with isotonic exercise, the muscle can develop maximal tension only at its optimal length.

Muscular Strength and Endurance

Resistance training programs can be designed to improve either muscular strength or muscular endurance. While there is considerable overlap in the training responses, there are several key differences. The sections below discuss how the principle of **specificity** applies to these two components of physical fitness.

Muscular Strength

Strength refers to the maximal tension or force produced by a muscle or muscle group. Strength is usually measured by determining how much weight can be lifted in a single effort. The one-repetition maximum (1 RM) test is determined through a trial-and-error procedure using either free weights (barbells and weights) or special machines (e.g., dynamometers, Hydra-gym, Nautilus, Universal apparatus). Most often 1 RM tests are completed for the following muscle groups: (a) the bench press for the muscles of the chest and upper arms; (b) the arm curl for the muscles on the anterior aspect of the upper arms; and (c) the leg press for the muscles of the upper legs and hips.

Programs designed specifically to develop muscular strength should use a high-intensity (80% – 90% of 1 RM), low-repetition format (less than eight repetitions), and the movements should be performed carefully at a controlled speed so that there is a consistent application of force throughout the movement. Good posture and body mechanics are extremely important in order to avoid injury, as is breathing properly and avoiding the **valsalva maneuver**. The valsalva maneuver occurs when the breath is held while a great deal of force is exerted. When the breath is held, the glottis in the back of throat is closed. Exerting force with the glottis closed results in an increase in pressure within the chest cavity (intrathoracic pressure). This increase in pressure squeezes down on the large veins in the

chest cavity, impeding venous return (blood flow back to the heart). If blood flow back to the heart is impeded, the heart has less blood to pump out. As a consequence, there is less flow of blood and oxygen to the brain, and sometimes dizziness and fainting may occur. It is generally recommended that people exhale when they are performing the concentric phase of a lift and inhale during the eccentric phase.

Movements requiring a high level of strength are performed primarily by the FT muscle fibers because they are capable of generating more force, and are primarily anaerobic in nature. Therefore, strength-training movements do not require or develop a high level of aerobic capacity because the muscles are using primarily the phosphagen (ATP-CP) system. Because strength training is relatively stressful on the connective tissues and muscular structures of the body, it is usually recommended that heavy strength training be performed only two or three times per week. It is important that the muscles and supporting structures be given time to recover sufficiently between workouts.

Muscular **hypertrophy** is often associated with a strength-development program. This hypertrophy is the result of an increase in both the number and size of individual muscle cells. The increase in size is due to a proliferation of actin and myosin myofilaments within the myofibrils, especially within the fast twitch muscle fibers. One common misconception is that women will develop "large" muscles if they strength-train. Generally women do not experience muscular hypertrophy to the same extent as men because the male hormone testosterone is important in synthesizing the contractile proteins. Nevertheless, women will increase substantially in strength in response to a progressive strength-training program.

Consistent with the **reversibility principle**, training adaptations will gradually decline if not reinforced by a "maintenance" program. With muscle disuse, as in paralysis, muscle **atrophy** or wasting occurs. To maintain strength gains and muscle size, lifting even once per week appears to be sufficient.

Muscular Endurance

Endurance refers to the ability to repeatedly contract a muscle or muscle group against resistance. Tests of muscular endurance usually involve selecting a fixed percentage of the maximum strength, 70% of the 1 RM, for example, and counting the number of repetitions that can be completed without resting. Sit-up or pull-up tests are other examples of muscular-endurance tests (not of strength tests, as often thought).

It is usually recommended that muscular-endurance training be conducted using a moderate-resistance (40% – 70% of 1 RM), high-repetition (10 – 50 repetitions) format. Be- cause this type of format is not as stressful to the muscles and connective tissue, muscular-endurance training programs can be completed as often as three to five times per week for maximum results. If training for a particular sport, the speed of contraction should be matched to the rate required during performance.

Training for muscular endurance is most specific to the ST muscle fibers and motor units. Because the contractions are carried out at a relatively low intensity, the slow twitch fibers rely primarily on aerobic metabolism. Training increases the concentration of the oxidative enzymes that extract oxygen from the blood, thus making energy production more efficient. An increase in tissue **vascularity,** or an increase in the number and size of blood vessels, often accompanies this type of program. Increased vascularity enhances blood supply and, consequently, oxygen delivery to the myofibrils. Regular participation in aerobic exercise generally enhances muscular endurance.

Flexibility

Flexibility refers to the ROM possible about a joint. Flexibility is often related to age: Young children are usually extremely flexible, while the elderly gradually lose much of the flexibility they had as younger adults. With specific flexibility training, the muscles and connective tissues adapt by elongating, thus increasing the range of motion.

ROM can be limited by the bony structure of a joint, the ligamentous structure of a joint, or the musculotendinous structure of the muscle(s) spanning the joint. The bony structure of a joint is a self-limiting factor that cannot be altered. A joint ligament (the fibrous band connecting bones) or joint capsule should not be stretched because to do so would lead to an unstable joint (joint laxity) and an increased risk of joint injury. Therefore, the only desirable way that range of motion can be altered is by gently stretching the musculotendinous structures controlling the movement of the joint. Sometimes these structures can become extremely taut, causing a reduction in the normal range of motion.

Flexibility may be related to the incidence of acute muscle injury due to strenuous exercise and also to **delayed onset muscle soreness (DOMS)**. Acute muscle injuries such as muscle pulls or tears are more likely to occur if the muscle fibers or surrounding tissues are so taut and inflexible that a sudden stretch causes tissue injury. The exact cause of DOMS, which occurs 24 – 48 hours after strenuous exercise, is not known. Current evidence suggests that it is caused by microscopic damage to muscle cell ultrastructure due to excessive mechanical force exerted by the muscle and connective tissues. DOMS is particularly associated with the eccentric phase of a movement, especially if the person is performing unaccustomed exercise. Stretching exercises performed before and after an exercise session may help to prevent soreness and also to relieve soreness when it does occur, but not all of the evidence suggests this.

There are three types of stretching to increase flexibility: static stretching, dynamic or ballistic stretching, and proprioceptive neuromuscular facilitation. **Static stretching** involves holding a static (nonmoving) position so that a joint is immobilized in a position that places the desired muscles and connective tissues passively at their greatest possible length. A static stretch position should be held for 30 – 60 seconds to achieve optimal results. Static stretching is best characterized as low-force, long-duration stretching and has repeatedly been shown

to produce good results with little muscle soreness. In fact, static stretching is commonly used to reduce muscle soreness. Little risk of physical injury exists if static stretching is performed as described.

Dynamic, or ballistic, stretching is characterized by rhythmic bobbing or bouncing motions representing relatively high-force, short-duration movements. **Ballistic stretching** motions, while seemingly effective, actually invoke **stretch reflexes** that oppose the desired stretching. Muscle stretch reflexes are involuntary motor responses controlled by the **muscle spindle**, a sensory organ located within the muscle. When a muscle spindle is stimulated, an impulse is propagated over a sensory nerve fiber. The nerve fiber synapses in the spinal cord with a motor neuron that returns to the muscle containing the muscle spindle (Figure 1.9a). This reflex causes the suddenly stretched muscle to respond with a corresponding contraction; the amount and rate of this contraction varies directly with the amount and rate of the movement causing the initial stretch. Thus, ballistic stretching evokes the opposite physiological re-

Figure 1.9
Simple muscle reflexes

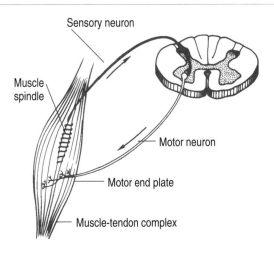

a. Simple muscle stretch reflex arc: The stretch of the muscle spindle causes reflex contraction.

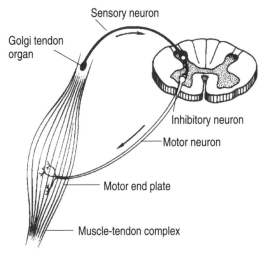

b. Simple inverse stretch reflex arc: The stretch of Golgi tendon organ causes reflex inhibition (relaxation).

sponse from that desired — an increase in muscle tension.

A firm static stretch, on the other hand, invokes an inhibition of the stretch reflex by stimulating another sensory organ (with a higher threshold level) called the **Golgi tendon organ**. When stimulated, this organ causes an inhibition not only of the muscle whose muscle spindle was stretched, but also of the entire muscle group (Figure 1.9b). Thus, static stretching brings about a reduction in muscle tension — the desirable physiological response. In addition, static stretching is safer than ballistic stretching because it does not impose a sudden, possibly injurious force upon the tissues.

A third type of stretching, **proprioceptive neuromuscular facilitation**, or **PNF**, is a technique originally developed for rehabilitative purposes in physical therapy. PNF involves statically stretching a muscle immediately after maximally contracting it against resistance. Carefully controlled experiments using PNF have generally found it to be superior to either static or **dynamic stretching**. However, it is not practical in the majority of cases as it requires a partner.

General flexibility exercises should be part of every physical fitness program and should be included in the warm-up and cool-down phase of every exercise session. Some general principles specific to the enhancement of flexibility include the following:

1. A very easy general warm-up (such as walking and swinging the arms) should precede specific stretching exercises to increase blood flow to the area.
2. Stretching exercises should be performed without bouncing or jerking, which may injure connective tissues and stimulate the stretch reflex.
3. Never attempt to stretch a muscle or muscle group beyond the normal range of motion.
4. All stretching should be done gently and only to the extent that muscle tension is perceived; stretching should not be painful.
5. Instructors should understand that their students will vary greatly in flexibility. Everyone is not equally flexible or equally responsive to flexibility training.

The Cardiovascular – Respiratory Systems

Cardiorespiratory endurance was defined earlier as the capacity of the heart and lung systems to deliver blood and, hence, oxygen to the working muscles during sustained exercise. Oxygen is used to produce ATP to perform low-to-moderate intensity exercise for long periods. One's capacity to perform aerobic exercise depends largely on the interaction of the cardiovascular system and the respiratory system to provide oxygen to the active cells so that carbohydrates and fatty acids can be converted to ATP for muscular contraction. These two systems are also important for the removal of metabolic waste products such as carbon dioxide and lactic acid and for the dissipation of the internal heat produced by metabolic processes.

There are three basic processes that must interact in order to provide adequate blood and nutrients to the tissues:

1. Getting oxygen into the blood — which is a function of **respiratory ventilation** coupled with the oxygen-carrying capacity of the blood.
2. Delivering oxygen to the active tissues — which is a function of cardiac output.

3. Extracting oxygen from the blood to complete the metabolic production of ATP — which is a function of the oxidative enzymes located within the active cells.

Oxygen-carrying Capacity

The oxygen-carrying capacity of blood is determined primarily by two variables: the ability to ventilate the lungs adequately and the hemoglobin content of the blood. Pulmonary **ventilation** is a function of both the rate and depth (**tidal volume**) of breathing. With the beginning of exercise, both tidal volume and breathing rate increase. This increase in ventilation volume brings more oxygen into the lungs, where it can be absorbed into the blood. In normal individuals, respiration does not limit exercise performance. However, individuals with **emphysema** (loss of elasticity of the lung tissue) or **asthma** (constriction of the breathing passages) cannot move enough air through their lungs to adequately oxygenate the blood. As a result, the blood leaving the lungs is not sufficiently loaded with oxygen, and exercise capacity is diminished.

Hemoglobin (Hb) is a protein molecule in red blood cells that is specifically adapted to bond (carry) oxygen molecules. When oxygen enters the lungs, it diffuses through the pulmonary membranes into the bloodstream where it binds to hemoglobin. The oxygen is then carried within the bloodstream throughout the body. Persons with low hemoglobin concentrations cannot carry as much oxygen in their blood as persons with high hemoglobin concentrations. For instance, in individuals with **anemia** (less than 12 g of Hb per 100 ml of blood), the blood's oxygen-carrying capacity is severely limited, and they fatigue very easily. In most healthy persons, however, the oxygen-carrying capacity of the blood is not a limiting factor in the performance of aerobic exercise. Regular aerobic exercise usually results in modest increases in both red blood cell and hemoglobin concentration.

Oxygen Delivery

Probably the most important factor in cardiovascular-respiratory endurance is the delivery of blood to the active cells, which is a function of **cardiac output**. Cardiac output is the product of **heart rate** (**HR**, beats per minute) and **stroke volume** (**SV**, the quantity of blood pumped per heart beat):

Cardiac output = HR x SV

At rest, cardiac output averages about 5 liters per minute. During maximal exercise this number can increase to up to 30 – 40 liters per minute in highly trained individuals. The increase in cardiac output is brought about by an increase in both HR and SV. HR generally increases in a linear fashion up to maximal levels (often estimated as 220 – age), while SV increases up to approximately 40% – 50% of an individual's maximal capacity and then plateaus. The increase in SV is brought about by increases in both venous return and an increase in the contractile force of the heart.

Also during exercise, blood flow patterns change according to metabolic need. Blood is shunted to the working muscles (to produce ATP for contraction) and to our skin (to dissipate the metabolic heat produced), while the amount of blood flowing to less active organs such as the kidney and intestinal tract decreases.

Blood pressure is also very important in blood flow distribution because it provides the driving force that pushes blood through the circulatory system. Blood pressure is influenced by many factors. **Systolic blood pressure** is a function of the force generated by the heart during its contractile phase (systole) and the resistance offered by the vessels to the blood flowing through them (peripheral resistance). Just as the strength of heart contractions can vary, some blood vessels (notably the smaller arteries called arterioles) can contract (**vasoconstriction**) or relax (**vasodilation**) and thus alter their resistance to blood flow, a fact important in determining patterns of blood flow. For example, during exercise vasoconstriction occurs in the vessels of inactive organs (such as the intestine), and vasodilation occurs in vessels of active organs (muscles), thus redirecting blood flow to areas of the body where it is most needed. Similar to HR, systolic blood pressure increases in a linear fashion throughout the range of exercise intensities.

Diastolic blood pressure is a measure of the pressure in the arteries during the relaxation phase (diastole) of the heart cycle. Because of the vasodilation of the blood vessels within the working muscles, more blood is allowed to enter the muscles. As a result, less blood is "trapped" on the arterial side of the circulation. Diastolic blood pressure usually stays the same or decreases slightly during exercise.

Oxygen Extraction

A third factor important in cardiovascular-respiratory endurance is the extraction of oxygen from the blood at the cellular level for the aerobic production of ATP. The amount of oxygen extracted is largely a function of muscle fiber type and the availability of specialized oxidative enzymes. As discussed earlier, the slow twitch muscle fibers are specifically adapted for oxygen extraction and utilization due to their high levels of oxidative enzymes. One of the most important adaptations to training is an increase in the number and size of the mitochondria, with a corresponding increase in the levels of oxidative enzymes used to aerobically produce ATP.

Acute Responses to Aerobic Exercise

Aerobic exercise is best characterized as large muscle, rhythmic activities (e.g., walking, jogging, aerobic dance, swimming, cross-country skiing) that can be sustained without undue fatigue for at least 10 to 15 minutes. Such movement patterns depend on the oxidative metabolic pathways to create ATP, and the goal of the body is to be in a **steady state**, where the energy needs are being met aerobically. The other metabolic pathways (the phosphagen system and anaerobic glycolysis) are used only minimally to produce energy for these types of activity.

Figure 1.10 highlights the changes that take place. When aerobic exercise begins, the body rapidly responds to increase the quantity of oxygen available to produce the ATP necessary to meet elevated metabolic demands. Cardiac output increases to deliver more blood to the active muscle cells. To meet this requirement, HR, SV, and systolic blood pressure increase immediately. Respiratory ventilation also increases to provide more oxygen to the red blood cells in the lungs.

The heavy bold line in Figure 1.10 indicates the level of **oxygen consumption** required at rest and the instantaneous increase that occurs with commencement of exercise (at upward arrow). The line returns to the resting level when exercise is abruptly stopped (at downward arrow). The *actual* oxygen consumption that results from the physiological responses to aerobic exercise is indicated by the sloping line in the figure. Notice that actual oxygen consumption does *not* immediately meet the physiological requirement for oxygen. Instead, an **oxygen deficit** occurs.

The physiological responses that occur with commencement of exercise take approximately two to four minutes to meet the increased metabolic demands for oxygen. During this time, the anaerobic metabolic systems — which are capable of producing energy more rapidly — produce the energy needed to carry out the exercise. During this period, the phosphagens are depleted, and excess lactic acid is produced. When the cardiorespiratory systems have fully responded, a new level of oxygen consumption is achieved. If the exercise intensity is not too high relative to the body's ability to provide oxygen to the muscles, a steady state is achieved.

With cessation of exercise, the requirement for oxygen abruptly returns to the initial resting level. Again, however, the body responds more slowly. As cardiac output, blood pressure, and respiratory ventilation return to resting levels, oxygen consumption slowly declines as well. This temporarily elevated level of oxygen consumption, called **oxygen debt**, "pays back" the oxygen deficit. This is also called **excess postexercise oxygen consumption** (**EPOC**). The energy produced during this time is used to replenish the depleted phosphagens, to eliminate accumulated lactic acid if it has not already been cleared from the blood, and to restore other homeostatic conditions.

Figure 1.10

Oxygen consumption during aerobic exercise

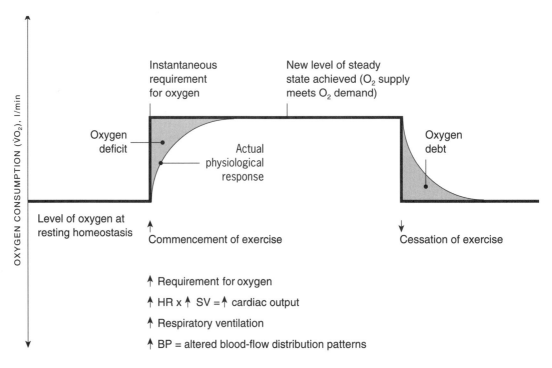

If exercise intensity is so high that the body cannot meet the metabolic demands of the muscles aerobically (i.e., not reach a steady state), the muscles have to depend on anaerobic metabolism for ATP production. When this occurs, one is said to have exceeded the **anaerobic threshold** (**AT**). When someone exceeds their AT, lactic acid accumulates very rapidly in the blood, the oxygen deficit and corresponding oxygen debt are extremely high, and exercise cannot be performed for more than a few minutes (Figure 1.11). It is also at this point that hyperventilation begins to occur. As the body tries to buffer the lactic acid (remove it from the system), one of the by-products is carbon dioxide (CO_2). CO_2 provides a powerful stimulus to the respiratory system, and the body increases respiration in an attempt to "blow off" the excess CO_2. This increase in respiration is often called the ventilatory threshold (VT) and is often used as an indirect indicator

of the AT. It is also at this point that muscle pain (the "burn" of lactic acid or oxygen deficiency) is experienced.

Guidelines for Improving Cardiovascular – Respiratory Endurance

When developing an exercise prescription, it is important to individualize the prescription for each client. There are three basic variables to consider when developing an exercise program to improve cardiovascular-respiratory endurance:

1. Exercise **intensity** — how hard to exercise.
2. Exercise **duration** — how long to exercise.
3. Exercise **frequency** — how often to exercise.

The following general recommendations are based upon well-established guidelines:

1. **Exercise intensity should be approximately 50% – 85% of maximal oxygen consumption ($\dot{V}O_2$ max) or HR reserve.** Below this range, little if any training stimulus is achieved. Above this

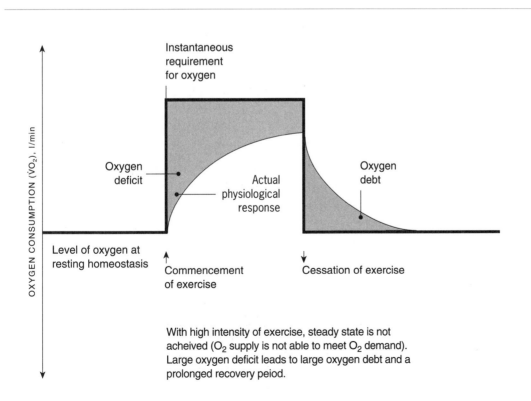

Figure 1.11
Oxygen consumption during anaerobic exercise

range of intensity, anaerobic processes must be relied on to contribute to total energy expenditure, and the resulting build-up of lactic acid limits how long people can maintain the exercise. Because measuring maximal oxygen consumption is so costly and time consuming, target HR zones have been established that adequately estimate exercise intensity in terms of maximal oxygen consumption. For aerobic exercise, HR is a fairly reliable indicator of how hard the body is working. The target zone of 50% – 85% of maximal oxygen consumption or maximal HR reserve is equivalent to 60% – 90% of maximal attainable HR. Chapter 5 describes two methods of calculating exercise target HR zones for aerobic exercise. When determining where to start people within the intensity continuum, remember that the starting exercise intensity will vary depending on the initial fitness level of the individual. You would probably want to start a sedentary, deconditioned person at the lower end of the target range (e.g., 50% – 60% of maximum), whereas you might start someone who is a regular exerciser at 70% – 80% of their maximum.

2. **Exercise duration may vary from 20 to 60 minutes of continuous aerobic activity.** The aerobic component of most aerobic exercise classes is 20 – 30 minutes. Duration refers to the actual time exercisers are within their target HR zones and does not include a warm-up or cool-down period. Exercise duration must again be individualized depending on client goals. If a student is not capable of completing 20 minutes of continuous exercise when first beginning an exercise program, this guideline can be set as an initial goal. If weight loss is a client's primary goal, a longer-duration (e.g., 60 minutes), low-intensity program may be most beneficial. For the average person, an exercise duration of 40 – 45 minutes within the target HR zone is adequate to meet their needs.

3. **Exercise frequency should be three – five days per week.** Three aerobic exercise sessions per week performed within the target HR zone for 20 minutes at each session should be considered a minimum guideline. A totally sedentary person will most likely experience a training stimulus with such a routine, but a more fit person will need to exercise more frequently — perhaps four – five days per week. Little additional benefit is achieved by exercising more than five days per week and most individuals will become bored if they exercise more frequently. Additionally, exercising more than five days per week greatly increases the chance of musculoskeletal injury.

Any program designed to improve cardiovascular endurance should apply the concept of progressive overload. **Overload** refers to the level of stress imposed on the physiological systems involved. For a training effect to occur, the system must be systematically stressed to a slightly higher level than it is normally accustomed. Applying the concept of progressive overload to cardiovascular endurance means gradually increasing the exercise intensity, the exercise duration, or the exercise frequency. As a general rule, exercise duration should be increased to target levels before exercise intensity is increased. Using jogging or running as an example, you may want to start with a specified distance and pace. After two weeks, increase the distance by about 10%. After another two weeks, increase the distance again. When the person has built up to their target distance, you can then increase the pace. This principle is the same for all forms of aerobic exercise.

Interval training involves exercising at high-intensity levels (80% – 100% of maximal HR) for relatively brief periods (usually 10 seconds to five minutes) with intervening rest or relief periods (walking, jogging) that allow HR to decline. Often the exercise periods are "anaerobic" rather than "aerobic." For athletes in training, interval training may offer an advantage because the higher intensity may more accurately simulate competitive conditions and result in increases in the anaerobic threshold. An athlete can thus maintain a faster pace before going into anaerobic metabolism. Generally, however, continuous exercise at lower levels of intensity is safer and more specific to the goals of most individuals. Continuous training is less stressful to the musculoskeletal system and, therefore, more appropriate for middle-aged and older adults.

Warm-up and Cool-down

The period of exercise at the desired target heart rate should be preceded by a warm-up of about five to 10 minutes. The warm-up should include stretching and limbering exercises to prepare the musculotendinous system for the exercises to be performed. Static stretching — holding a steady stretch with the desired muscles at their greatest possible length — is beneficial to joints and muscles and may help to prevent injuries and muscle soreness. Warm-up activities should also include large muscle movement to gradually increase HR, blood pressure, cardiac output, and respiratory ventilation to intermediate levels so that these mecha-

nisms are not suddenly taxed. A proper warm-up may also reduce the incidence of exercise-induced cardiac abnormalities such as **arrhythmias** (abnormal heart rhythms) or **ischemia** (lack of blood flow to the heart muscle).

It is important to cool down gradually after a period of vigorous exercise. Abruptly stopping exercise after a vigorous workout may allow a large quantity of blood to pool in the lower extremities, reducing venous return. As a result, cardiac output is reduced and blood flow to the brain is diminished, which may cause dizziness or faintness. It is best to provide a series of movements during the cool-down period that allows the muscles and cardiovascular – respiratory systems to gradually return to their pre-exercise levels. A gradual cool-down also aids in the removal of accumulated lactic acid and may prevent cardiac arrhythmias following strenuous exercise. When heart rates are near resting levels, muscle stretching and limbering exercises should again be performed to reduce the risk of developing DOMS. Probably the most effective time to perform flexibility exercises is when the muscles are warm and the body temperature is elevated after exercise.

Use of Hand or Ankle Weights with Aerobic Exercise

Individuals often seek ways to increase the intensity of their aerobic workout. Adding extra weight in the form of hand, wrist, or ankle weights increases the total mass that must be moved, so it seems logical that using extra weight would be beneficial in boosting the physiological demands of an activity. Research on the use of hand or wrist weights during a variety of different aerobic activities (e.g., walking, aerobic dance, step aerobics) is very consistent and indicates that the use of 1 – 3 pound (450 – 1350g) weights can increase heart rate by 5 – 10 beats per minute and oxygen consumption (as well as caloric expenditure) by about 5% – 15% compared to performing the same activity without weights. Weights greater than 3 pounds (1350g) are not generally recommended because they may put undue stress on the arm and shoulder muscles. Additionally, wrist weights are preferred over hand weights because they don't have to be gripped, which can cause an elevated blood pressure response in some people.

The beneficial effect of ankle weights is lower than that of either hand or wrist weights. Weights ranging from 1 to 3 pounds (450 – 1350g) can increase HR by an average of 3 – 5 beats per minute and oxygen consumption by 5% – 10% over unweighted conditions. A potential drawback to the use of ankle weights is that they may alter the biomechanics of the lower limbs, leading to injury. As a consequence, ankle weights are not generally recommended for use during actual aerobic activities.

Benefits of Aerobic Exercise for Healthy Participants

When performed appropriately, a regular program of aerobic exercise can have significant physiological benefits in as little as eight to 12 weeks. Changes to the cardiorespiratory system include improvements in cardiac efficiency (increased SV and a lower HR), increased respiratory capacity, and, ultimately, an increase in maximal oxygen consumption. These improvements provide individuals with a greater physiological reserve and allow them to perform everyday activi-

ties with less stress and strain. Regular exercise has also been shown to result in lowered blood pressure in moderately hypertensive individuals. This results in less work for the heart muscle and puts less stress on the blood vessels.

The benefits of aerobic exercise are not limited to the cardiovascular and respiratory systems. Recent studies have shown that weight-bearing exercise promotes improved bone density, an extremely important consideration in the prevention of osteoporosis after age 50 – 60, particularly in women. Improvements in the control of blood glucose and blood lipids (e.g., cholesterol, triglycerides) are also associated with consistent physical activity. One of the main reasons many people exercise is to control body weight. Exercise obviously burns calories, but, just as importantly, exercise serves to maintain or increase lean body mass, which is vital for maintaining resting metabolic rate. It is the decrease in muscle mass that contributes to the fall in metabolic rate as we age. And, finally, the psychological benefits of exercise cannot be overlooked. Exercise has long been associated with lower levels of anxiety and depression and a higher quality of life.

Benefits of Exercise for Persons with Chronic Disease

A well-planned aerobic exercise program can also provide significant health benefits to persons with chronic diseases such as adult-onset diabetes, osteoarthritis, obesity, pulmonary disease, and coronary heart disease.

Individuals with **adult-onset diabetes** (Type 2 diabetes) have difficulty utilizing glucose (carbohydrates) for energy, due to either a lack of insulin or the body's inability to utilize the available insulin (insulin resistance). Most of the time, individuals with Type 2 diabetes are overweight. Treatment of Type 2 diabetes usually involves a three-pronged approach: diet, weight loss, and exercise. Exercise enables carbohydrates to be used more effectively by promoting glucose uptake from the blood, thereby reducing insulin resistance. Exercise also helps to promote weight loss. Exercise programming for persons with Type 2 diabetes is rarely dangerous or difficult. Exercise for Type 1 diabetics is much more complex and is beyond the scope of this book. Any program of exercise for Type 1 diabetic patients must be performed under the guidance of a physician. The person with Type 1 diabetes needs to understand the interactions among exercise, glucose uptake, insulin, and carbohydrate consumption, because exercise can result in **hypoglycemia**, or hazardously low blood sugar, if done inappropriately.

Arthritis (osteoarthritis) is a gradual, progressive degeneration of joint structures that makes even normal movements painful. It has been speculated that high-impact exercise early in life contributes to the incidence of arthritis later on. However, research has found no association between exercise intensity and the incidence of arthritis, other than the tendency for arthritic pain to occur in areas of the body that have experienced earlier athletic injury. In fact, lifelong exercisers have been found to have less osteoarthritis than nonexercisers. Maintenance of good flexibility and developing moderate levels of muscular strength have been found to stabilize the joints and provide relief for the minor aches and pains of arthritis. An exercise program for arthritic patients should focus on nonweightbearing exercise modalities (e.g., stationary cycling, water-based exercise) and should avoid high-impact stress on the knees, hips, and lower back.

Obesity (the condition of having excess body fat) has become a major health-related problem in the industrialized world. Excess body weight is associated with a number of chronic diseases, including hypertension, diabetes, and coronary artery disease. The most effective way to lose body weight and body fat is through a sound program of caloric restriction and low-to-moderate intensity aerobic exercise. Dieting alone is not effective. While severe dieting can lead to weight loss, the loss is frequently from the lean body mass (mainly the muscles) rather than from the fat mass of the body, which results in a decrease in metabolic rate. An exercise program for the obese or overweight client should focus on burning the maximum number of calories per session and avoiding musculoskeletal injuries. Longer duration (building up to 45 – 60 minutes per day), low-to-moderate intensity (40% – 60% of maximum) exercise, performed 5 – 6 days per week should be the goal. Nonweightbearing or low-impact activities should also be stressed (e.g., walking, stationary cycling, water exercise).

People with pulmonary disease are severely limited by the amount of air they can move into and out of their lungs. The blood does not get adequately oxygenated and exercise capacity is very low. The most common forms of pulmonary disease are emphysema, **bronchitis**, and asthma. Emphysema and chronic bronchitis are usually the result of long-term cigarette smoking, whereas the exact cause of asthma is unknown. Asthma occurs when the bronchi (large breathing passages) become constricted (bronchospasm), and the onset of symptoms is usually related to irritants such as tobacco smoke, animal dander, and cold air. Some people also experience exercise-induced asthma (EIA). The most widely accepted hypothesis for the cause of EIA is that airway cooling irritates the lining of the respiratory tree and causes the bronchospasm. Previously it was thought that individuals with pulmonary disease should not exercise. However, a regular program of aerobic exercise has proven to decrease the amount of dyspnea (shortness of breath) in individuals with emphysema and bronchitis and increase their quality of life. People with asthma should also be encouraged to exercise and to have bronchodilator medications readily available if symptoms become severe. All patients with pulmonary disease should be under the care of a physician.

Coronary heart disease (CHD) involves partial or total closure of the coronary arteries, which results in symptoms or signs of ischemia (lack of blood flow to the heart muscle). The American Heart Association has identified a number of factors that increase the risk of cardiovascular disease. The primary risk factors are hypertension (elevated blood pressure), cigarette smoking, elevated blood lipid levels, and physical inactivity. Secondary risk factors include family history of heart disease, obesity, diabetes, being male, age over 65, and a high level of emotional stress. Obviously, little can be done to change one's age, gender, or family health history, but lifestyle changes can significantly alter the other risk factors. Regular participation in a well-planned aerobic exercise program has been shown to reduce high blood pressure, serum lipid levels, body fat, emotional stress, and cardiovascular mortality. Safety is a primary issue when exercising individuals with cardiac disease. Patients should be under the care of a physician and may require an exercise stress test to guide the exercise prescription.

Environmental Considerations When Exercising

Exercising under extreme environmental conditions can add significant stress to the cardiovascular system. Special precautions need to be taken when exercising in the heat or cold or at high altitude.

Exercising in the Heat

Considerable metabolic heat is produced during exercise. To reduce this internal heat load, venous blood is brought to the skin surface (peripheral vasodilation) to be cooled. When the sweat glands secrete water onto the skin, it is evaporated, which serves to cool the underlying blood. If environmental conditions are favorable, these mechanisms will adequately prevent the body temperature from rising more than about 2 – 3 degrees Fahrenheit, even during heavy exercise.

When exercising in the heat, however, dissipating internal body heat is difficult, and external heat from the environment may significantly add to the total heat load. This results in a higher heart rate than normal at any given level of exercise. For example, if someone walks at 3 miles per hour and their heart rate is normally 125 beats per minute, walking at the same speed in the heat may result in a heart rate of 135 – 140 beats per minute. Thus, exercisers (regardless of the type of exercise performed) need

Table 1.2
Heat Index

RELATIVE HUMIDITY %	TEMPERATURE (F°) (C° given in parentheses)										
	70 (21)	75 (24)	80 (27)	85 (29)	90 (32)	95 (35)	100 (38)	105 (41)	110 (43)	115 (46)	120 (49)
	APPARENT TEMPERATURE* (F°)										
0	64 (18)	69 (21)	73 (23)	78 (26)	83 (28)	87 (31)	91 (33)	95 (35)	99 (37)	103 (39)	107 (42)
10	65 (18)	70 (21)	75 (24)	80 (27)	85 (29)	90 (32)	95 (35)	100 (38)	105 (41)	111 (44)	116 (47)
20	66 (19)	72 (22)	77 (25)	82 (28)	87 (31)	93 (34)	99 (37)	105 (41)	112 (44)	120 (49)	130 (54)
30	67 (19)	73 (23)	78 (26)	84 (29)	90 (32)	96 (36)	104 (40)	113 (45)	123 (51)	135 (57)	148 (64)
40	68 (20)	74 (23)	79 (26)	86 (30)	93 (34)	101 (38)	110 (43)	123 (51)	137 (58)	151 (66)	
50	69 (21)	75 (24)	81 (27)	88 (31)	96 (36)	107 (42)	120 (49)	135 (57)	150 (66)		
60	70 (21)	76 (24)	82 (28)	90 (32)	100 (38)	114 (46)	132 (56)	149 (65)			
70	70 (21)	77 (25)	85 (29)	93 (34)	106 (41)	124 (51)	144 (62)				
80	71 (22)	78 (26)	86 (30)	97 (36)	113 (45)	136 (58)					
90	71 (22)	79 (26)	88 (31)	102 (39)	122 (50)						
100	72 (22)	80 (27)	91 (33)	108 (42)							

How to Use Heat Index
1. Across top locate temperature
2. Down left side locate relative humidity
3. Follow across and down to find Apparent Temperature
4. Determine Heat Stress Risk on chart at right.
Note: This Heat Index chart is designed to provide general guidelines for assessing the potential severity of heat stress. Individual reactions to heat will vary, in addition, studies indicate that susceptibility to heat disorders tends to increase with age. Exposure to full sunshine can increase Heat Index values by up to 15°F.

Apparent Temperature	Heat Stress Risk with Physical Activity and/or Prolonged Exposure
90° – 105° (32 – 41)	Heat cramps or heat exhaustion *possible*
105° – 130° (41 – 54)	Heat cramps or heat exhaustion *likely* Heatstroke *possible*
130° – 151° (54 – 66)	Heatstroke *highly likely*

*Combined index of heat and humidity and what it feels like to the body.

to decrease their absolute work load in the heat to stay within their prescribed target HR zone.

This elevated HR rate comes about primarily for two reasons. First, as the body tries to cool itself, the high degree of vasodilation in the vessels supplying the skin reduces venous return of blood to the heart and SV declines. The heart attempts to maintain cardiac output by elevating HR. Second, sweating results in a considerable loss of body water. If lost fluids are not replenished, dehydration eventually results, and blood volume declines. This will also decrease venous return to the heart. Again, the body responds with a higher HR to maintain cardiac output.

The most stressful environment to exercise in is a hot, humid environment. When the air contains a large quantity of water vapor, sweat will not evaporate readily. Since it is the evaporative process that cools the body, adequate cooling may not occur in humid conditions. Under these conditions, heat exhaustion and heat stroke become dangerous possibilities. Table 1.2 combines measures of heat and humidity into a simple-to-use **heat index**. The heat index provides guidelines regarding when exercise can be safely undertaken, and when it should be avoided.

Below are some additional tips for exercising in the heat:

1. **Begin exercising in the heat gradually.** Becoming acclimatized to exercising

Table 1.3
Windchill Factor Chart

Estimated wind speed (in mph) (km/h given in parentheses)	ACTUAL THERMOMETER READING (F°) (C° given in parentheses)											
	50 (10)	40 (4)	30 (-1)	20 (-7)	10 (-12)	0 (-18)	-10 (-23)	-20 (-29)	-30 (-34)	-40 (-40)	-50 (-46)	-60 (-51)
	EQUIVALENT TEMPERATURE (F°)											
calm	50 (10)	40 (4)	30 (-1)	20 (-7)	10 (-12)	0 (-18)	-10 (-23)	-20 (-29)	-30 (-34)	-40 (-40)	-50 (-46)	-60 (-51)
5 (8)	48 (9)	37 (3)	27 (-3)	16 (-9)	6 (-14)	-5 (-21)	-15 (-26)	-26 (-32)	-36 (-38)	-47 (-44)	-57 (-49)	-68 (-56)
10 (16)	40 (4)	28 (-2)	16 (-9)	4 (-16)	-9 (-23)	-24 (-31)	-33 (-36)	-46 (-43)	-58 (-50)	-70 (-57)	-83 (-64)	-95 (-71)
15 (24)	36 (2)	22 (-6)	9 (-13)	-5 (-21)	-18 (-28)	-32 (-36)	-45 (-43)	-58 (-50)	-72 (-58)	-85 (-65)	-99 (-78)	-112 (-80)
20 (32)	32 (0)	18 (-8)	4 (-16)	-10 (-23)	-25 (-32)	-39 (-39)	-53 (-47)	-67 (-55)	-82 (-63)	-96 (-71)	-110 (-79)	-124 (-87)
25 (40)	30 (-1)	16 (-9)	0 (-18)	-15 (-26)	-29 (-34)	-44 (-42)	-59 (-51)	-74 (-59)	-88 (-67)	-104 (-76)	-118 (-83)	-133 (-92)
30 (48)	28 (-2)	13 (-11)	-2 (-19)	-18 (-28)	-33 (-36)	-48 (-44)	-63 (-53)	-79 (-62)	-94 (-70)	-109 (-78)	-125 (-87)	-140 (-96)
35 (56)	27 (-3)	11 (-12)	-4 (-20)	-20 (-29)	-35 (-37)	-51 (-46)	-67 (-55)	-82 (-63)	-98 (-72)	-113 (-81)	-129 (-89)	-145 (-98)
40 (64)	26 (-3)	10 (-12)	-6 (-21)	-21 (-29)	-37 (-38)	-53 (-47)	-69 (-56)	-85 (-65)	-100 (-73)	-116 (-82)	-132 (-91)	-146 (-99)
(Wind speeds greater than 40 mph [64 km/h] have little additional effect.)	GREEN				YELLOW				RED			
	LITTLE DANGER (for properly clothed person). Maximum danger of false sense of security.				INCREASING DANGER Danger from freezing of exposed flesh.				GREAT DANGER			

in the heat takes approximately one week to 10 days. Start by exercising for short periods of time each day.

2. **Always wear lightweight, well-ventilated clothing.** Cotton materials are cooler; most synthetics retain heat. Wear light-colored clothing if exercising in the sun; white reflects heat better than other colors.

3. **Never wear impermeable or non-breathable garments.** The notion that wearing rubber suits or nonbreathable garments adds to weight loss is a myth. Wearing impermeable clothing is a dangerous practice that could lead to significant heat stress and heat injury.

4. **Replace body fluids as they are lost.** Drink lots of fluids at regular intervals while exercising. Don't wait until thirst occurs because thirst is not an adequate indicator of the need to replace body fluids. It is generally recommended that 1 – 2 cups of water be consumed before exercise and at least 1 cup every 15 – 20 minutes during exercise in the heat.

5. **Recording daily body weights is an excellent way to prevent accumulative dehydration.** For example, if 5 pounds (2.25 kg) of body water is lost after aerobic exercise, this water should be replaced before exercising again the next day. If lost water has not been regained, exercise should be curtailed until the body is adequately rehydrated.

Exercising in the Cold

The major problems encountered when exercising in the cold are associated with an excessive loss of body heat, which can result in hypothermia or frostbite. Additionally, the cold can also cause a generalized vasoconstriction that can increase peripheral resistance and blood pressure. This may cause problems in people who are hypertensive or who have heart disease. Following exercise, chilling can occur quickly if the body surface is wet with sweat and heat loss continues.

Heat loss from the body becomes greatly accelerated when there is a strong wind. The wind chill factor can be quite significant. Similar to the heat index chart mentioned previously, Table 1.3 provides the various combinations of temperature and wind velocity that can be used as guidelines when deciding if it is safe to exercise in the cold.

Below are some additional tips for exercising in the cold:

1. **Wear several layers of clothing.** By layering clothing, garments can be removed and replaced as needed. When exercise intensity is high, remove outer garments. Then, during periods of rest, warm-up, cool-down, or low-intensity exercise, put them back on. A head covering is also important because considerable body heat radiates from the head.

2. **Allow for adequate ventilation of sweat.** Sweating during heavy exercise can soak inner garments. If evaporation does not readily occur, the wet garments will continue to drain the body of heat during rest periods, when retention of body heat is important.

3. **Select garment materials that allow the body to give off body heat during exercise and retain body heat during inactive periods.** Cotton is a good choice for exercising in the heat because it soaks up sweat readily and allows evaporation; for those same reasons, however, cotton is a poor choice for exercising in the cold. Wool is an excellent choice when exercising in the cold because even when it is wet it maintains body heat. Newer, synthetic materials (e.g., polypropylene) are also excellent choices, as they wick sweat away from the body, thus preventing heat loss. When wind chill is a problem, nylon materials are good for outerwear. Gore-Tex®-like materials, although much more expensive than nylon, are probably the best choice for outerwear because they can break the wind, are waterproof, and allow moisture to move away from the body.

4. **Replace body fluids in the cold, just as in the heat.** Fluid replacement is also vitally important when exercising in cold air. Large amounts of water are lost from the body during even normal respiration; this effect becomes magnified when exercising.

Exercising at Higher Altitudes

At moderate-to-high altitudes, the **partial pressure*** of oxygen in the air is reduced. Because there is less pressure to drive the oxygen molecules into the blood in the lungs, the oxygen-carrying capacity of the blood is reduced. Therefore, a person exercising at high altitude will not be able to deliver as much oxygen to the exercising muscles, and exercise intensity will have to be reduced (compared to sea level) to keep the HR in a target zone.

---

* Partial pressure is the pressure of each gas in a multiple gas system such as air, which is composed of nitrogen, oxygen, and carbon dioxide.

Signs and symptoms of altitude sickness include shortness of breath, headache, lightheadedness, and nausea. Generally, altitude sickness can be avoided by acclimatizing oneself properly. This means gradually increasing exercise and activity levels over the span of two to three days. Using a prolonged warm-up and cool-down and incorporating into the regimen shorter, more frequent exercise sessions at a lower intensity should help most people become accustomed to exercising at higher altitudes.

Summary

This chapter is designed to provide the exercise instructor with basic principles of exercise physiology. Considerable space is devoted to the presentation of aerobic and anaerobic metabolism because the principle of specificity clearly dictates that physiological adaptations are specific to encountered stresses. The exercise instructor must understand the various methods of applying progressive overload and the physiological adaptations that result from this. Too often the exercising public falls victim to the poor advice of exercise teachers, coaches, and other "experts," who fail to apply the concept of exercise specificity because they simply do not understand basic principles.

A large amount of information has been given in a relatively small amount of space. The emphasis has been on basic understanding rather than on detailed explanation. Students of this material are strongly encouraged to seek further knowledge of exercise physiology and the principles of physical fitness and human movement through more advanced study.

Suggested Reading

Alter, M.J. (1996). *Science of Flexibility*. 2nd ed. Champaign, Ill.: Human Kinetics.

American College of Sports Medicine. (1995). *Guidelines for Exercise Testing and Prescription*. 5th ed. Baltimore: Williams and Wilkins.

American College of Sports Medicine. (1998). Position Stand: The Recommended Quantity and Quality of Exercise for Developing and Maintaining Cardiorespiratory and Muscular Fitness and Flexibility in Healthy Adults. *Medicine & Science in Sports & Exercise,* 30, 975 – 991.

Fleck, S.J. & Kraemer, W.J. (1997). *Designing Resistance Training Programs*. Champaign, Ill.: Human Kinetics.

Howley, E.T. & Franks, B.D. (1997). *Health Fitness Instructor's Handbook*. 3rd ed. Champaign, Ill.: Human Kinetics.

Plowman, S.A. & Smith, D.L. (1997). *Exercise Physiology for Health, Fitness, and Performance*. Boston: Allyn and Bacon.

Chapter 2

In This Chapter:

Rod A. Harter, Ph.D., A.T.C., is an associate professor and program director of athletic training education in the Department of Exercise and Sport Science at Oregon State University in Corvallis. Dr. Harter is a certified athletic trainer and a fellow of the American College of Sports Medicine. His areas of specialization are human anatomy, sports medicine, and biomechanics.

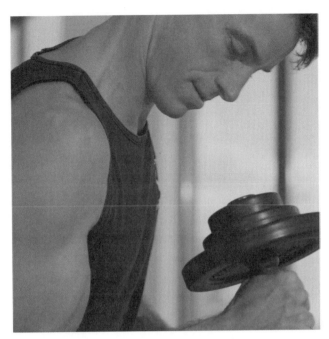

Fundamentals of Anatomy and
Applied Kinesiology

By Rod A. Harter

This chapter is divided into two sections; the first part provides an overview of the functional anatomy of five major systems operating within the human body: the cardiovascular system, the respiratory system, the nervous system, the skeletal system, and the muscular system. The second part is dedicated to kinesiology, the specialized study of the science of human movement. Anatomy is a broad science concerned with the study of the structure of the body and the relationships of the body parts to one another. A fundamental understanding of human anatomy is required of the group fitness instructor, whose professional responsibilities include exercise programming designed to help clients achieve their personal fitness goals.

Kinesiology combines aspects of physics, classical mechanics, physiology, and functional anatomy to help explain what causes human movement and is included in this text to provide you with information about how to make group fitness activities efficient, injury-free, and more specific to the targeted muscles. The objective of this chapter is to explain how the component parts of the body work together to provide the stability and **mobility** needed for effective human movement in sport, recreation, and the activities of daily living.

Anatomical Terminology

When studying anatomy for the first time, you may encounter descriptive or functional terms that are unfamiliar. Use of the correct anatomical terms for position, location, and direction is essential when describing a particular movement, exercise, or activity to a client or colleague.

Most anatomical terms have their roots in the Latin and Greek languages, and are usually quite descriptive. For example, many muscle names tell of the muscle's location, shape, or action. To illustrate this point, let us use the anterior tibialis muscle as our example. Anterior means "toward the front" while tibialis refers to the tibia, the larger of the two bones in the lower leg. In this case, by knowing the meanings of the root words, you now understand both the anatomical term and the location of this muscle — the anterior tibialis muscle is found on the front part of the tibia. Other important terms that describe anatomical positions are defined in Table 2.1. To help you avoid having to refer continually to a medical dictionary to define the terms used throughout this chapter, a summary of commonly used anatomical terms is presented in Table 2.2. A representation of anatomical position is given in Figure 2.1, along with the anatomical planes of motion.

Table 2.1
Anatomical, Directional, and Regional Terms

Term	Definition	Term	Definition
Anterior (ventral)	Toward the front	Palmar	The anterior or ventral surface of the hands
Posterior (dorsal)	Toward the back	Sagittal plane	A longitudinal (imaginary) line that divides the body or any of its parts into right and left halves
Superior	Toward the head		
Inferior	Away from the head		
Medial	Toward the midline of the body	Mediolateral axis	The transverse axis of rotation about which sagittal plane movement occurs; perpendicular to the sagittal plane
Lateral	Away from the midline of the body		
Proximal	Toward the attached end of the limb, origin of the structure, or midline of the body		
Distal	Away from the attached end of the limb, origin of the structure, or midline of the body	Frontal plane	A longitudinal (imaginary) section that divides the body into anterior and posterior halves
Cervical	Regional term referring to the neck	Anteroposterior axis	The front-to-back axis of rotation about which frontal plane movement occurs; perpendicular to the frontal plane
Thoracic	Regional term referring to the portion of body between the neck and the abdomen; also known as the chest (thorax)		
Lumbar	Regional term referring to the low back; the portion between the abdomen and the pelvis	Transverse plane	Also known as the horizontal plane; an imaginary line that divides the body or any of its parts into superior and inferior halves
Plantar	The sole or bottom of the foot	Longitudinal axis	The vertical axis of rotation about which transverse plane motion occurs; perpendicular to the transverse plane
Dorsal	The top surface of the foot and hands		

Table 2.2
Common Anatomical Terminology

Root	Meaning	Term	Definition
Arthro	Joint	Arthritis	Inflammation in a joint
Bi	Two, both	Bilateral	On both sides
Brachium	Arm	Brachialis	Muscle of the arm
Cardio	Heart	Cardiology	The study of the heart
Cephalo	Head	Cephalic	Pertaining to the head
Chrondro	Cartilage	Chondroectomy	Excision of a cartilage
Costo	Rib	Costochondral	Pertaining to a rib and its cartilage
Dermo	Skin	Dermatitis	Inflammation of the skin
Hemo, hemat	Blood	Hemorrhage	Internal or external bleeding
Ilio	Ilium	Ilium	The wide, upper part of the pelvic bone
Myo	Muscle	Myocitis	Inflammation of a muscle
Os, osteo	Bone	Osteopenia	Loss of bone mineral
Pulmo	Lung	Pulmonary artery	Vessel that brings blood to the lungs
Thoraco	Chest	Thorax	Chest
Tri	Three	Triceps brachii	Three-headed muscle on the arm

In the following sections, the functions of the five major systems in the human body most pertinent to exercise and physical activity will be reviewed in a summary manner. These systems are the cardiovascular system, the respiratory system, the nervous system, the skeletal system, and the muscular system.

Cardiovascular System

Oxygen is required for energy production, and thus sustains cellular activity (cellular metabolism) in the human body. A by-product of this cellular activity is carbon dioxide. High levels of carbon dioxide in the cells produce acidic conditions that are very poisonous to cells; thus, excess carbon dioxide must be eliminated rapidly. The cardiovascular and respiratory systems are primarily responsible for this function. The cardiovascular system is composed of the blood, the blood vessels, and the heart. The cardiovascular system distributes oxygen and nutrients to the cells, carries carbon dioxide and metabolic wastes from the cells,

Figure 2.1
Anatomical reference position and planes of motion

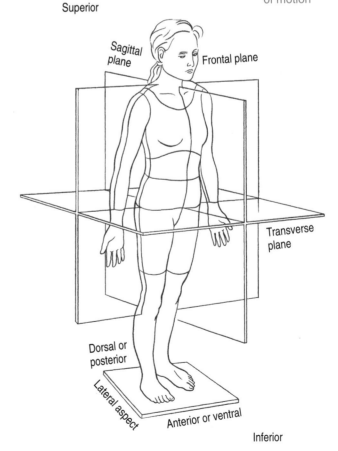

protects against disease, helps regulate body temperature, and prevents serious blood loss after injury through the formation of clots.

Blood is the only fluid tissue in the body and is composed of two parts: formed elements, which include different types of living blood cells — white blood cells, red blood cells, and platelets — and plasma, the nonliving liquid portion of blood. Plasma is about 92% water and 8% dissolved solutes. There are more than 100 different types of dissolved solutes in plasma; the most abundant of these are plasma proteins. In adults, blood accounts for about 8% of body weight; an average-size healthy woman has about 4 to 5 liters, while an average-size healthy man has approximately 5 to 6 liters of blood.

Types of Blood Vessels

There are two types of blood vessels: **arteries,** which carry blood away from the heart, and **veins,** which transport blood toward the heart. Arteries are thicker than veins, and their muscular walls help propel

Figure 2.2

Major arteries
of the body
(anterior view)

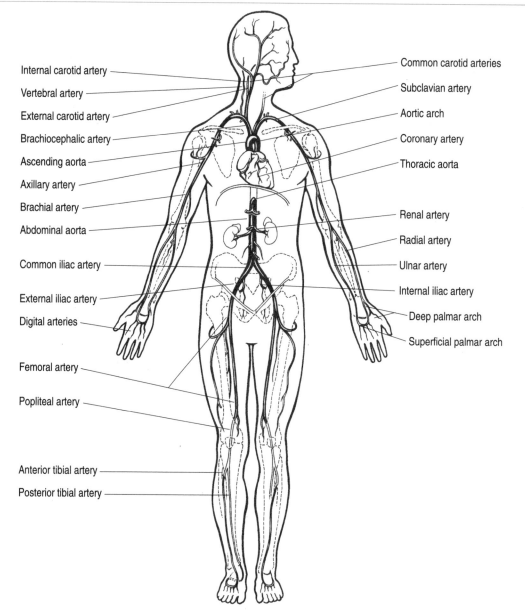

Internal carotid artery
Vertebral artery
External carotid artery
Brachiocephalic artery
Ascending aorta
Axillary artery
Brachial artery
Abdominal aorta
Common iliac artery
External iliac artery
Digital arteries
Femoral artery
Popliteal artery
Anterior tibial artery
Posterior tibial artery

Common carotid arteries
Subclavian artery
Aortic arch
Coronary artery
Thoracic aorta
Renal artery
Radial artery
Ulnar artery
Internal iliac artery
Deep palmar arch
Superficial palmar arch

blood (Figure 2.2). Unlike arteries, veins contain valves that prevent blood from flowing backward. The largest arteries are those nearest the heart; as blood flows further away from the heart, the arteries branch into smaller arteries called **arterioles,** which deliver the blood to the even smaller **capillaries**. These microscopic blood vessels branch to form an extensive network throughout the **distal** tissues. The critical exchange of nutrients and metabolic waste products takes place here in the capillary beds. Depleted of oxygen and nutrients on the way from the heart to the periphery, capillary blood reaches the end of the line and now begins the long journey back to the heart via small vessels called **venules**. Within our closed circulatory system, the venules are a continuation of the capillaries, and these tiny structures ultimately join together to form veins. As the blood is carried closer and closer to the heart, the veins become larger, carrying a greater volume of blood (Figure 2.3).

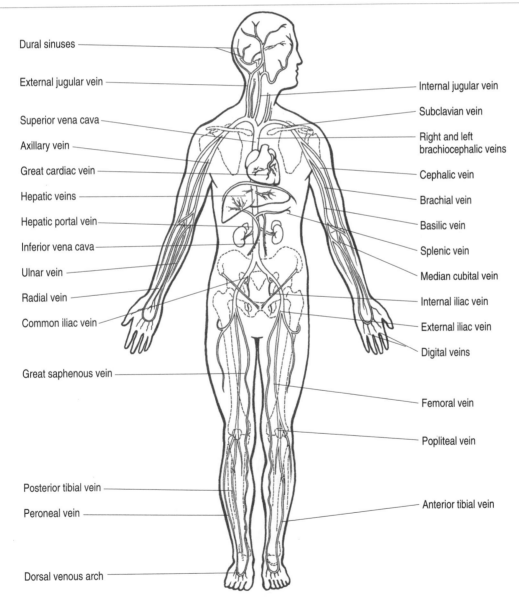

Figure 2.3
Major veins of the body (anterior view)

Dural sinuses
External jugular vein
Superior vena cava
Axillary vein
Great cardiac vein
Hepatic veins
Hepatic portal vein
Inferior vena cava
Ulnar vein
Radial vein
Common iliac vein
Great saphenous vein
Posterior tibial vein
Peroneal vein
Dorsal venous arch

Internal jugular vein
Subclavian vein
Right and left brachiocephalic veins
Cephalic vein
Brachial vein
Basilic vein
Splenic vein
Median cubital vein
Internal iliac vein
External iliac vein
Digital veins
Femoral vein
Popliteal vein
Anterior tibial vein

The Heart

The human heart is a hollow, muscular organ at the center of the cardiovascular system. In the adult, the heart is about the same size as the closed fist and lies to the left of center, behind the sternum and between the lungs. The heart itself is divided into four chambers that receive circulating blood. The two upper chambers are called the right and left **atria**, while the two lower chambers of the heart are known as the right and left **ventricles** (Figure 2.4).

The heart is a series of four separate pumps: two primer pumps, the atria, and two power pumps, the ventricles. Knowledge of the sequence of blood flow through the heart is fundamental to understanding the cardiovascular system. The right atrium receives blood from all parts of the body except the lungs. The **superior** vena cava, the large vein that drains blood from body parts superior to the heart (head, neck, arms) and its counterpart, the **inferior** vena cava, which brings blood from the parts of the body inferior to the heart (legs, abdominal region), transport blood to the right atrium. During contraction of the heart, blood accumulates in the right atrium. With relaxation of the heart, blood from the right atrium flows into the right ventricle, which during contraction pumps it into the pulmonary trunk. The pulmonary trunk then divides into right and left pulmonary arteries, which transport blood to the lungs, where carbon dioxide is released and oxygen is acquired. This freshly oxygenated blood returns to the heart via four pulmonary veins that empty into the left atrium. The blood then passes into the left ventricle; during contraction of the heart it is pumped from here into the ascending **aorta**. From this point the blood is distributed to all body parts (except the lungs) by several large arteries.

Respiratory System

The respiratory system supplies oxygen, eliminates carbon dioxide, and helps regulate the acid-base balance (pH) of the body. The respiratory system is composed of the lungs and the series of passageways (e.g., mouth, throat, trachea, and

Figure 2.4
Structure of the heart and flow of blood within it

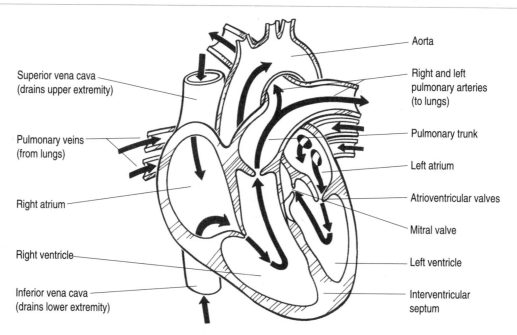

Superior vena cava
(drains upper extremity)

Pulmonary veins
(from lungs)

Right atrium

Right ventricle

Inferior vena cava
(drains lower extremity)

Aorta

Right and left
pulmonary arteries
(to lungs)

Pulmonary trunk

Left atrium

Atrioventricular valves

Mitral valve

Left ventricle

Interventricular
septum

bronchi) leading to and from the lungs. The process of **respiration** is the overall exchange of gases (e.g., oxygen, carbon dioxide, and nitrogen) between the atmosphere, the blood, and the cells.

There are three general phases of respiration: external, internal, and cellular. External respiration is the exchange of oxygen and carbon dioxide between the atmosphere and the blood within the large capillaries in the lungs. Internal respiration involves the exchange of those gases between the blood and the cells of the body. Cellular respiration involves the utilization of oxygen and the production of carbon dioxide by the metabolic activity within cells. When the body is at rest, air enters the respiratory system via the nostrils and is warmed as it passes through a series of nasal cavities lined by mucous membrane covered with cilia (small hairs) that filter out small particles. From the nasal cavity, inspired air next enters the pharynx (throat), which lies just **posterior** to the nasal and oral (mouth) cavities. The pharynx serves as a passageway for air and food and also provides a resonating chamber for speech sounds. During vigorous physical activity, mouth breathing tends to predominate, and air taken in via the mouth is not filtered to the same extent as air taken in through the nostrils.

The larynx, or voice box, is the enlarged upper (**proximal**) end of the trachea (windpipe). The larynx conducts air to and from the lungs via the pharynx. An easy landmark for locating the larynx is the thyroid **cartilage** or Adam's apple. The trachea is a tubular airway approximately 4.5 inches long (about 12 cm) kept open by a series of C-shaped cartilages that have a function similar to the wire rings in a vacuum cleaner hose. The trachea extends from the larynx

to approximately the level of the fifth thoracic vertebra, where it divides into the right and left **primary bronchi**. After this division, each primary bronchus then enters a lung and divides into smaller secondary bronchi, one for each lobe of the lung (five in total). The secondary bronchi branch into many tertiary bronchi, and these branch several times further, eventually forming tiny terminal **bronchioles**. The terminal bronchioles have microscopic branches called respiratory bronchioles that, in turn, subdivide into several alveolar ducts (plural = **alveoli**). The actual exchange of respiratory gases, such as oxygen and carbon dioxide, between the lungs and the blood occurs at this anatomic level. Lungs contain an estimated 300 million alveoli that provide an extremely large surface area (approximately 230 square feet or 70 square meters) for the exchange of gases. The continuous branching of the trachea resembles a tree trunk and its branches and is commonly referred to as the **bronchial tree** (Figure 2.5).

The final components of the respiratory system are the lungs, paired, cone-shaped organs lying in the thoracic cavity. The right lung has three lobes, while the left lung has only two. The diaphragm is the muscle that forms the floor of the thoracic cavity, contracts during inspiration, and relaxes to allow expiration. The lungs are separated by a space known as the mediastinum, which contains, most notably, the heart, the esophagus (the tube that connects the throat with the stomach), and a portion of the trachea.

Nervous System

The nervous system is the body's control center and network for internal communication. Of primary importance to the group fitness instructor are the nervous system's functions of stimulating and controlling movement. A skeletal muscle cannot contract until it receives a stimulus from either an internal source (e.g., a nerve impulse) or an external source (e.g., electrical muscle stimulation treatment). Without central control, coordinated human movements are impossible.

Our nervous system is divided into two parts according to location: the central nervous system and the peripheral nervous system. The central nervous system (CNS), comprised of the brain and the spinal cord, is totally enclosed within bony structures. The skull protects the brain, while the spinal cord is protected by the vertebral canal of the spinal column. The CNS is the control center of the nervous system, since it receives input from the peripheral nervous system, integrates this information, and formulates appropriate responses to the input. The peripheral nervous system (PNS) is made up of nerves that connect the extremities and their **receptors** within the CNS. The PNS includes 12 pairs of cranial nerves, two of which arise from the brain, while the remaining 10 pairs begin in the brain stem. The PNS also includes 31 pairs of spinal nerves that originate from the spinal cord. The spinal nerves include eight cervical pairs, 12 thoracic pairs, five lumbar pairs, five sacral pairs, and one coccygeal pair (Figure 2.6). These nerves are named and

Figure 2.5

a. Upper and lower respiratory pathways

b. Enlargement of the transition from terminal bronchiole into alveoli

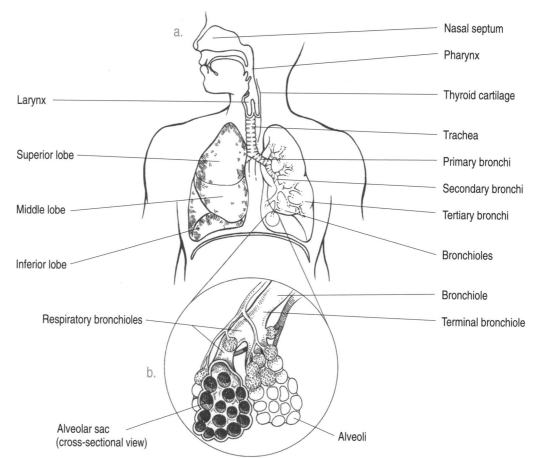

a.

Larynx

Superior lobe

Middle lobe

Inferior lobe

Respiratory bronchioles

b.

Alveolar sac (cross-sectional view)

Nasal septum

Pharynx

Thyroid cartilage

Trachea

Primary bronchi

Secondary bronchi

Tertiary bronchi

Bronchioles

Bronchiole

Terminal bronchiole

Alveoli

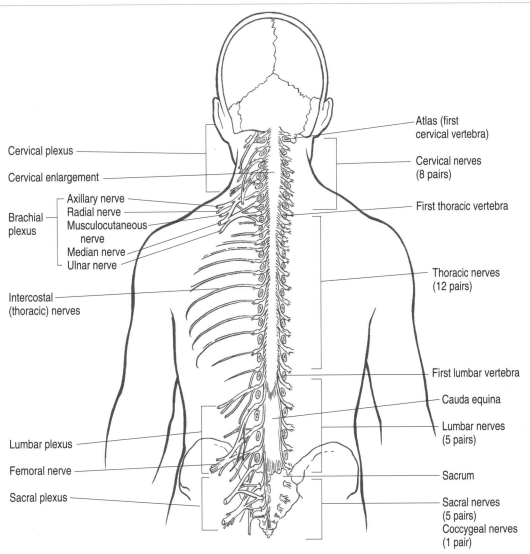

Cervical plexus

Cervical enlargement

Brachial plexus
- Axillary nerve
- Radial nerve
- Musculocutaneous nerve
- Median nerve
- Ulnar nerve

Intercostal (thoracic) nerves

Lumbar plexus

Femoral nerve

Sacral plexus

Atlas (first cervical vertebra)

Cervical nerves (8 pairs)

First thoracic vertebra

Thoracic nerves (12 pairs)

First lumbar vertebra

Cauda equina

Lumbar nerves (5 pairs)

Sacrum

Sacral nerves (5 pairs)
Coccygeal nerves (1 pair)

numbered according to region and the vertebral level at which they emerge from the spinal cord. For example, the third lumbar nerve (written L3) exits the spinal cord at the level of the third lumbar vertebra.

The anterior branches of the second through twelfth thoracic spinal nerves (T2 to T12 nerve roots) innervate muscles and other structures such as the internal organs individually. In all other cases, the anterior branches of the spinal nerves combine with adjacent nerves to form one of the four networks of nerves or plexuses. There are four major nerve plexuses in the human body:

the cervical plexus, the brachial plexus, the lumbar plexus, and the sacral plexus. The C1 through C4 nerve roots join to create the cervical plexus, which innervates the head, neck, upper chest, and shoulders. The nerves of the brachial plexus (C5 to T1) provide motor and sensory functions for the shoulder all the way down to the fingers of the hand. The L1 to L4 nerve roots, which form the lumbar plexus, innervate the abdomen, groin, genitalia, and anterolateral aspect of the thigh, while the sacral plexus (L4 to S4) supplies the large muscles of the posterior thigh and the entire lower leg, ankle, and foot. Table 2.3 provides

**Table 2.3
Selected Spinal Nerve Roots and
Major Muscles Innervated**

Nerve Root	Muscles Innervated
C3	Trapezius, longus capitis, longus cervicis, scalenus medius
C4	Diaphragm, trapezius, levator scapulae, scalenus anterior and medius
C5	Biceps brachii, deltoid, rhomboid major and minor, supraspinatus, infraspinatus
C6	Serratus anterior, latissimus dorsi, brachioradialis, extensor carpi radialis longus and brevis, extensor carpi ulnaris, supinator
C7	Triceps brachii, flexor carpi radialis, flexor carpi ulnaris
C8	Extensor pollicis longus and brevis, adductor pollicis longus
T1	Intrinsic muscles of the hand (lumbricals, interossei)
L2	Psoas major and minor, adductor magnus, adductor longus, adductor brevis
L3	Rectus femoris, vastus lateralis, vastus medialis, vastus intermedius, psoas major and minor
L4	Tibialis anterior, tibialis posterior
L5	Extensor hallucis longus, extensor digitorum longus, peroneus longus and brevis, gluteus maximus, gluteus medius
S1	Gastrocnemius, soleus, biceps femoris, semitendinosus, semimembranosus, gluteus maximus
S2	Gluteus maximus, flexor hallucis longus, flexor digitorum longus
S4	Bladder, rectum

a summary of the primary spinal nerve roots that supply the major muscles innervated by each of these plexuses.

The cells that comprise the nervous system carry messages called nerve impulses that originate in either the CNS or in specialized nerve cells called receptors. Receptors are located throughout the body; different types of receptors are sensitive to pain, temperature, pressure, and changes in body position. Sensory nerve cells carry the impulses from the peripheral receptors to the spinal cord and brain. Motor nerve cells car-

ry impulses away from the CNS to respond to the perceived changes in the body's internal or external environment.

Neurological Factors Affecting Movement

Voluntary human movement is regulated and controlled by complex interactions within our central and peripheral nervous systems. The three major types of sensory input come from the visual (eyes), vestibular (inner ear), and somatic (body) sensory systems. Of particular interest is the feedback received in the CNS from somatic sensory receptors found in muscles, tendons, ligaments, joint capsules, and skin. These sensory organs are collectively known as **proprioceptors** and they gather information about body position and the direction and velocity of movement.

Effective learning and performance of the movement patterns taught by group fitness instructors depend on input from the client's sensory pathways to his or her brain. The brain interprets this sensory information and a specific motor response is formulated in regard to the magnitude, direction, and rate of change of body movement. Sensory receptors can provide a conscious or **kinesthetic awareness** of body and limb position; you see first-hand evidence of this neurological capability when your clients follow your lead, mirroring you perfectly. Kinesthesis is the conscious awareness of the position of body parts and the amount and velocity of joint movement. This information comes primarily from the proprioceptors located in the muscles, tendons, ligaments, and joint capsules. This type of perception allows a person to initiate and modify movement patterns; it also affects his or her perception of posture. When poor posture is habitual, the person may perceive a wrong alignment as being correct.

To change that perception, additional input must be given to the sensory receptors. For example, to correct a rounded shoulders (humpback) posture, the person must repeatedly perform retraction of the shoulder blades throughout the day.

When performing a complex physical activity, such as an inclined bench press, the central and peripheral nervous systems work together to initiate, guide, and monitor all aspects of the specific activity. In this example, the nerve receptors in the periphery, located in the arm and shoulder region, provide continuous information (feedback) to the CNS regarding the amount of resistance encountered, limb position, pressure sensed on the palms of the hands, and so on. This communication between central and peripheral nervous systems, utilizing the motor and sensory nerve pathways, is essential for us to learn, modify, and successfully perform both simple and complex physical activities.

Reflex Activity

Sensory receptors are also involved in unconscious reflexes that deserve brief mention here. Two important types of proprioceptors are located in our muscles (muscle spindles) and tendons (Golgi tendon organs [GTOs]). Muscle spindles are sensitive to high levels and/or rapid increases in tension within the muscle and respond to this stimulus by triggering the **stretch reflex**, a protective activation of the muscle being stretched in order to prevent injury. Similarly, the GTOs located in the proximal and distal tendons of a muscle respond to high (dangerous) levels of tension, but their reflex action is to induce relaxation within their resident muscle, diminishing the amount of tension in the tendon and preventing injury. Both reflex actions are protective and have important

applications for the group fitness instructor utilizing stretching exercises as part of the warm-up and cool-down phases of a class. Activation of the stretch reflex can and should be avoided by performing slow, controlled, static stretching techniques. Conversely, the GTO reflex is a desired response during flexibility exercises and is activated by holding a static stretch position for six to 10 seconds, causing the GTOs to fire and inhibit the muscle being stretched, thus permitting additional **range of motion** and stretching.

Skeletal System

The human skeletal system (Figure 2.7) can be divided into two sections: the **axial skeleton**, 80 bones that comprise the head, neck, and trunk; and the appendicular skeleton, 126 bones that form the extremities (Table 2.4). The 206 bones that form the human skeleton perform five basic, yet very important functions. First, the skeletal system provides protection for many of the vital organs, such as the heart, brain, and spinal cord. Second, the skeleton provides support for the soft tissues so that erect posture and the form of the body can be maintained. Third, the bones provide a framework of **levers** to which muscles are attached. When particular muscles are stimulated, long bones act as levers to produce movement. Fourth, the red marrow of bone is responsible for the production of certain blood cells, namely, red blood cells, some types of white blood cells, and platelets. Fifth, bones serve as storage areas for calcium, phosphorus, potassium, sodium, and other minerals. Due to their high mineral content, bones often remain intact for thousands of years after death. Fat is also

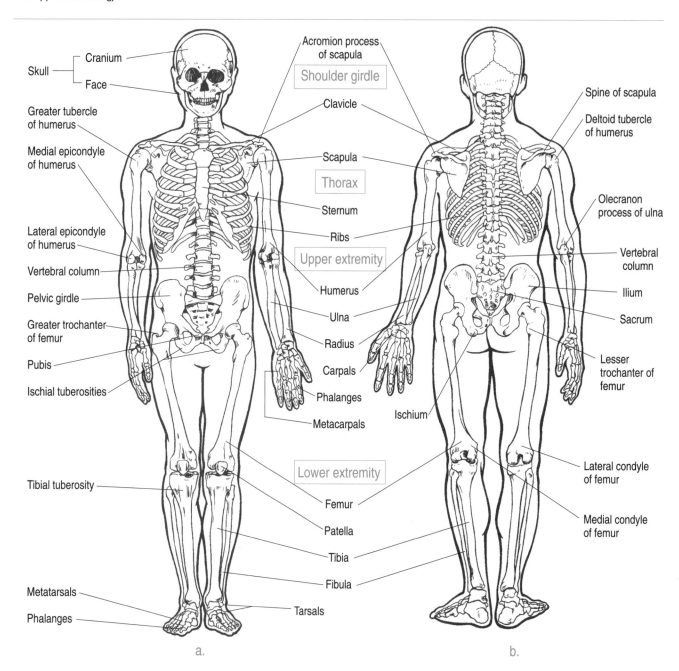

Skull — Cranium / Face
Greater tubercle of humerus
Medial epicondyle of humerus
Lateral epicondyle of humerus
Vertebral column
Pelvic girdle
Greater trochanter of femur
Pubis
Ischial tuberosities

Acromion process of scapula
Shoulder girdle
Clavicle
Scapula
Thorax
Sternum
Ribs
Upper extremity
Humerus
Ulna
Radius
Carpals
Phalanges
Metacarpals

Tibial tuberosity

Lower extremity
Femur
Patella
Tibia
Fibula

Metatarsals
Phalanges
Tarsals

Spine of scapula
Deltoid tubercle of humerus
Olecranon process of ulna
Vertebral column
Ilium
Sacrum
Lesser trochanter of femur
Lateral condyle of femur
Medial condyle of femur

Ischium

a.

b.

Figure 2.7

Skeletal system
a. anterior view

b. posterior view

stored within the middle section of long bones in the medullary cavity (Figure 2.8).

Bones may also be classified according to their shape: long, short, flat, irregular, or sesamoid. Long bones are those in which the length exceeds the width and the thickness. Most of the bones in the lower and upper extremities are long bones, including the femur, tibia, fibula, and metatarsals in the lower limb, and the humerus, radius, ulna, and metacarpals in the upper extremity. Each long bone has a shaft called a **diaphysis** and two ends that are usually wider than the shaft, known as **epiphyses** (singular = epiphysis). During our childhood and adolescent years, these cartilaginous epiphyses are active as growth plates that permit normal longitudinal bone growth

Table 2.4
Bones in the Axial and Appendicular Skeletons

Axial Skeleton	Number of Bones
Skull	
Cranium	8
Face	14
Hyoid	1
Vertebral Column	26
Thorax	
Sternum	1
Ribs	24
(Auditory ossicles)*	6
	80

Appendicular Skeleton	Number of Bones
Lower Extremity	
Phalanges	28
Metatarsals	10
Tarsals	14
Patella	2
Tibia	2
Fibula	2
Femur	2
Pelvic Girdle	
Hip or pelvis (Os coxae = ilium, ischium, and pubis)	2
Shoulder Girdle	
Clavicle	2
Scapula	2
Upper Extremity	
Phalanges	28
Metacarpals	10
Carpals	16
Radius	2
Ulna	2
Humerus	2
	126

*NOTE: The auditory ossicles, three per ear, are not considered to be part of the axial or appendicular skeletons, but rather a separate group of bones. They were placed in the axial skeleton group for convenience.

to take place. By the time the human skeleton fully matures at young adulthood (age range, 18 to 21 years), the epiphyses have changed from cartilage, become fully ossified bone, and no further longitudinal growth in long bones takes place.

The outer surface of the diaphysis of a long bone is surrounded by a **connective tissue** sheath called **periosteum** (see Figure 2.8).

The periosteum has two layers, an outer layer that serves as an attachment site for muscles and tendons and an inner layer that, when disrupted by fracture, signals the release of osteoblasts (bone-forming cells) to create new bone and repair the fracture. The anatomical complement to the periosteum is the **endosteum**, a soft-tissue lining of the internal surface of the diaphysis in the medullary canal. The primary function of the endosteum is to resorb old and/or unneeded bone through the action of osteoclasts (bone-resorbing cells). Throughout much of our lifetime, the ongoing, typically balanced activity of the osteoblasts and osteoclasts results in the remodeling of our bones and helps to sustain the circumferential dimension of long bones. On reaching middle age and, for women specifically, menopause, significant changes in reproductive hormone levels (estrogen) negatively affect metabolic activity in bone. In time, these changes may cause severe reductions in bone mineral density (osteopenia) and, ultimately, osteoporosis.

Short bones have no long axis and are approximately equal in length and width. This type of bone is found in the hands (carpals) and the feet (tarsals). Flat bones are partially described by their name; they are thin but usually bent or curved rather than flat. The bones of the skull, the ribs, the sternum, and the scapulae (shoulder blades) are examples. Irregular bones are bones of various shapes that do not fall into these other categories. The hip bones, the **vertebrae**, and many of the bones of the skull are examples. Sesamoid bones, literally "seed-like" bones, comprise the fifth small but important type of bone and are embedded within a tendinous structure. This type of bone (e.g., the patellar) increases the efficiency of the muscle in which it is located

Figure 2.8
Long bone gross
anatomy

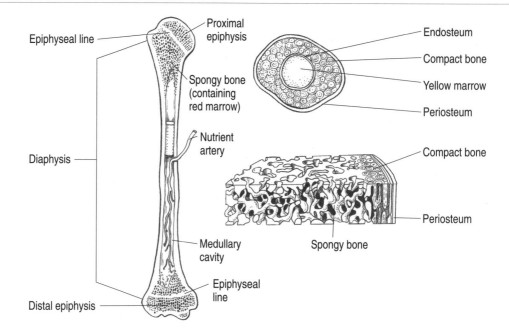

by improving the mechanical advantage of the muscle at that joint.

Bone contains an inorganic component composed of mineral salts, primarily calcium and potassium, and an organic component made of **collagen**, a complex protein that is found in various forms in bone and other connective tissues. According to **Wolff's Law**, bone is capable of adjusting its strength in proportion to the amount of stress placed on it. When young, healthy people participate in exercise programs for extended periods of time, their bones can become more dense through increased deposition of mineral salts and the number of collagen fibers. On the other hand, if bones are not subjected to mechanical stresses, as in individuals with sedentary lifestyles or in the absence of gravitational loading, such as in space flight or nonweightbearing exercises, bones will become less dense over time as mineral is withdrawn from bone. An easy way to remember this important law is with the saying, "form follows function." Simply stated, the form that bone will take (strong or weak) is

in direct response to the recent demands placed on that bone. When Wolff's Law was written in 1892, little if anything was known about the influences that genetics, nutrition, hormonal levels (estrogen and testosterone), and tobacco and alcohol use have on bone. Our present day understanding of these and other factors points out the limitations of the century-old Wolff's Law.

This knowledge has important implications for the group fitness instructor who must have the bone health of his/her client in mind when creating specific conditioning and resistance-exercise programs. As a group fitness instructor you should emphasize the positive influence on bone health as one of the main reasons for your clients to begin or continue with their regular participation in physical activity. Since the low levels of the hormone estrogen that accompany **amenorrhea** (two or less menstrual periods per year) and menopause in women lead to substantial bone mineral loss, it is important that you assist your clients in developing strength building programs. Additionally, you should encourage your post-menopausal clients to discuss estrogen replacement with their physicians.

Axial Skeleton

As previously stated, the axial skeleton consists of the 80 bones that form the skull, the vertebral column, and the thorax (chest). This portion of the skeletal system provides the main structural support for the body while also protecting the central nervous system and vital organs in the thorax (heart, lungs, etc.). Of primary importance is the adult vertebral column, consisting of 33 vertebrae divided into five groups and named according to the region of the body in which they are located. The upper seven are **cervical vertebrae**, followed in descending order by 12 **thoracic vertebrae**, five **lumbar vertebrae**, five sacral vertebrae fused into one bone as the sacrum, and four coccygeal vertebrae fused together into one bone called the **coccyx**. The sacral vertebrae and coccygeal vertebrae become fused in the adult, so there are only 24 movable vertebrae (Figure 2.9).

Appendicular Skeleton

The appendicular skeleton is composed of the bones of the lower and upper limbs and the bones by which the legs and arms attach to the axial skeleton — the pelvic (hip) and pectoral (chest) girdles. The pelvic girdle consists of two large hip bones known collectively as the os coxae, each side consisting of an ilium, an ischium, and a pubis (see Figure 2.7). The two pectoral girdles, each consisting of a clavicle (collarbone) and scapula (shoulder blade), attach the bones of the upper extremities to the axial skeleton at the sternum. Since the sternoclavicular joints are the only direct bone-to-bone links between the upper extremities and the axial

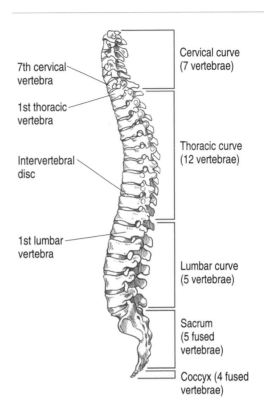

Figure 2.9
Vertebral column (lateral view)

7th cervical vertebra

1st thoracic vertebra

Intervertebral disc

1st lumbar vertebra

Cervical curve (7 vertebrae)

Thoracic curve (12 vertebrae)

Lumbar curve (5 vertebrae)

Sacrum (5 fused vertebrae)

Coccyx (4 fused vertebrae)

skeleton, several tradeoffs exist from this configuration. Most important, the pectoral girdle does not provide very strong support for the upper extremity. However, the girdle does permit a wide range of movements at the shoulder, making it the most mobile joint in the body.

Articulations (Joints)

An **articulation**, or joint, is the point of contact or connection between bones or between bones and cartilage. Ligaments, the dense, fibrous strands of connective tissue that link together the bony segments, maintain the stability and integrity of all joints. Some joints permit large ranges of motion in several directions, while other joints permit virtually no motion at all. The various joints in the body can be classified into two general categories according to (1) the structure of the joints and (2) the type of movement allowed by the joints.

Structural Classification of Joints

When classifying joints according to their structure, two main characteristics differentiate the types of joints: (1) the type of connective tissue that holds the bones of the joint together and (2) the presence or absence of a joint cavity. There are three major structural categories of joints: fibrous, cartilaginous, and synovial. Fibrous joints have no joint cavity and include all joints in which the bones are held tightly together by fibrous connective tissue. Very little space separates the ends of the bones of these joints; as a result, little or no movement occurs. Examples include the joints, or sutures, between the bones of the skull, the joint between the distal tibia and fibula, and the joint between the radius and ulna (Figure 2.10).

Figure 2.10

Example of a fibrous joint — distal tibio-fibular joint

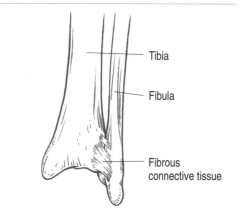

As the name implies, cartilaginous joints connect bones that are slightly separated by an intervening cartilage. No joint cavity exists and, similar to fibrous joints, little or no motion is possible. Familiar examples include the joints formed by the cartilages that connect the ribs to the sternum (breastbone) and intervertebral disks that separate the bodies of vertebrae that comprise the spinal column (Figure 2.11).

The vast majority of the joints in the human body are synovial joints. These joints all have a space, or joint cavity, between the bones forming the joint. Having more space between bones allows for greater amount of movement to occur at that joint. The capacity for movement of synovial joints is limited by the shapes of the bones of the joint and the soft tissues such as ligaments, joint capsules, tendons, and muscles that surround the joint. Synovial joints have five distinguishing features that set them apart structurally from the other types of joints. First, as previously described, all synovial joints have a joint cavity. Second, a ligamentous joint capsule made of dense, fibrous connective tissue surrounds each synovial joint. Third, the ends of the bones in synovial joints are covered with a thin layer of articular cartilage. This articular cartilage is made of hyaline ("glass-like") cartilage, and while it covers the surfaces of the articulating bones, the hyaline cartilage does not attach the bones together. Fourth, the inner surface of the joint capsule is lined with a thin synovial membrane. The synovial membrane's primary function is the secretion of synovial fluid, the fifth and final unique characteristic of all synovial joints. Synovial fluid acts as a lubricant for the joint, and provides nutrition to the articular cartilage. Normally, only a very small amount of synovial fluid (one or two teaspoonfuls) is present in

Figure 2.11

Example of a cartilaginous joint — sternocostal joint

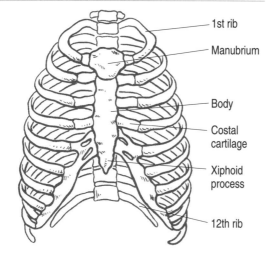

even the largest joints, such as the knee and shoulder. However, acute injury to, or overuse of, these synovial joints can stimulate the synovial membrane to secrete excessive fluid, typically producing pain, swelling, and decreased range of motion.

In addition to these five features, some synovial joints have fibrocartilage disks called menisci (singular = meniscus). An important weightbearing joint like the knee has two menisci. At the knee and other major joints, fibrocartilages help to absorb shock, increase joint stability, aid in joint nutrition by directing the flow of synovial fluid, and increase the joint contact area, thereby decreasing the pressure (load per unit area) on the weightbearing structures. Injury to a fibrocartilage changes the load bearing pattern and shock absorptive capabilities in that joint and can accelerate the wear and tear on joint surfaces and lead to premature degenerative joint disease.

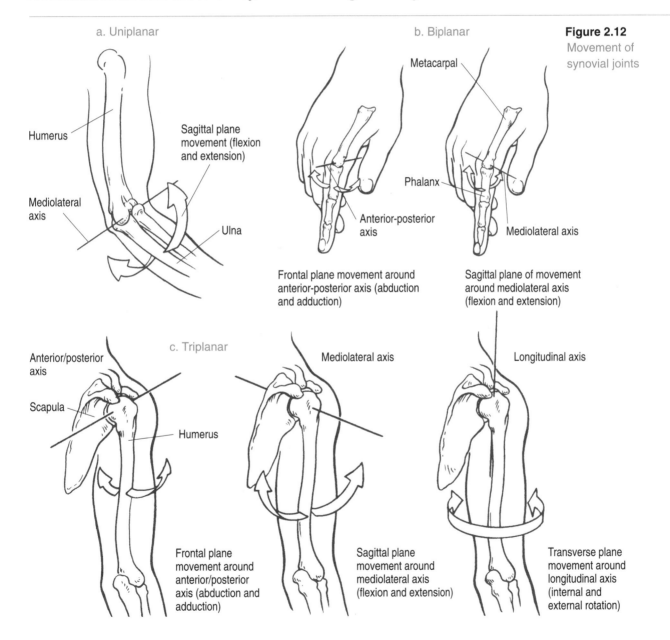

Figure 2.12
Movement of synovial joints

a. Uniplanar

Humerus

Sagittal plane movement (flexion and extension)

Mediolateral axis

Ulna

b. Biplanar

Metacarpal

Phalanx

Anterior-posterior axis

Mediolateral axis

Frontal plane movement around anterior-posterior axis (abduction and adduction)

Sagittal plane of movement around mediolateral axis (flexion and extension)

c. Triplanar

Anterior/posterior axis

Scapula

Humerus

Mediolateral axis

Longitudinal axis

Frontal plane movement around anterior/posterior axis (abduction and adduction)

Sagittal plane movement around mediolateral axis (flexion and extension)

Transverse plane movement around longitudinal axis (internal and external rotation)

Types of Movement of Synovial Joints

The functional classification of synovial joints is based upon the degree and type of movement they allow. Recall our earlier discussion of the anatomical planes of motion used to describe the actions of the body (see Figure 2.1). In order for a joint to move in a given plane, there must typically be an axis of rotation. An axis of rotation is an imaginary line perpendicular to the plane of movement about which a joint rotates. Due to their configuration, many joints have several axes of rotation, enabling bones to move in the various planes or directions.

Joints with one axis of rotation can only move in one plane and are known as uniplanar joints. These uniplanar joints are also known as hinge joints, in that hinges typically work only in one plane. The ankle (talo-crural) and the elbow (ulnohumeral) joints are examples of uniplanar joints (Figure 2.12a). Some joints have two axes of rotation, permitting motion in two planes that are at right angles to one another. These biplanar joints include a category of synovial joints known as condyloid joints, formed by the rounded, widened ends (condyles) of the two articulating bones. Condyloid joints allow full motion in one plane and have limited range of motion in a second plane. The knee (tibiofemoral), the joints of the hand and fingers (metacarpal-phalangeal), and the joints of the foot and toes (metatarsal-phalangeal joints), are all examples of condyloid joints (Figure 2.12b). Triplanar joints have three axes of motion and permit movement in three planes. Examples include the hip joint and the shoulder (glenohumeral), both of which are ball-

Table 2.5
Major Joints in the Body

Region/Joint	Type	Number of Axes of Rotation	Movement(s) Possible
Lower Extremity			
Metatarsophalangeal	Synovial (condyloid)	2	Flexion and extension; abduction and adduction; circumduction
Ankle	Synovial (hinge)	1	Plantar flexion and dorsiflexion
Between distal tibia and fibula	Fibrous	0	No voluntary motion possible
Knee (tibia and femur)	Synovial (condyloid)	2	Flexion and extension; internal and external rotation
Hip	Synovial (ball and socket)	3	Flexion and extension; abduction and adduction; circumduction; internal and external rotation
Upper Extremity			
Metacarpophalangeal	Synovial (condyloid)	2	Flexion and extension; abduction and adduction; circumduction
Thumb	Synovial (saddle)	3	Flexion and extension; abduction and adduction; circumduction; opposition and reposition
Wrist	Synovial (ellipsoid)	2	Flexion and extension; abduction and adduction; circumduction
Radioulnar	Synovial (pivot)	1	Pronation and supination
Elbow (ulna and humerus)	Synovial (hinge)	1	Flexion and extension
Shoulder (glenohumeral)	Synovial (ball and socket)	3	Flexion and extension; abduction and adduction; circumduction; internal and external rotation
Ribs and sternum	Cartilaginous	0	Slight movement possible (respiration)

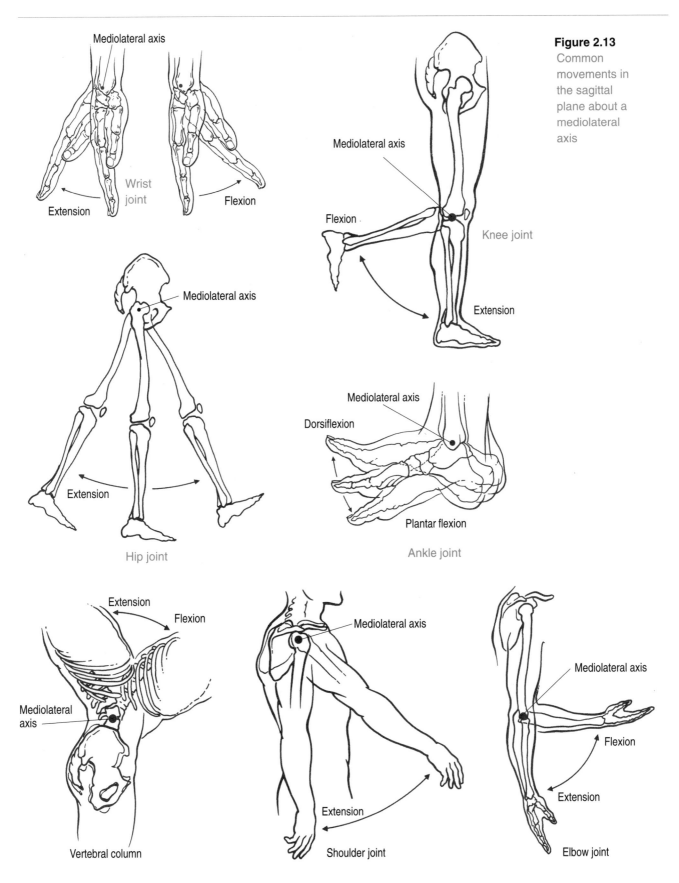

Figure 2.13
Common movements in the sagittal plane about a mediolateral axis

Figure 2.14

Common movements
in the frontal plane
about an anteropos-
terior axis

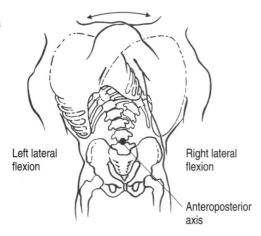

Left lateral
flexion

Right lateral
flexion

Anteroposterior
axis

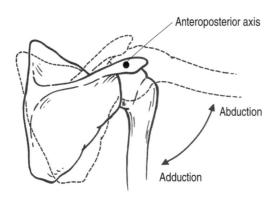

Anteroposterior axis

Abduction

Adduction

Glenohumeral joint

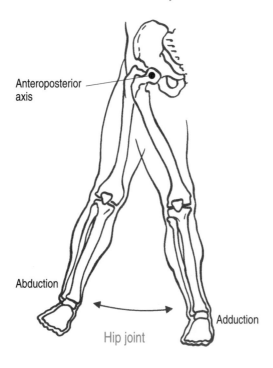

Anteroposterior
axis

Abduction

Adduction

Hip joint

and-socket joints, and the thumb (the first metacarpal-phalangeal), which is a saddle joint (Figure 2.12c). A summary of the major joints in the body, classified by type and movements possible at each, is presented in Table 2.5.

Human Movement Terminology

Human motion occurs in three dimensions as body parts rotate about the joints. **Flexion** usually involves a decrease in the angle between the anterior surfaces of articulating bones, whereas **extension** most often describes an increase in this angle. Flexion and extension both occur in the **sagittal plane** and this fundamental movement occurs at most of the synovial joints (Figure 2.13). **Abduction** is a **lateral** movement away from the midline of the body. When the arm or leg is moved away from the midline of the body, abduction occurs. **Adduction** is the return motion from abduction and involves movement of the body part toward the midline of the body, to regain anatomical position. Abduction and adduction movements occur in the **frontal plane** and are possible at many joints, some examples of which are presented in Figure 2.14. **Rotation** at a joint occurs in the **transverse plane** about a longitudinal axis and is described as being either **internal rotation** or **external rotation** of the bone involved. The hip, shoulder, and joints of the spine are among the joints most frequently requiring rotation for the performance of the activities of daily living (Figure 2.15).

At some synovial joints, the fundamental movements are given specialized names in order to clarify their action; these are summarized in Table 2.6. Forearm **supination** and **pronation** are motions that

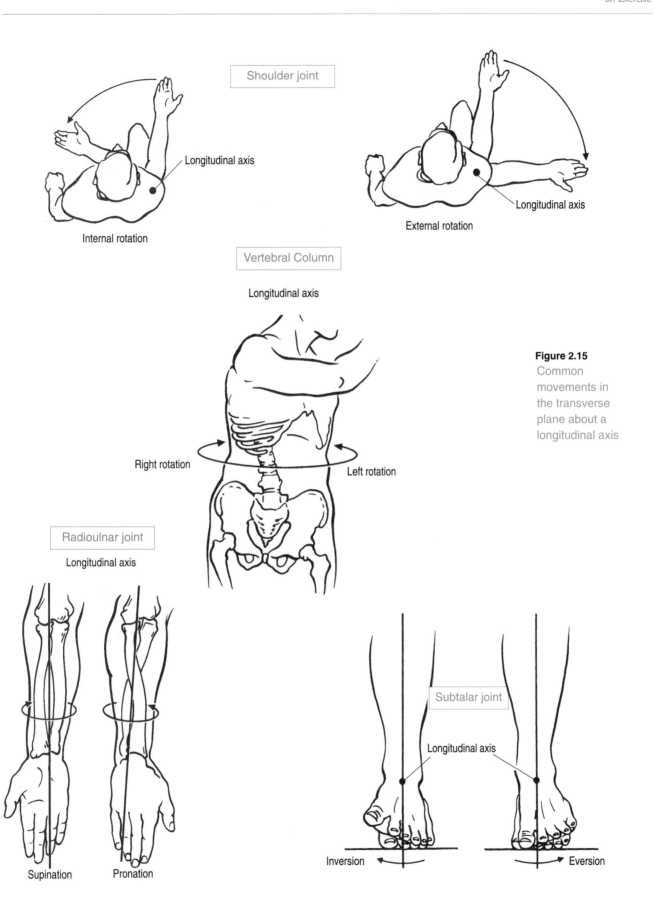

Shoulder joint

Longitudinal axis

Internal rotation

Longitudinal axis

External rotation

Vertebral Column

Longitudinal axis

Right rotation

Left rotation

Figure 2.15
Common movements in the transverse plane about a longitudinal axis

Radioulnar joint

Longitudinal axis

Supination

Pronation

Subtalar joint

Longitudinal axis

Inversion

Eversion

Table 2.6
Fundamental Human Movements (from Anatomical Position)

Plane	Action	Definition
Sagittal	Flexion	Decreasing the angle between two bones
	Extension	Increasing the angle between two bones
	Dorsiflexion	Moving the top of the foot toward the shin (occurs only at the ankle joint)
	Plantar flexion	Moving the sole of the foot downward; "pointing the toes" (only at the ankle)
Frontal	Abduction	Motion away from the midline of the body
	Adduction	Motion toward the midline of the body
	Elevation	Moving to a superior position
	Depression	Moving to an inferior position
	Inversion	Lifting the medial border of the foot (only at the subtalar joint)
	Eversion	Lifting the lateral border of the foot (only at the subtalar joint)
Transverse	Internal rotation	Inward or medial turning about the vertical axis of bone
	External rotation	Outward or lateral turning about the vertical axis of a bone
	Pronation	Rotating the forearm internally (palm down position)
	Supination	Rotating the forearm laterally from the elbow (palm-up position)
	Horizontal flexion	From a 90-degree abducted arm position, the humerus is brought in the toward the midline of the body in the transverse plane
	Horizontal extension	The return movement of the humerus from horizontal flexion
Multiplanar	Circumduction	Motion that describes a "cone"; combines flexion, abduction, extension, and adduction in sequence
	Opposition	Thumb movement unique to humans and primates

occur in the transverse plane. Supination is a term that specifically describes the external rotation of the forearm (radioulnar joint,) which causes the palm to face anteriorly. The radius and the ulna are parallel in this position, which is the anatomical or reference position for the forearms (see Figure 2.1). Pronation describes the internal rotation of the forearm that causes the radius to cross diagonally over the ulna and the palms to face posteriorly. **Circumduction** is a biplanar movement that involves the sequential combination of flexion, abduction, extension, and adduction. Circumduction is possible at the shoulder, hip, wrist, and spinal joints, among others.

Muscular System

While our bones and joints provide the structural framework for the body, the system most directly affected by exercise is the muscular system, through the coordinated activation and relaxation of specific muscles that enable us to move. There are three types of human muscle tissue: cardiac, visceral, and skeletal. Cardiac muscle tissue forms the walls of the heart and its contractile activity is involuntary by nature. The second type, visceral (smooth) muscle, is found in the walls of internal organs like the stomach and intestines and in blood vessels. Visceral muscle activity is also involuntary, and thus it is not under conscious control. Skeletal muscle tissue is attached to bones by tendons and is typically named according to its location, function, or size. Skeletal muscle is voluntary muscle; that is, it can be made to contract by conscious effort. While all three types of muscle have vital functions, the structure and function of skeletal muscles warrant further discussion. Both ends of a skeletal muscle are attached to bone via tendons (cords of inelastic connective tissue). In some cases, skeletal muscles are attached to bone by an aponeurosis, a broad, flat type of tendon. The wide, flat insertion of the rectus abdominis is an excellent example of an aponeurosis.

There are more than 600 muscles in the human body, but only the major muscles will be discussed in this chapter. Muscles are named according to their location (posterior tibialis, subscapularis), shape (deltoid, trapezius, rhomboid), action (extensor digitorum longus, adductor magnus), number of divisions (biceps brachii, triceps brachii, quadriceps femoris), bony attachments (coracobrachialis, iliocostalis), and size relationships (gluteus maximus, gluteus medius, gluteus minimus). In addition, several muscles have the descriptive terms "longus" (long) or "brevis" (short) in their names.

When skeletal muscle is stimulated by an impulse from its motor nerve, it performs one function: it develops tension (**force**). There are three ways in which a muscle can achieve this: by shortening and producing joint movement (**concentric** muscle action), by lengthening and controlling the motion (**eccentric** muscle action), or by staying the same length and creating no joint motion (**isometric** muscle action). Generally speaking, concentric muscle actions occur when the direction of movement is opposite the pull of gravity, and eccentric muscle actions occur when the direction of motion is the same as the force of gravity.

From a functional perspective, most muscles are arranged on the trunk and extremities in opposing pairs. That is, when one muscle is acting to achieve a desired movement, it is referred to the **agonist**; the muscle that opposes the action of the agonist is known as the **antagonist**. For example, during the upward phase of a bent knee curl-up, the abdominal muscles are acting concentrically as agonists to produce flexion of the trunk, while the erector spinae group of muscles of the back are elongated in an eccentric mode as antagonists. At most joints several muscles work together to perform the same anatomical function; these muscles are functionally known as **synergists** (syn = together; erg = work). For the example just given, the synergistic actions of the rectus abdominis, external oblique, and internal oblique produce flexion of the trunk.

Perhaps the most difficult and often confusing aspect of functional anatomy is the fact that any given skeletal muscle can perform different, exactly opposite functions, depending on the circumstances and desired human movement. Most anatomy books only describe the concentric function(s) of a muscle, ignoring the motions produced when that same muscle acts eccentrically. A squat exercise and the quadriceps femoris, the very large and familiar muscle that covers the anterior thigh, illustrate this point nicely. Focusing our attention on the knee, the downward phase of a squat requires knee flexion while the upward phase involves knee extension. From reading this chapter you will learn that the quadriceps, when acting concentrically, are the main knee extensors and that the hamstrings are the primary knee flexors. However, since the direction of movement in the downward phase of the squat is the same direction as gravity, the observed knee flexion movement is controlled by an eccentric (lengthening) action of the quadriceps. During the upward phase of the squat, the quadriceps shorten concentrically to produce powerful extension of the knee, overcoming gravity and pushing the body upward in the direction opposite of gravity's pull. During this one simple exercise, we see how the quadriceps acted as both a knee flexor and knee extensor, and how the only role the hamstrings had at the knee was that of the antagonist, rather than agonist. Every skeletal muscle has this same functional capability, producing exactly opposite movements when it shortens and lengthens.

The greatest amount of muscle force (tension) is generated during eccentric muscle actions, followed by isometric and then concentric muscle actions. Voluntary, coordinated maximal or submaximal efforts produce muscle actions that may or may not result in joint movement. Locomotion (walking, running) is the result of the complex, combined functioning of the bones, joints, nerves, and muscles. Isometric muscle actions enable the maintenance of posture in stationary positions (e.g., sitting and standing). As a by-product of performance of the activities of daily living, muscles produce heat, important in maintaining normal body temperature.

Muscles of the Lower Extremity

The major links of the lower extremity are the (1) ankle joint formed by the distal tibia, distal fibula, and talus; (2) knee joint composed of the tibiofemoral and patellofemoral joints; and (3) hip joint linking the femur with the hip (coxal) bone. When compared to the muscles of the upper extremity, the muscles of the lower extremity tend to be larger and more powerful. Many of the muscles of the lower extremity cross two joints, either the hip and the knee, or the knee and the ankle. The major muscles of the lower extremity that act at more than one joint are listed in Table 2.7.

Muscles That Act at the Ankle and the Foot

The muscles of the leg are grouped into four compartments that are divided by fibrous interosseous membranes (inter = between; os = bone) between the tibia and

Table 2.7
Actions of Major Lower Extremity Multijoint Muscles

Muscle	Hip	Knee	Ankle
Rectus femoris	Flexion	Extension	————
Biceps femoris	Extension (long head) External rotation	Flexion External rotation	————
Semitendinosus	Extension Internal rotation	Flexion Internal rotation	————
Semimembranosus	Extension Internal rotation	Flexion Internal rotation	————
Gracilis	Adduction Internal rotation	Flexion Internal rotation	————
Sartorius	Flexion External rotation	Flexion Internal rotation	————
Gastrocnemius	————	Flexion	Plantar flexion

fibula (Figure 2.16). The anterior tibial compartment muscles act concentrically to extend the toes and dorsiflex the ankle. These muscles include the anterior tibialis, extensor digitorum longus, and extensor hallucis longus (Figure 2.17). The muscles of the lateral tibial compartment are known as the peroneals (peroneus longus and peroneus brevis) and act to cause **eversion** (abduction) of the foot and assist in plantarflexion of the ankle (Figure 2.18). The posterior muscles of the leg are contained in two separate spaces — the superficial and deep posterior tibial compartments. The largest muscles of the calf (soleus and gastrocnemius), along with the much smaller plantaris, are located in the superficial posterior tibial compartment. The deep posterior tibial compartment contains the posterior tibialis, flexor hallucis longus, flexor digitorum longus, and the popliteus (Figure 2.19). The primary functions of these posterior muscles include plantarflexion of the ankle, flexion of the toes, and **inversion** of the foot. The popliteus has no function at the ankle or foot, but instead plays a vital role by initiating knee flexion. The largest tendon in the body, the Achilles tendon, found in the superficial posterior compartment, connects the gastrocnemius and soleus via one common tendon to the calcaneus (heel bone). The origins, insertions, primary functions, and examples of exercises to develop the muscles that act at the ankle and the foot are presented in Table 2.8.

Muscles That Act at the Knee Joint

The muscles that cross the tibiofemoral (knee) joint can be divided into three functional groups based upon their location in one of the muscular compartments of the thigh. While the lower leg has four separate

Figure 2.16
Contents of the muscular compartments of the lower leg

Anterior compartment
• Tibialis anterior
• Extensor digitorum longus
• Extensor hallucis longus

Tibia

Fibula

Deep posterior compartment
• Tibialis posterior
• Flexor digitorum longus
• Flexor hallucis longus

Superficial posterior compartment
• Soleus
• Gastrocnemius
• Popliteus
• Plantaris

Lateral compartment
• Peroneus longus
• Peroneus brevis

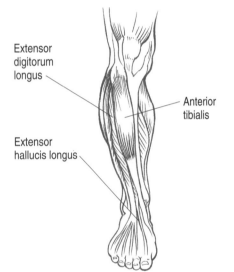

Figure 2.17
Anterior compartment muscles of the lower leg; primary muscles for dorsiflexion and inversion

Extensor digitorum longus

Anterior tibialis

Extensor hallucis longus

Figure 2.18
Lateral compartment muscles of the lower leg; primary muscles for eversion

Peroneus longus

Peroneus brevis

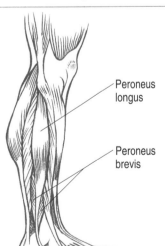

**Table 2.8
Major Muscles That Act at the Ankle and Foot**

Muscle	Origin	Insertion	Primary Function(s)	Sample Exercises
Anterior tibialis	Proximal 2/3 of lateral tibia	Medial aspect of 1st cuneiform and 1st metatarsal	Dorsiflexion at ankle; inversion at foot	Cycling with toe clips, resisted inversion (with dorsiflexion)
Peroneus longus	Head of fibula and proximal 2/3 of lateral fibula	Inferior aspects of medial tarsal (1st cuneiform) and 1st metatarsal	Plantar flexion at ankle; eversion at foot	Resisted eversion of foot; walking on inside of foot
Peroneus brevis	Distal 2/3 of lateral fibula	Base of the 5th metatarsal	Plantar flexion at ankle; eversion at foot	Resisted eversion of foot with rubber tubing; walking on inside of foot
Gastrocnemius	Posterior surfaces of femoral condyles	Posterior surface of calcaneus via Achilles tendon	Plantar flexion at ankle	Hill running, jumping rope, toe raises with barbell on shoulder, cycling, stair-climber machine, in-line skating
Soleus posterior surfaces of tibia and fibula	Proximal 2/3 of via Achilles tendon	Posterior surface of calcaneus	Plantar flexion at ankle	Virtually the same as for gastrocnemius; bent-knee toe raises with resistance
Posterior tibialis	Posterior surface of tibia-fibular interosseous membrane	Lower medial surfaces of medial tarsals and metatarsals	Plantar flexion at ankle; inversion at foot	Resisted inversion of foot with surgical tubing with plantar flexion

muscular compartments, the thigh has three distinct compartments, each innervated by a different peripheral nerve (Figure 2.20). The anterior compartment is supplied by the femoral nerve, the posterior compartment by the sciatic nerve, and the **medial** compartment by the obturator nerve.

The four major muscles on the front of the thigh are located in the anterior compartment; the primary function of these muscles is to extend the knee. These muscles are typically grouped together and referred to as the quadriceps femoris, although each muscle has its own individual name: rectus femoris, vastus medialis, vastus intermedius, and vastus lateralis. The quadriceps femoris muscle inserts into the proximal tibia at the tibial tuberosity via the patellar tendon (Figure 2.21).

Figure 2.19

Superficial and deep posterior tibial compartment muscles; primary muscles for plantarflexion

a. Superficial posterior compartment muscles
b. Deep posterior compartment muscles

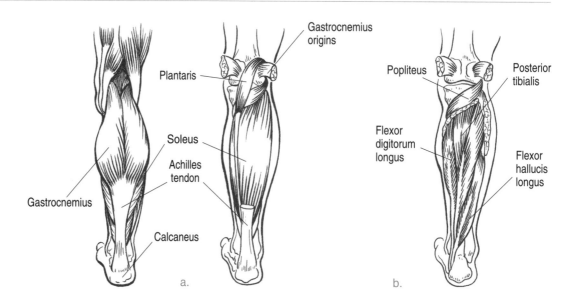

The muscles found in the posterior compartment of the thigh are the biceps femoris, semitendinosus, and semimembranosus. These muscles, collectively known as the hamstrings, cross the knee joint and cause flexion of the leg. This large group of muscles has a common origin at the ischial tuberosity. Below the knee, the biceps femoris attaches laterally, while the semitendinosus and semimembranosus attach on the medial aspect of the tibia (Figure 2.22). Given these attachment sites, the biceps femoris is an external rotator, while the semitendinosus and semimembranosus are internal rotators of the knee (when it is flexed). Between the hamstring tendons lies the popliteal space, a triangular area on the posterior-medial aspect of the knee joint.

The third major group of muscles that act at the knee is located in the medial compartment of the thigh and includes two of the three muscles in the pes anserine ("goose's foot") group (Figure 2.23). The pes anserine group got its name from the flat, web-shaped common tendon of attachment of the sartorius, the gracilis, and the previously mentioned semitendinosus. These muscles are grouped together because of their common site of insertion on the medial tibia, just below the knee. The sartorius, the longest muscle in the body, originates on the ilium and courses diagonally across the anterior aspect of the thigh to its insertion on the proximal tibia. Even though the sartorius is an anterior thigh muscle, its concentric action causes flexion of the knee, functioning like the hamstrings. As a group, the three pes anserine muscles internally rotate the tibia when the knee is flexed. The origins, insertions, primary functions, and examples of exercises to develop the major muscles that act on the leg are presented in Table 2.9.

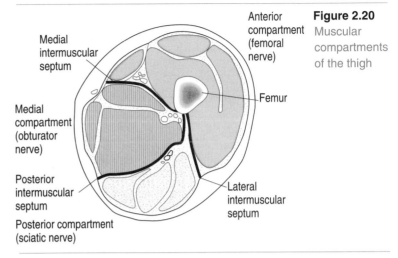

Figure 2.20
Muscular compartments of the thigh

Anterior compartment (femoral nerve)
Medial intermuscular septum
Medial compartment (obturator nerve)
Posterior intermuscular septum
Posterior compartment (sciatic nerve)
Femur
Lateral intermuscular septum

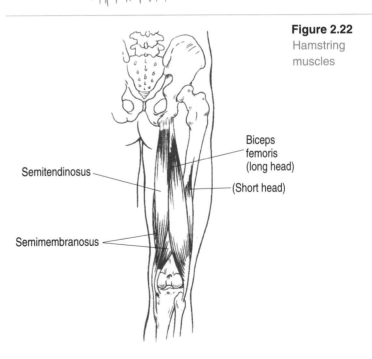

Figure 2.21
Quadriceps femoris muscle

Rectus femoris
Vastus lateralis
Vastus intermedialis
Vastus medialis

Figure 2.22
Hamstring muscles

Semitendinosus
Semimembranosus
Biceps femoris (long head)
(Short head)

Table 2.9
Major Muscles that Act at the Knee Joint

Muscle	Origin	Insertion	Primary Function(s)	Sample Exercises
Rectus femoris	Anterior-inferior spine of ilium	Superior aspect of patella and patellar tendon	Extension (most effective when the hip is extended)	Cycling, leg press machine, squat, vertical jumping, stair climbing, jumping rope, plyometrics
Vastus lateralis, intermedius, and medialis	Proximal 2/3 of anterior femur at midline	Patella and tibial tuberosity via the patellar tendon	Extension (particularly when the hip is flexed)	Same as for rectus femoris, resisted knee extension, in-line skating, cross-country skiing
Biceps femoris	Ischial tuberosity	Lateral condyle of tibia and head of fibula	Flexion and external rotation	Jumping rope, hamstring curls with knee in external rotation
Semitendinosus	Ischial tuberosity aspect of tibia	Proximal anterior-medial	Flexion and internal rotation	Essentially the same as for biceps femoris; hamstring curls with knee in internal rotation
Semimembranosus	Ischial tuberosity	Posterior aspect of medial tibial condyle	Flexion and internal rotation	Same as semitendinosus

Muscles That Act at the Hip Joint

Most of the muscles that act at the hip joint have their origins on the pelvis and the bulk of the muscle tissue is located on the thigh. Recall the three muscular compartments of the thigh presented in Figure 2.20. At the anterior aspect of the hip, the psoas major and the psoas minor muscles arise from the transverse processes of the five lumbar ver-

tebrae. These two muscles, along with the iliacus, have a common attachment on the lesser trochanter of the femur and work together as powerful flexors of the thigh. This group of three muscles is collectively known as the iliopsoas. The rectus femoris is the only muscle of the quadriceps femoris group that crosses the hip joint; it also causes flexion of the thigh (see Figure 2.21).

Figure 2.23

Pes anserine muscles: sartorius, gracilis, and semitendinosus

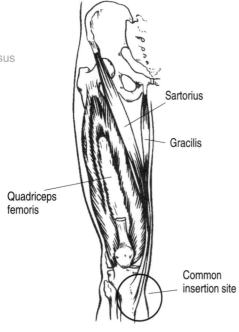

Sartorius

Gracilis

Quadriceps femoris

Common insertion site

a. Anterior view

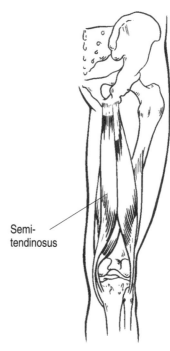

Semi-tendinosus

b. Posterior view

Posteriorly, several muscles combine to give shape to the buttocks and serve as powerful mobilizers of the hip joint. The largest and most superficial of the three is the gluteus maximus, which extends and externally rotates the hip. The gluteus maximus is a very large muscle that has fibers that lie superior and inferior to the hip joint; when the superior (upper) fibers are stimulated, they cause hip abduction. Activation of the inferior (lower) fibers of the gluteus maximus pulls the hip toward midline (adduction). Underlying the gluteus maximus are the gluteus medius and the gluteus minimus, which combine to abduct and internally rotate the hip. Also on the posterior aspect of the thigh are the hamstring muscles (biceps femoris, semitendinosus, semimembranosus), which function to extend the hip joint (see Figure 2.22).

The muscles located in the medial compartment of the thigh are named for both their function and their size. The adductor magnus, adductor longus, and adductor brevis work together to adduct the hip joint. In addition, the gracilis and pectineus muscles are synergists for adduction of the hip (Figure 2.24). The origins, insertions, primary actions, and examples of exercises to develop the major muscles that act at the hip are presented in Table 2.10.

Muscles That Act on the Trunk

This discussion of the muscles of the trunk will include only the major muscles associated with the spinal column and the walls of the abdomen. Concentric actions of these muscles results primarily in sagittal plane motion, (flexion and extension of the trunk).

Table 2.10
Major Muscles That Act at the Hip Joint

Muscle	Origin	Insertion	Primary Function(s)	Sample Exercises
Iliacus	Inner surface of the ilium and base of sacrum	Lesser trochanter of femur	Flexion and external rotation	Straight-leg sit-ups, running with knees lifted up high, leg raises
Psoas major and psoas minor	Transverse processes of all 5 lumbar vertebrae	Lesser trochanter of femur	Flexion and external rotation	Essentially same as iliacus
Rectus femoris	Anterior-inferior spine of ilium	Superior aspect of patella and patellar tendon	Flexion	Running, leg press, squat, jumping rope
Gluteus maximus	Posterior 1/4 of iliac crest and sacrum	Gluteal line of femur and iliotibial band	Extension and external rotation	Cycling, plyometrics, jumping rope, squats, stair-climbing machine
Gluteus medius and minimus	Lateral surface of ilium	Greater trochanter of femur	Abduction	Side-lying leg raises, walking, running
Biceps femoris	Ischial tuberosity	Lateral condyle of tibia and head of fibula	Extension	Cycling, hamstring curls with knee in external rotation
Semitendinosus	Ischial tuberosity	Proximal anterior-medial aspect of tibia	Extension	Essentially the same as for biceps femoris; hamstring curls with knee in internal rotation
Semimembranosus	Ischial tuberosity	Posterior aspect of medial tibial condyle	Extension	Same as semitendinosus
Adductor magnus	Pubic ramus and ischial tuberosity	Medial aspects of femur rotation adduction exercises	Adduction and external manual resistance	Side-lying bottom leg raises;
Adductor brevis and longus	Pubic ramus and ischial tuberosity	Medial aspects of femur	Adduction, flexion, and internal rotation	Side-lying bottom leg raises, resisted adduction

Figure 2.24
Medial thigh compartment muscles responsible for hip adduction

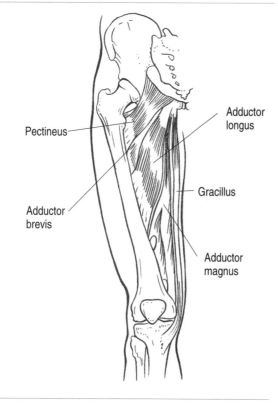

Pectineus

Adductor brevis

Adductor longus

Gracillus

Adductor magnus

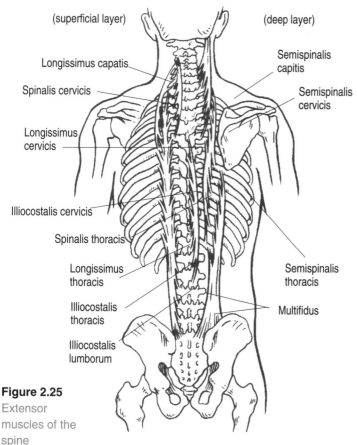

(superficial layer)

(deep layer)

Longissimus capatis

Spinalis cervicis

Longissimus cervicis

Illiocostalis cervicis

Spinalis thoracis

Longissimus thoracis

Illiocostalis thoracis

Illiocostalis lumborum

Semispinalis capitis

Semispinalis cervicis

Semispinalis thoracis

Multifidus

Figure 2.25
Extensor muscles of the spine

The three major muscles responsible for extension of the vertebral column, from lateral to medial are the iliocostalis, the longissimus, and the spinalis. These are better known by their functional group name — erector spinae. Each of the three columns of muscles in this group has a subdivision name based on the particular portion of the spinal column to which it attaches. For example, the iliocostalis muscle has three divisions: iliocostalis lumborum (in the lumbar region of the spine), iliocostalis thoracis (in the thoracic region of the spine), and iliocostalis cervicis (in the cervical or neck region of the spine) (Figure 2.25). The erector spinae muscles are assisted by the semispinalis (thoracis, cervicis, capitis) and multifidus muscles. When these muscles act bilaterally (right and left side muscles stimulated at the same time), their concentric action produces extension of the spine. Unilateral concentric action of the erector spinae muscles will produce **lateral flexion** to that side.

The anterior walls of the abdominal cavity are supported entirely by the strength of the muscles located there, for there are no bones to uphold this region. To make up for the lack of a skeletal framework, the three layers of muscles in the abdominal wall run in different directions, providing additional support (Figure 2.26). In the outermost (superficial) layer is the external oblique muscle, the fibers of which run anteriorly downward and toward the midline. In the second layer, the fibers of the internal oblique muscle run posteriorly and downward. An easy way to remember the orientation of these two muscles is to picture the fibers of the external oblique running into the front pockets of your slacks and the fibers of the internal oblique running diagonally into the rear pockets. Unilateral (one side) contraction of

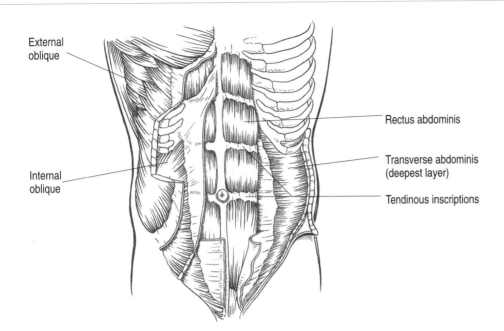

Figure 2.26
Muscles of the abdominal wall

External oblique

Rectus abdominis

Transverse abdominis (deepest layer)

Internal oblique

Tendinous inscriptions

the lateral fibers of the obliques (external and internal) produces lateral flexion of the spinal column on that side. Trunk rotation to the right is produced by the simultaneous activation of the left external oblique and the right internal oblique muscle; the opposite combination (right external oblique, left internal oblique) will produce left trunk rotation. Bilateral (both sides) concentric muscle action of the external and internal obliques will flex the trunk and compress the abdominal cavity.

The deepest of the three muscular layers of the abdominal wall contains the transverse abdominis muscle. The fibers of this thin muscle run horizontally, encircling the abdominal cavity; stimulation of this muscle compresses the abdomen but produces no anatomical motion (see Figure 2.26).

The rectus abdominis is a narrow, flat, superficial muscle on the anterior aspect of the abdominal wall that flexes the vertebral column; its fibers run vertically from the pubis to the rib cage. The rectus abdominis is crossed by three transverse fibrous bands

called tendinous inscriptions (see Figure 2.26). The origins, insertions, primary functions, and examples of exercises to develop the muscles that act on the trunk are presented in Table 2.11.

Muscles of the Upper Extremity

As a group fitness instructor studying the musculature of the upper extremity, you must know the anatomical motions (and the muscles responsible for producing these movements) at the four major links of the upper body. Specifically, these four joints are the wrist joint, composed of the distal radius and ulna and proximal carpal bones; the elbow joint, formed by the union of the olecranon process of the ulna and the distal humerus; the shoulder joint, consisting of the proximal humerus and the glenoid fossa of the scapula; and the scapulothoracic articulation. The connection between the scapula and the thorax is not a bony joint, per se, but more an important functional, soft tissue (muscle and fascia) link between the scapula and the trunk. Similar to the lower

Table 2.11
Major Muscles that Act at the Trunk

Muscle	Origin	Insertion	Primary Function(s)	Sample Exercises
Rectus abdominis	Pubic crest	Cartilage of 5th through 7th ribs and xiphoid process	Flexion and lateral flexion of the trunk (unilateral action)	Bent-knee sit-ups, partial curl-ups, good posture, pelvic tilts
External oblique	Anteriolateral borders of lower 8 ribs	Anterior 1/2 of ilium, pubic crest, and anterior fascia	Flexion, lateral flexion, and rotation of the trunk	Twisting bent-knee sit-ups (rotation opposite), curl-ups
Internal oblique	Iliac crest	Cartilage of last 3–4 ribs	Flexion, lateral flexion, and rotation of the trunk	Twisting bent-knee sit-ups (rotation same side), and curl ups
Transverse abdominis	Iliac crest, lumbar fascia, and cartilages of last 6 ribs	Xiphoid process of sternum, anterior fascia, and pubis	Compresses abdomen	No motor function
Erector spinae	Posterior iliac crest and sacrum	Angles of ribs, transverse processes of all ribs	Extension of trunk	Squat, dead lift, prone back extension exercises, good standing posture

extremity, there are many muscles in the upper extremity that act at two joints; these muscles are identified in Table 2.12.

Muscles That Act at the Wrist

The muscles that act at the wrist joint can be grouped according to their origin and function. The flexor-pronator muscles originate on the medial epicondyle of the humerus, and cause flexion of the wrist and pronation (palm facing down) of the forearm (radius and ulna). The primary wrist flexors are the flexor carpi radialis, palmaris longus, and flexor carpi ulnaris (Figure 2.27a). The palmaris longus muscle is absent in approximately 10% of the population. The major pronators of the forearm are the pronator teres at the elbow and the pronator quadratus at the wrist (Figure 2.27b). The antagonist muscles to the flexor-pronators are the extensor-supinator muscles, which arise from a common tendon on the lateral humeral epicondyle and, as their group name indicates, produce extension of the wrist and supination of the forearm. The major wrist extensors are the extensor carpi radialis longus and the extensor carpi ulnaris (Figure 2.27c). Simply enough, the supinator muscle (with substantial syn-

Table 2.12
Actions of Major Upper Extremity Multijoint Muscles

Muscle	Shoulder	Elbow	Forearm	Wrist
Biceps brachii	Flexion	Flexion	Supination	----------
Brachioradialis	----------	Flexion	Pronation, supination	----------
Triceps brachii	Extension (long head)	Extension	----------	----------
Flexor carpi radialis	----------	Flexion	----------	Flexion, abduction
Flexor carpi ulnaris	----------	Flexion	----------	Flexion, adduction
Extensor carpi radialis longus and brevis	----------	Extension	----------	Extension
Extensor carpi ulnaris	----------	Extension	----------	Extension, adduction

ergistic help from the biceps brachii) is responsible for supination of the forearm (see Figure 2.27b). The origins, insertions, primary functions, and examples of exercises to develop the muscles that act at the wrist and forearm are presented in Table 2.13.

Muscles That Act at the Elbow Joint

As you may recall, the elbow (ulnohumeral) joint is a hinge joint, and as such, permits motion in only one plane. In the case of the elbow, that one plane is the sagittal plane, and the only motions that occur in the sagittal plane are flexion and extension. The flexors of the elbow, the biceps brachii, brachialis, and brachioradialis, are located on the anterior aspect of the arm (humerus) (Figure 2.28). The triceps brachii is the major extensor of the elbow joint and is located on the posterior aspect of the arm. As its name suggests, the triceps have three heads or origins — one on the scapula and two on the proximal hu-

merus. All three heads converge and insert via a common tendon into the olecranon process of the ulna (Figure 2.29). The origins, insertions, primary functions, and examples of exercises to develop the muscles that act at the elbow joint are listed in Table 2.14.

Muscles That Act at the Shoulder Joint

As mentioned previously, the shoulder (glenohumeral) joint is the most mobile joint in the body. We will concern ourselves with only the nine major muscles that cross the shoulder joint and act on the arm (humerus). The two largest muscles, the pectoralis major and the latissimus dorsi, have their origins on the thorax. The pectoralis major has several important functions at the shoulder: the clavicular portion of the pectoralis major causes flexion, while its sternal fibers produce shoulder extension in the sagittal plane; adduction in the frontal plane; and internal rotation in the transverse plane (see Figure

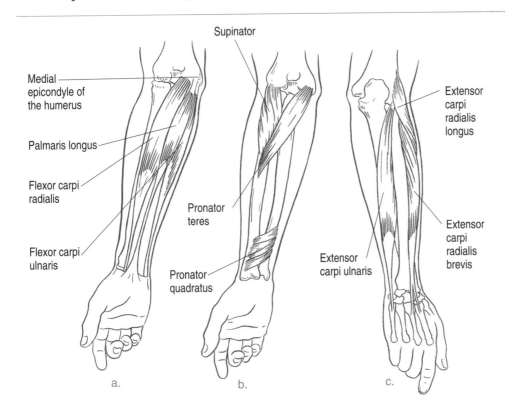

Figure 2.27

Muscles of the forearm and wrist

a. Wrist flexors
b. Forearm pronators
c. Wrist extensors

Supinator

Medial epicondyle of the humerus

Palmaris longus

Flexor carpi radialis

Flexor carpi ulnaris

Pronator teres

Pronator quadratus

Extensor carpi radialis longus

Extensor carpi radialis brevis

Extensor carpi ulnaris

a.

b.

c.

Table 2.13
Major Muscles That Act at the Wrist

Muscle	Origin	Insertion	Primary Function(s)	Sample Exercises
Flexor carpi radialis	Medial epicondyle of humerus	2nd and 3rd metacarpals	Flexion	Wrist curls against resistance; grip strengthening exercises; baseball and softball, racquet sports, particularly racquetball and badminton
Flexor carpi ulnaris	Medial epicondyle of humerus	5th metacarpal	Flexion	Same as flexor carpi radialis
Extensor carpi radialis longus	Lateral epicondyle of humerus	2nd metacarpal	Extension	"Reverse" wrist curls, racquet sports, particularly tennis
Extensor carpi ulnaris	Lateral epicondyle of humerus	5th metacarpal	Extension	Same as extensor carpi radialis longus

2.28). The latissimus dorsi arises posteriorly from the pelvis and lumbar and lower thoracic vertebrae. Interestingly, due to its medial insertion on the arm, the latissimus shares two functions with the pectoralis major. While the latissimus dorsi is a prime extensor of the shoulder joint, it complements the pectoralis as an adductor and internal rotator of the arm (Figure 2.30).

The remaining muscles that act at the shoulder joint have their origins on the scapula itself. The superficial deltoid muscle is located on the superior aspect of the shoulder joint and resembles its name in several ways. The deltoid muscle is shaped like a triangle (Greek letter delta = Δ) and is divided in three functional sections. The anterior deltoid fibers flex and internally rotate the shoulder. The middle portion of the deltoid is a primary abductor of the glenohumeral joint. The posterior deltoid fibers extend the shoulder as well as produce external rotation when activated (see Figures 2.28 and 2.30).

The rotator cuff muscles, a group of four relatively small muscles, are functionally very important (Figure 2.31). These muscles act to oppose the pull of gravity and stabilize the humeral head by pulling it inward and slightly downward into the glenohumeral joint. For this reason, the rotator cuff muscles are sometimes referred to as the compressor cuff, in that they compress the humeral head in against the glenoid fossa of the scapula. The four rotator cuff muscles are easily remembered with the acronym SITS: the supraspinatus, which abducts the arm; the infraspinatus and teres minor, which externally rotate the arm; and the subscapularis. As its name describes, the subscapu-

Figure 2.28
Superficial musculature of the anterior chest, shoulder, and arm (humerus)

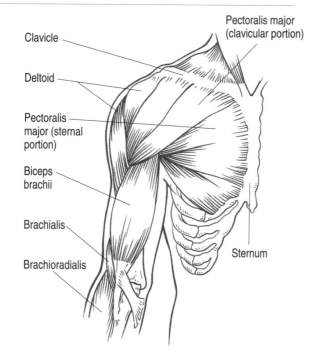

Clavicle

Deltoid

Pectoralis major (sternal portion)

Biceps brachii

Brachialis

Brachioradialis

Pectoralis major (clavicular portion)

Sternum

Table 2.14
Major Muscles That Act on the Elbow

Muscle	Origin	Insertion	Primary Function(s)	Sample Exercises
Biceps brachii	Long head from tubercle above glenoid cavity; short head from coracoid process of scapula	Radial tuberosity and bicipital aponeurosis	Flexion at elbow; supation at forearm	"Curling" with barbell, rowing machine, chin-ups, rock climbing, upright "rows" with barbell
Brachialis	Anterior humerus	Ulnar tuberosity and coronoid process of ulna	Flexion at elbow	Same as for biceps brachii
Brachioradialis	Distal 2/3 of lateral condyloid ridge of humerus	Radial styloid process	Flexion at elbow	Same as for biceps brachii
Triceps brachii	Long head from lower edge of glenoid cavity of scapula; lateral head from posterior humerus; short head from distal 2/3 of posterior humerus	Olecranon process of ulna	Extension at elbow	Push-ups, dips on parallel bars, bench press, military press, reverse curls
Pronator teres	Distal end of medial humerus and medial aspect of ulna	Middle 1/3 of lateral radius	Flexion at elbow; pronation at forearm	Pronation of forearm with dumbbell

laris is located on the inferior surface of the scapula, and internally rotates the arm. The origins, insertions, primary functions, and examples of exercises designed to develop the muscles that cross the shoulder joint are presented in Table 2.15.

The rotator cuff muscles are frequently injured due to errors in training (e.g., general overuse, improper or insufficient warm-up, and excessive repetitions of shoulder abduction with internal rotation). Inflammation of the rotator cuff commonly results in a painful

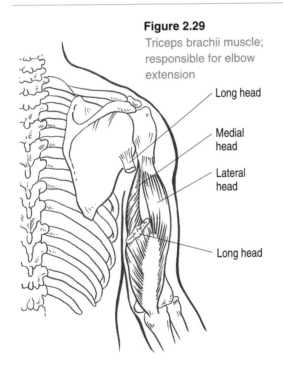

Figure 2.29

Triceps brachii muscle; responsible for elbow extension

Long head

Medial head

Lateral head

Long head

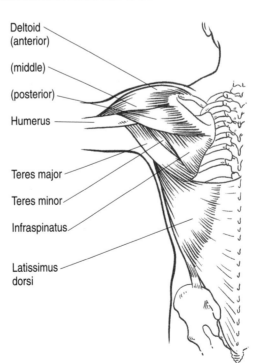

Deltoid (anterior)

(middle)

(posterior)

Humerus

Teres major

Teres minor

Infraspinatus

Latissimus dorsi

Figure 2.30

Superficial musculature of the superior and inferior shoulder joint; prime movers for shoulder abduction (deltoid) and adduction (latissimus dorsi and teres major)

**Table 2.15
Major Muscles Thˆat Act at the Shoulder**

Muscle	Origin	Insertion	Primary Function(s)	Sample Exercises
Pectoralis major	Clavicle, sternum, and first six costal cartilages	Greater tubercle of humerus	Flexion; adduction; internal rotation	Push-ups, pull-ups, incline bench press, regular bench press, climbing a rope, all types of throwing, tennis serve
Deltoid	Anterolateral clavicle, border of the acromion, and lower edge of spine of the scapula	Deltoid tubercle of humerus on mid-lateral surface	Abduction: entire muscle; anterior fibers: flexion, internal rotation; posterior fibers: extension, external rotation	Lateral "butterfly" (abduction) exercises with dumbbells, anterior deltoid has similar functions as the pectoralis major
Latissimus dorsi	Lower six thoracic vertebrae, all lumbar vertebrae, crests of ilium and sacrum, lower four ribs	Medial side of intertubercular groove of humerus	Extension; adduction; internal rotation	Chin-ups, rope climbing, dips on parallel bars, rowing, any exercise that involves pulling the arms downward against resistance, e.g., "lat" pulls on exercise machine
Rotator cuff	Various aspects of scapula	All insert on greater tubercle of humerus except for the subscapularis, which inserts on the lesser tubercle of humerus	Infraspinatus and teres minor:external rotation; subscapularis: internal rotation; supraspinatus: abduction	Exercises that involve internal and external rotation, e.g., tennis serve, throwing a baseball, internal and external rotation exercises from prone/supine position with dumbbells

condition known as impingement syndrome in which the irritated rotator cuff muscles, their tendons, and the nearby bursa sacs are compressed between the humeral head and the acromion process of the scapula when the arm is abducted. The group fitness instructor who recommends exercise regimens that include repeated overhead arm motions, such as swimming, resistance training, and racquet sports should closely monitor client performance in order to avoid inducing shoulder impingement syndrome.

Figure 2.31
Rotator cuff muscles
a. Anterior view of subscapularis
b. Posterior view of supraspinatus, infraspinatus, and teres minor

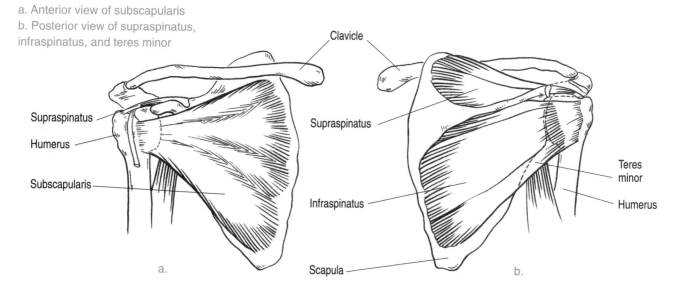

Muscles That Act at the Scapulothoracic Articulation

The primary function of the muscles and fascia that make up the soft tissue connection between the scapula and the trunk is to stabilize the scapula during movement of the arm (humerus). The four major muscles that anchor the scapula to the thorax are named according to their shape (trapezius, rhomboid major, and rhomboid minor) and function (levator scapula) (Figure 2.32). Due to its shape and the varied directions of pull of its fibers, the superficial trapezius muscle has several different functions. The upper portion of the trapezius is responsible for **elevation** of the scapula, (e.g., shrugging the shoulders). The middle section of the trapezius has horizontally directed fibers, resulting in adduction of the scapula when stimulated. The fibers of the lower portion of the trapezius are angled downward toward their attachment on the thoracic vertebrae. Concentric action of the lower trapezius primarily results in **depression** and adduction of the scapula.

Deep to the trapezius are the rhomboids (major and minor), which work in unison to produce adduction and slight elevation of the scapula (see Figure 2.32). Good muscle tone in the rhomboids will help maintain good upper back posture, and thereby help avoid the "rounded shoulders" posture. The levator scapula muscle runs from the upper cervical vertebrae to the medial border of the scapula and, together with the upper part of the trapezius, elevates the scapula. The origins, insertions, primary functions, and examples of exercises to develop the muscles of the scapulothoracic articulation are listed in Table 2.16.

Overview of Kinesiology

Kinesiology, as it is known to exercise scientists, physical education teachers, and allied health practitioners, involves the study of human movement from a physical science perspective. A common way for professors to describe **kinesiology**

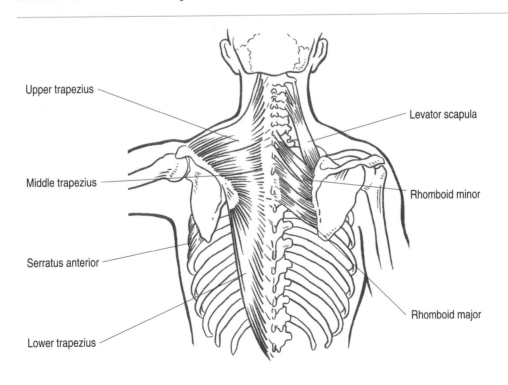

Figure 2.32
Superficial and deep muscles that act at the scapulothoracic articulation

Upper trapezius

Middle trapezius

Serratus anterior

Lower trapezius

Levator scapula

Rhomboid minor

Rhomboid major

Table 2.16
Major Muscles That Act at the Scapulothoracic Articulation

Muscle	Origin	Insertion	Primary Function(s)	Sample Exercises
Trapezius	Occipital bone, spines of cervical and thoracic vertebrae	Acromion process and spine of scapula	Upper: elevation of scapula; Middle: adduction of scapula; Lower: depression of scapula	Upright rowing, shoulder shrugs with resistance
Levator scapula	Upper four or five cervical vertebrae	Vertebral border of scapula	Elevation of scapula	Shoulder shrugs with resistance
Rhomboid major and minor	Spines of seventh cervical through fifth thoracic vertebrae	Vertebral border of scapula	Adduction and elevation of scapula	Chin-ups, supported dumbbell bent-over row

to their students is to have them imagine the human body as a living machine designed for the performance of work. In order to accomplish this work, there must be a meaningful, purposeful integration of the anatomical, neurological, and physiological systems in accordance with the physical laws of nature. An understanding of kinesiology provides you with a framework with which to analyze the vast multitude of human movements, and to make decisions and judgments regarding the safety and effectiveness of any particular movement and its role in the accomplishment of a specific fitness or personal goal of a client.

In this context, kinesiology can provide you with the tools to analyze movement and its subcomponents in order to increase function, improve efficiency, and prevent injury. To use these tools, consider the body's daily activities, postures, and the mechanical stresses it undergoes in these positions. Next, identify possible areas of weakness or tightness caused by those habitual positions and activities. Then, design activities to improve the body's function under those specific conditions. The result will be a balanced fitness program that not only includes cardiovascular endurance, but also muscular balance, neutral postural alignment, and good body mechanics.

Biomechanical Principles of Movement

As an area of study, biomechanics involves the application of mechanics to living organisms (chiefly human beings) and the study of the effects of the forces applied. The analytical process within biomechanics can either be quantitative or qualitative; to accurately analyze human movement, one must first understand the physical laws that apply to the motion of all objects. While Sir Isaac Newton is perhaps best known for his realization of the law of gravitation through observation of an apple falling from a tree to the ground, his formulation of the three important natural laws that govern motion is his greatest contribution to science.

Law of Inertia

Newton's first law of motion is the **law of inertia**, which states that a body at rest will stay at rest and that a body in motion will stay in motion (with the same direction and velocity) unless acted upon by an external force. A body's inertial characteristics are proportional to its mass. Therefore, it is more difficult to start moving a heavy object than a light one. Similarly, if two objects are moving at the same velocity, it requires more effort to stop or slow the heavier object than the lighter one.

Law of Acceleration

The **law of acceleration**, Newton's second law, states that the force (F) acting on a body in a given direction is equal to the body's mass (m) multiplied by the body's acceleration (a) in that direction ($F = ma$). Newton's second law also relates to a moving body's momentum, in that a body's linear momentum is equal to its mass multiplied by its velocity. For a given mass, the application of additional force will accelerate the body to a higher velocity, thus creating greater momentum. For a given velocity, linear momentum (M) will be increased if the mass of the body is increased. Angular momentum is governed by similar principles, only the motion performed is about an axis. If one of your clients is using an 8-lb. dumbbell to perform biceps curls to slow tempo music, there will be less momentum produced than when moving that same weight at a faster tempo. If the tempo of movement to the music (velocity = v) is held constant, but your client switches to a dumbbell with greater mass (m), the momentum ($M = mv$) will increase accordingly.

Law of Reaction

Newton's third law, the **law of reaction**, states that every **applied force** is accompanied by an equal and opposite reaction force. Thus, for every action there is an equal and opposite reaction. This law has bearing on the impact forces (ground reaction forces) that the body must absorb during activities such as step aerobics, jogging, and plyometrics. According to Newtonian principles, the ground exerts a force against the body equal to the force that the body applies to the ground as we walk, jog, or sprint. Step aerobics remains a popular group fitness activity even though its participants sustain a significant number of overuse injuries. Athletic shoes designed specifically for step aerobics have added cushioning in the metatarsal region of the foot where much of the vertically directed ground reaction force is concentrated. A recent study of step aerobic exercise indicated that significantly smaller magnitude ground reaction forces occurred with a 6-inch step when compared to 8-inch and 10-inch step heights (Maybury & Waterfield, 1997). Little difference in ground reaction forces existed between the 8-inch and 10-inch step heights; these findings suggest that participants should use a lower step height to reduce the risk of an overuse injury to the lower limb.

Understanding of the anatomical and biomechanical factors that affect muscles and create movement is crucial for effective exercise design and program implementation. The next step in this process is to apply these principles to identify the individual and collective contributions of muscles through an analytical process. Leonardo da Vinci, perhaps the premier anatomist in all of history, simplified the study of functional anatomy for all of us when he likened human tendons to "cords attached to skeletons." If you can remember a muscle's location, its attachment sites, and its lines of pull (i.e., the orientation of the muscle fibers as they cross a particular joint) then you'll have a clear understanding of the anatomical motions that muscle produces. It may be beneficial to view human movement similar to how a puppeteer manipulates the strings of a puppet to cause movement; the "strings" that produce our motion are the tendons connected to the muscles that have been activated by our CNS. The following sections of this chapter contain numerous examples of common movements produced during exercise by the muscles of the lower and upper extremities.

Kinesiology of the Lower Extremity

In this chapter, movements of the lower extremity are defined as those of the hip, knee, and ankle joints. The normal ranges of motion for these joints are presented in Figure 2.33. The following sections provide details regarding the functions of spe-

Figure 2.33

Lower extremity movements and range of motion

a. Hip flexion range of motion without pelvic rotation 120°; extension (to 0°)

b. Hip extension and hyperextension (<20°)

c. Range of motion for rotation at the hip

d. Range of motion for hip abduction

e. Range of motion of the knee; flexion-extension and hyperextension

f. Ankle range of motion with knee flexed

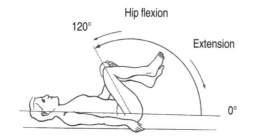

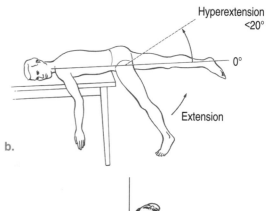

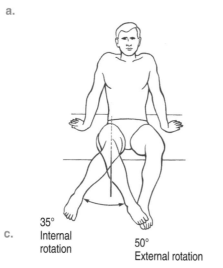

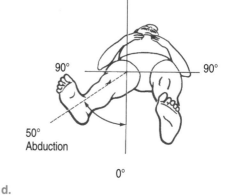

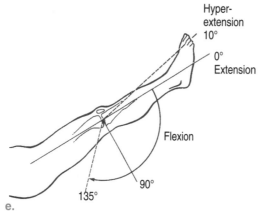

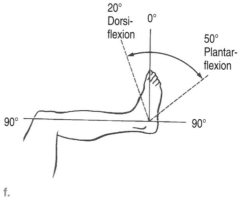

cific muscles in the lower extremity and examples of exercises to develop strength and improve flexibility.

Anterior Hip Muscles: Hip Flexors

The primary hip flexors are the iliopsoas, rectus femoris, sartorius, and tensor fasciae latae. These muscles act synergistically to cause hip flexion, as in a straight leg raise or knee lift. They also act eccentrically to control hip extension, such as in the downward phases of a straight leg raise or knee lift.

The iliopsoas is actually three muscles, the psoas major, the psoas minor (absent in about 10% of us), and the iliacus, that function as one unit. The iliacus gets its name from its origin on the inner surface of the ilium of the hip and inserts into the lesser trochanter of the femur. The psoas major and psoas minor originate on the transverse processes of the five lumbar vertebrae, and attach to the femur at the lesser trochanter. Given the origin of the psoas, it must create a large force to raise or lower the mass of a straight leg. In most people the abdominals are not strong enough to balance the force created by the psoas to keep the spine in neutral position during a straight leg lift. This is one reason why straight-leg sit-ups and leg-lowering exercises are not recommended. Because of its origin at the lumbar spine, psoas tightness (inflexibility) or hypertrophy can result in passive **hyperextension** of the lumbar spine (lordosis). Tightness in the iliopsoas can be attributed to a lack of stretching exercises, and poor standing and sitting postures.

To stretch the iliopsoas, have the client stand in a forward lunge position with one knee flexed and foot flat, and the heel of the other leg off the floor (Figure 2.34). Instruct them to concentrically activate their abdominals and flex the lumbar spine and hold

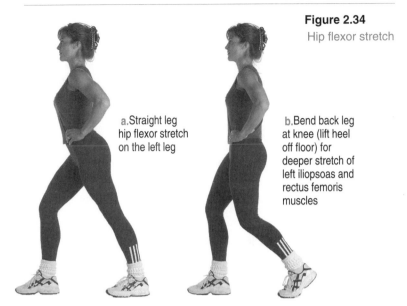

Figure 2.34
Hip flexor stretch

a.Straight leg hip flexor stretch on the left leg

b.Bend back leg at knee (lift heel off floor) for deeper stretch of left iliopsoas and rectus femoris muscles

this position for at least 10 seconds. Careful observation of this activity is important, as the tendency is to hyperextend the lumbar spine during this stretch, putting unwanted compressive loads on the joints of the lumbar spine. To strengthen the iliopsoas, use the abdominals to tilt the pelvis posteriorly from a supine position in order to stabilize the low back, and then lift one leg at a time (knee straight) upward against gravity (Figure 2.35).

The rectus femoris is the only one of the four muscles of the quadriceps femoris that crosses the hip joint. This muscle works at both the knee and hip; concentric action of the rectus femoris results in hip flexion, knee

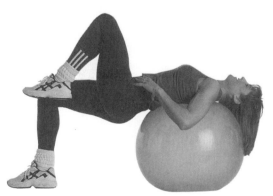

Figure 2.35
Advanced hip flexors (iliopsas) strengthening exercise; may perform with knee extended for greater resistance

extension, or both simultaneously. The best exercise to strengthen this muscle is the standing straight leg raise. To stretch the rectus femoris, perform the iliopsoas lunge stretch then lower the body so that the back knee bends (Figure 2.34b).

The sartorius is the longest muscle in the body, originating from the anterior superior iliac spine (ASIS) and inserting onto the medial tibia, just below the knee. This multi-joint muscle flexes, abducts, and externally rotates the hip while flexing and internally rotating the knee. Just lateral to the sartorius is the tensor fasciae latae (TFL), a short muscle with a very long tendon that combines with the lower fibers of the gluteus maximus. The TFL has the ASIS as its origin, and inserts at the iliotibial tract on the lateral tibia below the knee.

Posterior Hip Muscles: Hip Extensors

The primary hip extensors are the hamstrings (biceps femoris, semitendinosus, and semimembranosus) and the gluteus maximus. Working concentrically, these muscles extend the hip joint against gravity, such as during a prone leg lift. They are also activated to control eccentric hip flexion (e.g., motion during the downward phase of a squat or lunge) (Figure 2.36).

During normal walking and other low-intensity movements, the hamstrings are the **prime movers** for hip extension, as there is little activity in the gluteus maximus. With higher intensity activities (e.g., stair climbing, sprinting, and stationary cycling) for which greater hip ranges of motion and more powerful hip extension are required, the gluteus maximus plays the primary role. Most of the activities in a step aerobics class recruit the gluteus maximus for hip extension in addition to the always-active hamstrings, but other group activities, such as indoor cycling, jumping rope, and power walking on hilly terrain, also recruit the gluteus. If your client has "buns of steel" as one of his or her fitness goals, be sure to include moderate- to higher-intensity activities that extend and hyperextend the hip. One guideline for choosing activities that involve the gluteus maximus is to select exercises that require approximately 90 degrees of hip flexion — these activities tend to be more vigorous and require firing of the gluteus maximus to provide the extra force needed to help the hamstrings accomplish the task.

Lateral Hip Muscles: Hip Abductors and External Rotators

The abductors and external rotators of the hip are found posterior and lateral to the hip joint in the area known as the buttocks. The three gluteal muscles (gluteus medius, gluteus minimus, and the superior fibers of the gluteus maximus) are the primary hip abductors and are assisted by the tensor fasciae latae (Figure 2.37). The origins of these muscles are superior to the joint; therefore, when these muscles shorten concentrically, the hip

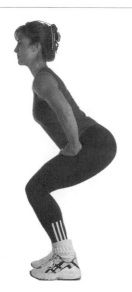

Figure 2.36

Eccentric action of the gluteus maximus and hamstrings control the downward (hip flexion) phase of the squat is pulled away from the midline of the body into abduction. Recall that the function of a muscle depends on the orientation (line of pull) of its fibers in relation to the joint at which it is acting. The gluteus maximus and gluteus medius cover such large areas of the joint that one portion of the each muscle is capable of producing an anatomical motion opposite that of another portion. Each of these muscles has a primary action that is performed by all portions of the muscle. The primary function of the gluteus maximus is hip extension, while the main action of the gluteus medius is abduction. Some fibers of the gluteus maximus cross the hip superior to the central axis of the joint, and others cross inferior to the functional axis of the joint. This means that those fibers of the gluteus maximus superior to the axis will produce abduction, while the inferior fibers will cause adduction. The anterior portion of the gluteus medius acts concentrically to cause internal rotation and the posterior fibers produce external rotation.

There are six external rotators of the hip located deep to the gluteus maximus. From superior to inferior, these muscles are the piriformis, superior gemellus, obturator internus, obturator externus, inferior gemellus, and the quadratus femoris (Figure 2.38). The orientation of the muscle fibers in this group is horizontal and this, coupled with their position posterior to the joint, makes them efficient external rotators of the hip. When the hip is extended, the gluteus maximus also functions as an external rotator. To stretch the external rotator muscles, have the client lay flat on her or his back and pull their flexed knee and hip diagonally across the body (Figure 2.39). This position involves adduction and internal rotation, which effectively stretches these muscles.

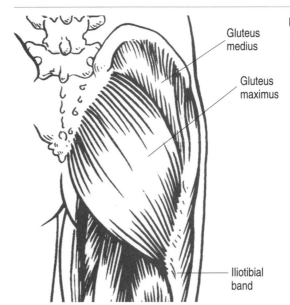

Figure 2.37
Superficial gluteal muscles of the hip

Gluteus medius
Gluteus maximus
Iliotibial band

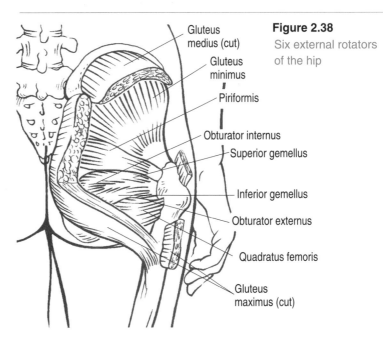

Figure 2.38
Six external rotators of the hip

Gluteus medius (cut)
Gluteus minimus
Piriformis
Obturator internus
Superior gemellus
Inferior gemellus
Obturator externus
Quadratus femoris
Gluteus maximus (cut)

An understanding of concentric and eccentric muscle actions is critical for proper design of exercise programs. Recall the previous discussion of the rules for determining what type of muscle action is occurring. If the movement direction is opposite the pull of gravity, the active muscle is working concentrically; if the direction of movement is the same as the pull of gravity, then the muscle is working eccentrically. However,

Figure 2.39

Stretching of the deep external rotators of the left hip. Keep shoulders and back flat; pull flexed hip and knee across torso.

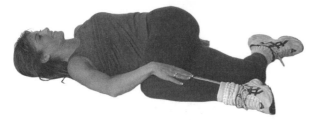

when gravity is "eliminated" during movements that occur parallel to the mat, each muscle group acts concentrically to produce the desired motion. When resistance is added through the use of elastic tubing, the same principles apply in all planes of motion; concentric muscle actions occur if the movement increases the resistance in the elastic tubing, and eccentric muscle actions occur if the motion decreases the resistance offered by the tubing.

Figure 2.40 employs hip abduction and adduction exercises to provide four examples of how body position can modify the influence of gravity. In Figure 2.40a, side-lying leg lifts are depicted. The initial action is hip abduction against gravity's pull. Therefore, the hip abductors are acting concentrically as agonists. In the downward phase of the leg lift, the hip joint action is adduction. The joint motion occurs slowly in the same direction as the gravity's pull; therefore, the hip abductors are working eccentrically as agonists to control hip adduction.

Figure 2.40b shows a supine hip abduction/adduction exercise with the hips flexed, knees extended, and feet in the air; the initial action that occurs is abduction of the hip joints as the legs move farther apart. Since the movement occurs in the same direction as the force of gravity, the hip

adductors control the motion via eccentric muscle action. To bring the legs back together again in a vertical position, the hip adductor muscles work concentrically against the pull of gravity.

In the third example (Figure 2.40c), hip abduction and adduction are performed from a supine position, effectively eliminating the force of gravity as a source of resistance. From this position, the motions occur neither against nor in the same direction as gravity but perpendicular to the pull of gravity. There is a concentric action of the hip abductors when the extended legs move apart and a concentric action of the hip adductors when the legs are moved back together.

In the final example (Figure 2.40d), elastic tubing is added to the exercise described in the previous paragraph. Concentric muscle actions of the hip abductors occur when the client moves her legs away from midline, increasing the resistance in the elastic tubing. Conversely, eccentric muscle actions occur in the hip abductors during the return to the starting position (adduction), against the force supplied by the elastic band at the lower leg.

Medial Hip Muscles: Hip Adductors and Internal Rotators

The muscles that produce adduction and interior rotation are located anterior, inferior, and medial to the hip joint. In this case, the muscle names clearly indicate function; the major adductors are the adductor magnus, adductor longus, and adductor brevis. Because of the anatomy of the hip, these muscles sometimes function as internal rotators and sometimes as external rotators. The most important internal rotators of the hip are the adductor muscles and the gluteus medius and minimus. Figure 2.40 provides several good examples of exercises that recruit the adductors of the hip.

The inner thigh is an area of concern for many female clients. Many want to lose the fat deposits that have accumulated along the medial thigh and develop greater muscle strength ("tone") in their adductors. It is important to educate your clients with the knowledge that spot-reduction of fat does not work, regardless of what they see on infomercials on television. To decrease body fat stores along the inner thigh or anywhere else in the body, caloric expenditure must consistently exceed caloric intake. Irrespective of gender, participation in physical activity for 30 minutes a day for most days of the week will help decrease body-fat percentage and increase the percentage of lean mass (e.g., muscles and tendons) in the body.

Anterior Knee Muscles: Knee Extensors

The large muscle on the front of the thigh, the quadriceps femoris, controls knee extension when acting concentrically. As the Latin roots of its name implies, the quadriceps is composed of four different muscles that act together to extend the knee. Three of the four muscles — the vastus lateralis, vastus medialis, and vastus intermedius — originate on the proximal femur. The rectus femoris, the only one of the quadriceps that acts at the hip, acts concentrically to produce hip flexion, a function made possible by its origin on the anterior inferior iliac spine. The quadriceps muscles combine distally to form the patellar tendon, within which the patella is found. The patella is the largest sesamoid bone in the body and acts like a pulley to increase the mechanical advantage

Figure 2.40
Concentric and eccentric hip muscle actions

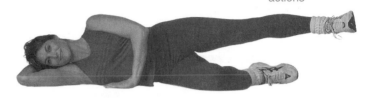

a. Side-lying leg lifts; abductors work concentrically in the upward phase and eccentrically in the downward phase

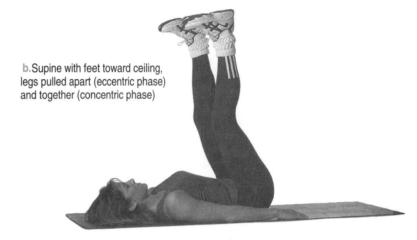

b. Supine with feet toward ceiling, legs pulled apart (eccentric phase) and together (concentric phase)

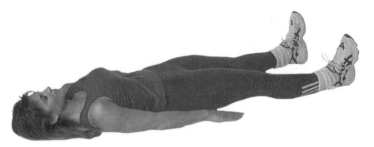

c. Moving apart: concentric of hip abductors; moving together: concentric of hip adductors

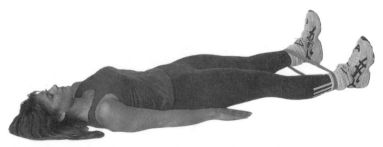

d. Concentric (legs apart) and eccentric (legs together) actions of the hip abductors with elastic resistance

of the quadriceps by as much as 30% at some knee joint angles.

During relaxed standing there is little activity in the quadriceps, with most of the weight borne on the knee joint surfaces. When the lower limb is in a weightbearing position, the quadriceps act eccentrically to permit knee flexion (e.g., flexing the knee slowly when moving from a standing position to a seated position). In the activities of daily living, strong quadriceps are needed for lifting heavy objects, climbing stairs, and during power walking. Squats, lunges, and stepping are important elements in preparing the quadriceps for daily functioning. Some experts say that the safest approach in a group exercise class setting is to set the limit on knee flexion in the weightbearing knee at 90 degrees.

Posterior Knee Muscles: Knee Flexors

The primary knee flexors are the hamstrings muscle group (semitendinosus, semi-

membranosus, and biceps femoris); their functional characteristics were discussed previously with the hip extensors. The sartorius, popliteus, gastrocnemius, and gracilis are secondary knee flexors (see Figures 2.19 and 2.23). The popliteus plays the most unique role of these muscles in that it is responsible for initiating knee flexion and "unlocking" the knee from its extended position.

To stretch the hamstrings effectively, position the muscle in hip flexion and knee extension. From a standing position, put the foot of the leg to be stretched on a step and slowly bend forward at the waist, keeping a flat back (neutral spine position). This isolates the stretch to the hamstring and avoids overstressing the erector spinae muscles. To increase the intensity of the stretch, have the client flex the knee and hip of the limb not being stretched (Figure 2.41).

Anterior Leg Muscles: Dorsiflexors

The muscles in the anterior compartment of the lower leg (see Figures 2.16 and 2.17) are the anterior tibialis, extensor hallucis longus, and extensor digitorum longus. These muscles are collectively responsible for controlling **dorsiflexion** of the ankle. These muscles also act eccentrically during locomotor activities, such as walking and running, to lower the foot to the ground with control. Without the vital eccentric action of the dorsiflexor muscles as dynamic shock absorbers, the foot would slap the ground with each stride or impact. Given that the ground reaction forces during running are three to five times one's body weight with each stride and that there are approximately 1500 to 1800 strides (ground impacts) per mile (1.6 km), the importance of the shock absorption role of these muscles cannot be overstated.

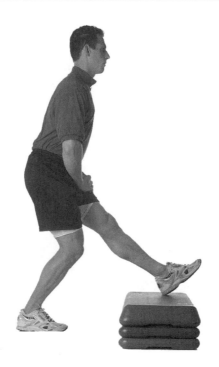

Figure 2.41
Standing hamstring stretch; hands should be used for balance — do not apply pressure to the knee

The anterior tibialis inserts on the medial aspect of the foot and combines with the posterior tibialis to serve as the prime movers for inversion of the foot. A common method of warming these muscles prior to impact activities is to perform toe tapping, either straight ahead or side-to-side.

Posterior Leg Muscles: Plantar Flexors

The large superficial muscles of the posterior tibial compartment (see Figures 2.16 and 2.19) are the primary plantar flexors of the ankle joint. While more easily palpated and visible than the underlying soleus muscle, the gastrocnemius is actually the smaller of the two. These muscles combine distally to form the Achilles tendon, the largest tendon in the body, which attaches to the calcaneus. The gastrocnemius, as mentioned previously, acts at both the knee and the ankle; the soleus acts only at the ankle joint. Indeed, there are eight muscles that act as synergists for **plantar flexion**, evolutionary evidence of the importance of the plantar flexion force production. The remaining six muscles, specifically the posterior tibialis, flexor hallucis longus, flexor digitorum longus, plantaris, peroneus longus, and peroneus brevis, play secondary functional roles in producing the propulsion force required for human locomotion.

The gastrocnemius and soleus muscles are often inflexible, particularly among clients who wear high heels. To stretch the two-joint gastrocnemius, the hip and knee should be extended and the ankle should be in a dorsiflexed position while the heel remains on the ground. To stretch the soleus, a similar posture is assumed, except that the knee is flexed to about 20 degrees to isolate the soleus. These stretches can be performed while seated or lying down, but more commonly are performed against a real or imagined wall (i.e., the "wall stretch") (Figure 2.42), or by utilizing a step aerobics bench.

Lateral Leg Muscles: Evertors

The peroneus longus and peroneus brevis are muscles found in the lateral tibial compartment (see Figures 2.16 and 2.18) that are responsible for eversion of the foot (i.e., pulling the foot laterally in the frontal plane). The tendons of these muscles curve around behind the lateral malleolus and attach on the foot. Both muscles play secondary roles as plantar flexors at the ankle due to their posterior location relative to the axis of motion of the talo-crural (ankle) joint. These muscles are active during virtually all locomotor activities to provide dynamic stability at the sub-talar joint, acting eccentrically to prevent the joint from rolling too far into inversion and possibly causing a sprain.

Figure 2.42

Stretching of the gastrocnemius (rear leg) and soleus (front leg) muscles

Gastrocnemius stretch

Soleus stretch

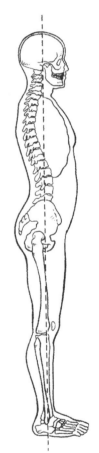

Figure 2.43

Neutral spinal alignment with slight anterior curve at neck and low back and posterior curve in the thoracic region

Figure 2.44
Range of motion of
the thoracic and
lumbar spine

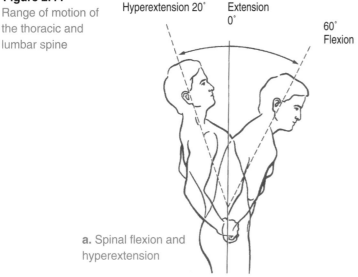

Hyperextension 20°   Extension 0°   60° Flexion

a. Spinal flexion and hyperextension

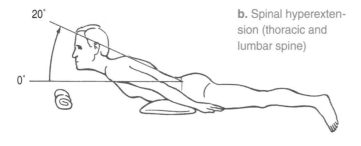

20°   0°

b. Spinal hyperextension (thoracic and lumbar spine)

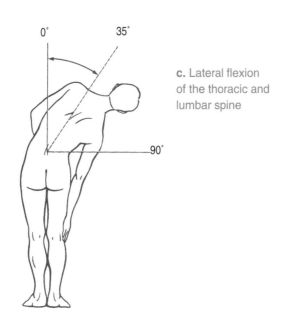

0°   35°   90°

c. Lateral flexion of the thoracic and lumbar spine

Kinesiology of the Spine and Pelvis

Posture and the Neutral Spine

Given the wide variation of human body shapes, sizes, and types, there is a general lack of agreement about what comprises ideal posture. The spine of a fully grown adult has three naturally occurring curves: two slight anterior curves at the neck and low back and one slight posterior curve in the thoracic region (Figure 2.43). This **neutral spine position** requires the mathematical balance of 12 vertebrae curved in the anterior direction (the seven cervical plus the five lumbar vertebrae) with the 12 thoracic region vertebrae curved in the posterior direction. The normal ranges of motion of the thoracic and lumbar spine are presented in Figure 2.44.

You can assess muscular balance by having a client stand in anatomical position and observing him or her from the back and from the side. If a person stands in this neutral alignment and is viewed from the rear, a plumb bob suspended from above would pass through the midline of the skull, the center of the vertebral column over the spinous processes, the vertical crease between the buttocks, and touch the ground midway between the feet. Group fitness classes can promote good posture and muscular balance by having clients perform all activities with a neutral spine alignment. Effective cueing and correction techniques, combined with verbal and visual feedback, help clients to be more aware of their posture. Good posture is a neuromuscular skill that can be reacquired through repetition and practice.

The position of the pelvis plays a major role in the determination of the forces applied at the lumbar spine. If the lumbar spine is correctly aligned with regard to the pelvis, and the pelvis is properly balanced in relation to the legs, then the forces applied to the low back can be reduced. To achieve this balance requires good muscle strength and flexibility on both sides of the trunk — the trunk and hip flexors anteriorly and the trunk and spine extensors posteriorly (Figure 2.45).

Abnormal and Fatigue-related Postures

Deviations from neutral spine position can be temporary or permanent; muscle spasm and pain following a soft-tissue injury to the back, fatigue, or muscular imbalance may cause these deviations. When applied at the appropriate time with the correct dosage (frequency, intensity, and duration), exercise can help alleviate each of these conditions. Some postural deviations are structural (bony) in nature, and typically do not respond to exercise. The three most common abnormal postures are lordosis, kyphosis, and scoliosis.

Lordosis is an excessive anterior curvature of the spine that typically occurs at the low back, but may also occur at the neck (Figure 2.46a). The lay term for lordosis of the lumbar spine is "swayback," a condition marked by protruding buttocks and weak abdominal muscles. Lordotic or swayback posture has been associated with low back pain, a condition commonly experienced by late term pregnant women and middle aged persons with large concentrations of abdominal fat. Lordotic posture will cause an anterior tilting of the pelvis, placing tension on the anterior longitudinal ligaments of the spine and compression on the posterior part of the intervertebral discs. If this posture is maintained over weeks and months, the back extensor and hip flexor muscles will adapt by losing their extensibility, and the hamstring

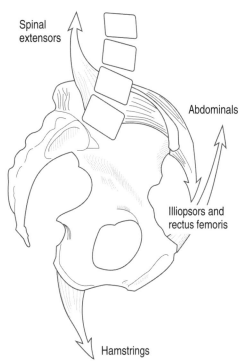

Figure 2.45
Muscular control of the pelvis by the abdominal and hip flexors (iliopsoas) anteriorly and the spinal extensors (erector spinae) and hamstrings posteriorly

and abdominal muscles will lengthen, becoming more lax and further decreasing their control of the pelvis. Unlike obesity, pregnancy has a finite beginning and end, and most back pain and changes in posture associated with pregnancy are resolved postpartum. The overweight or obese client with swayback presents a significant challenge to the group fitness instructor. To correct the anterior pelvic tilt position associated with lumbar lordosis, focus on strengthening the client's abdominal and hip extensor (hamstring) muscles, while stretching the hip flexors (iliopsoas) and spine extensors (erector spinae).

Kyphosis is an excessive posterior curvature of the spine, typically seen in the thoracic region (Figure 2. 46b). The presence of kyphosis will give the client a characteristic "humpback," with associated rounded shoulders, a sunken chest, and forward head with neck hyperextension. Kyphosis is a common postural abnormality among older persons with osteoporosis. In some instances, the rounded shoulders posture is caused by weakness or disuse atrophy of the muscles that control scapular movement — the rhomboids and trapezius. Varying levels of success have been found with strengthening programs intended to correct this postural deformity.

Scoliosis is an excessive lateral curvature of the spine, more prevalent among women than men. With scoliosis, the pelvis and shoulders often appear uneven and the vertebrae may rotate, causing a posterior shift of the rib cage on one side (Figure 2.46c). If a client has one of these three postural abnormalities and cannot actively assume a neutral spine posture, refer him or her to a physician.

A temporary lordosis (in standing position) or kyphosis (in sitting position) may occur every day when clients are tired — so-called fatigue postures. Fatigue postures cause physical stress, muscle imbalance, and eventually pain. Over time, the bones of the spine may adapt to these postures, causing skeletal (rather than soft tissue) deviations that become irreversible.

Muscular Balance and Imbalance

When muscular balance is present, the neutral spine position can occur. However, a problem in one muscle group often creates problems in the opposing muscle group. If one muscle group is too tight (inflexible), it may pull the body out of neutral position, causing increased stress and a tendency toward im-

Figure 2.46
Postural deviations

a. Lordosis: Increased anterior lumbar curve from neutral

b. Kyphosis: Increased posterior thoracic curve from neutral

c. Scoliosis: Excessive lateral spinal curve with possible vertebral rotation

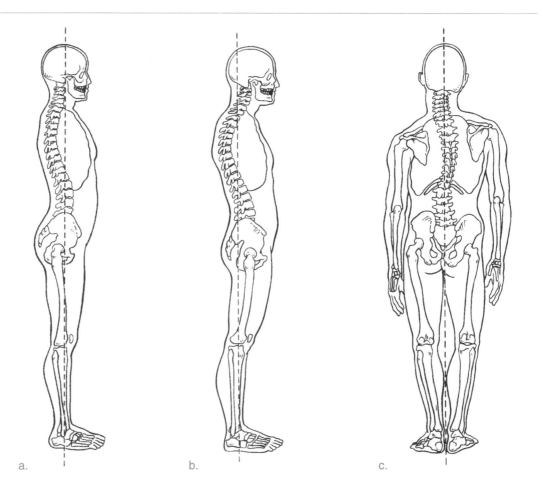

a.   b.   c.

balance on the opposite side of the body. Conversely, if a particular muscle group is weakened from injury or fatigue, the body will fall out of alignment in the opposite direction.

The term muscular balance refers to the symmetry of the interconnected components of muscle and connective tissue. Specifically, muscular balance involves (1) equal strength and flexibility on the right and left sides of the body (bilateral symmetry); (2) proportional strength ratios in opposing (agonist/antagonist) muscle groups, although they may not be exactly equal; and (3) a balance in flexibility, in that normal ranges of motion are achieved but not exceeded.

One example of agonist/antagonist muscle imbalance is the relationship between the erector spinae and the abdominal muscles. Very commonly, the abdominals are overmatched by the muscles that extend the trunk and neutral spine is lost. Persons with localized low back pain from mechanical causes (no intervertebral disk or spinal nerve involvement) are typically given abdominal strengthening rehabilitation exercises to regain muscular control of the pelvis and balance with the erector spinae.

While not involving the spine, a frequent muscular imbalance affects the function of the quadriceps and hamstrings. In untrained individuals, the naturally occurring size of the quadriceps is about twice that of the hamstrings, creating an imbalance in the agonist/antagonist relationship. With regular training, the ratio of hamstrings-to-quadriceps size and strength improves, but hamstring strains remain an all too frequent result of this muscular imbalance. Similarly, strength differences are often present between dominant and nondominant limbs, particularly in the upper extremity. One method to counteract this is to have clients perform

unilateral resistance exercises with dumbbells, isolating the right and left sides, rather than using a barbell to perform the same activity.

Trunk Flexors: Abdominal Muscles

The abdominal muscles are found on the anterior and lateral surfaces of the trunk, and they flex, laterally flex, and rotate the trunk. Trunk flexion occurs in the sagittal plane, right and left lateral flexion occurs in the frontal plane of motion, and right and left trunk rotation occurs in the transverse plane. The abdominal muscle group is composed of the rectus abdominis, the external oblique, the internal oblique, and the transverse abdominis (see Figure 2.26). The transverse abdominis, found in the deepest layer of abdominal muscle, supports and compresses the viscera and has no voluntary motor function. Therefore, only the remaining three anterior trunk muscles will be discussed further.

The fibers of rectus abdominis are superficial and run longitudinally from the lower part of the chest to the pubic bone. Synergistic concentric actions of the right and left rectus abdominis muscles produce flexion of the trunk, as in the upward phase of an abdominal curl or crunch. While the anatomical movement during the return (downward) phase of the crunch is trunk extension, it is the eccentric muscle actions of the right and left rectus abdominis muscles (trunk flexors) that control the slow return to the mat. Unilateral concentric activation of the right or left rectus abdominis will result in lateral flexion of the trunk. The most effective exercises to develop this muscle are posterior pelvic tilts, supine abdominal curls, straight reverse abdominal curls (eccentric action

Figure 2.47
Abdominal strength and
endurance exercises

a. Abdominal crunch for external obliques

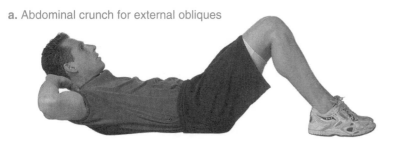

b. Abdominal curl for rectus abdominus and obliques

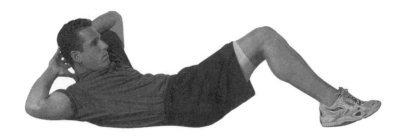

c. Side-lying torso raise
for internal and external
obliques

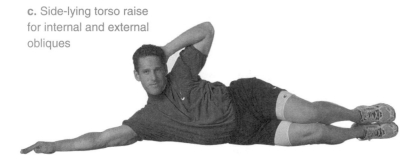

emphasized), and abdominal crunches (Figure 2.47a).

Also in the superficial layer of trunk muscles are the external obliques. These muscles originate on the ribs and attach to the iliac crest and the aponeurosis of the rectus abdominis; their fibers run diagonally downward and forward, as if into the front pockets of your pants. When the right and left external obliques act together concentrically, they produce trunk flexion. Right and left sides

can be activated independently to cause lateral flexion and, when combined with concentric action of the opposite internal oblique, produce trunk rotation to the opposite side. An example is the oblique (twisting) abdominal curl (Figure 2.47b), with the shoulder taken toward the opposite hip. The best exercises for the external obliques are supine pelvic tilts, straight abdominal curls with the hips and knees partially extended to create more resistance, oblique abdominal curls, and straight and oblique reverse abdominal curls (e.g., lifting the knees overhead until the buttocks leave the floor).

The internal oblique muscles are found deep to the external obliques, and their fibers run diagonally downward and posteriorly, as if into the back pockets of your pants. Their functions include flexion, lateral flexion, and rotation of the trunk to the same side. Effective exercises to tone and strengthen the internal obliques are supine pelvic tilts, oblique abdominal curls, straight and oblique reverse abdominal curls, and side-lying torso raises (Figure 2.47c).

There are several effective methods of increasing the resistance and loading pattern during abdominal exercises; one such variation is to change body positions relative to gravity (e.g., partial abdominal curl on an incline bench (head down) rather than on a flat mat). Another variation is to change the end of the muscle that is stabilized and the one that is moved (e.g., perform abdominal curls with the shoulders lifted, then change to a reverse curl with the hips lifted). You can also emphasize endurance training for the abdominals by holding an abdominal curl at various points in the arc of motion while having the client perform exercises for the hip adductors or flexors.

Trunk Extensors: Erector Spinae Group

The erector spinae group of muscles, formed by the iliocostalis, longissimus, and spinalis, when acting bilaterally and concentrically, will produce trunk extension and hyperextension. These muscles also act eccentrically to control flexion of the spine from a standing position, as in bending over to pick up the morning newspaper. When the erector spinae muscles are stimulated unilaterally, they cause lateral flexion to that same side. In normal standing posture, the level of activity in these muscles is quite low.

Exercises that are effective to strengthen this muscle group include the prone trunk hyperextension lift (Figure 2.48a), and, from a kneeling (all-fours) position, simultaneous lifting of the opposite arm and leg (Figure 2.48b). The latter exercise causes the erector spinae muscles to function as stabilizers of the spine to maintain neutral position. For clients seeking more advanced challenges, incorporate a stability ball into the exercise program to develop balance and proprioception along with trunk extensor strength (Figure 2.49).

To stretch the erector spinae group, have clients lie on a mat in a supine position with posterior pelvic tilt and gently pull either one or both knees to their chest with their arms, holding this position for at least 10 seconds (Figure 2.50). The posterior pelvic tilt position flattens the anterior (lordotic) curve in the lumbar region of the spine and places the erector spinae on stretch.

Kinesiology of the Upper Extremity

Upper-extremity segments include the head and neck, shoulder girdle (scapulothoracic articulation),

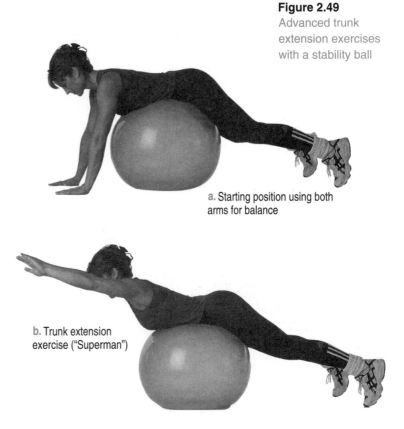

Figure 2.48
Basic and intermediate difficulty strength exercises for the trunk extensors

a. Prone hyperextension

b. Lift the opposite arm and leg simultaneously while keeping the spine in neutral.

Figure 2.49
Advanced trunk extension exercises with a stability ball

a. Starting position using both arms for balance

b. Trunk extension exercise ("Superman")

Figure 2.50
Flexibility exercises for the
erector spinae muscles in supine
position with posterior pelvic tilt

a. Single knee to
shoulder

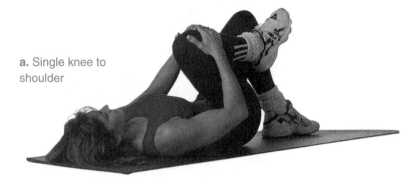

b. Double knee
to chest

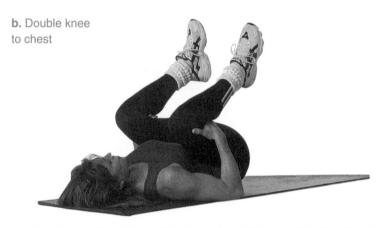

Figure 2.51
The four articulations of the
shoulder joint complex

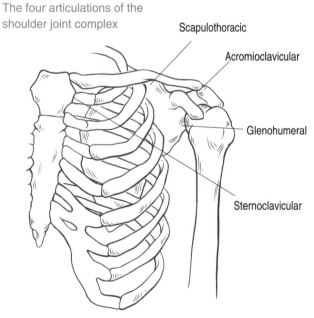

Scapulothoracic

Acromioclavicular

Glenohumeral

Sternoclavicular

shoulders, elbows, wrists, and hands. Tables 2.13 through 2.16 present a summary of the muscles in each of these regions, their origins and insertions, primary function(s), and specific examples of exercises involving these muscles. Prior to discussion of the functional relationships of the muscles in the upper extremity, the terms shoulder joint complex, glenohumeral joint, and shoulder girdle must be differentiated. The term **shoulder joint complex** describes the coordinated functioning of four separate upper extremity segments: the sternoclavicular joint (S/C), the junction of the sternum and the proximal clavicle; the acromioclavicular joint (A/C), the junction of the acromion process of the scapula with the distal clavicle; the glenohumeral joint (G/H), the ball and socket joint composed of the glenoid fossa of the scapula and the humeral head; and the scapulothoracic articulation (S/T), the muscles and fascia connecting the scapulae to the thorax (Figure 2.51). The more general term shoulder girdle, used in context, is synonymous with the formal anatomical term, **scapulothoracic articulation**.

Each of the true bony joints in the shoulder complex (S/C, A/C, and G/H) are synovial joints that permit large ranges of movement in all three anatomical planes. Add to this the coupling of the G/H joint with the S/T articulation and the result is the most mobile joint in the body. Therefore, many motions are possible at the G/H joint: flexion and extension in the sagittal plane, abduction and adduction in the frontal plane, circumduction in a combination of the sagittal and frontal planes, internal and external rotation, and horizontal flexion and extension in the transverse plane (Figure 2.52).

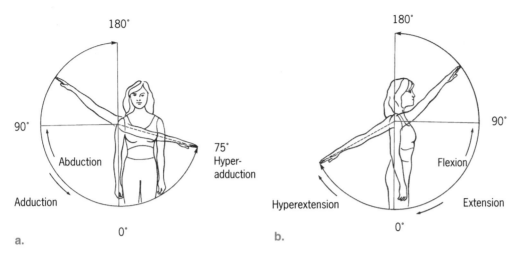

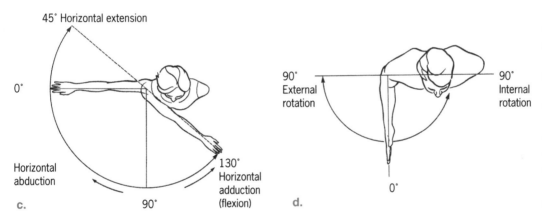

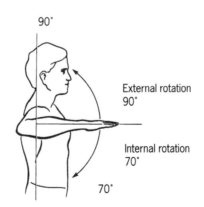

Figure 2.52
Shoulder joint range
of motion

a. Shoulder
abduction 180°,
adduction (to 0°);
hyperadduction 75°
(frontal plane)

b. Shoulder range
of motion in sagittal
plane: flexion 180°;
extension (to 0°);
hyperextension 60°

c. Shoulder range
of motion in the trans-
verse plane: horizon-
tal adduction (flexion)
130°; horizontal ab-
duction (to 0°); hori-
zontal extension 45°

d. Shoulder rotation
range of motion in
the transverse plane
(shoulder is adducted
to 0°): extend rotation
90°; internal rotation
90°

e. Shoulder rotation
range of motion in the
sagittal plane/trans-
verse plane viewed
from the external
(outward) rotation 90°,
internal rotation 70°
(shoulder joint is
abducted to 90°)

The scapulothoracic articulation and the glenohumeral joints work together to produce coordinated flexion and extension and abduction and adduction. This relationship is referred to as **scapulohumeral rhythm** and, throughout the range of motion possible in flexion/extension and abduction/adduction, a ratio of approximately 2 degrees of G/H motion for every 1 degree of S/T motion exists. Translated to absolute terms, to achieve 180 degrees of flexion or abduction, approximately 120 degrees of motion occurs at the glenohumeral joint and 60 degrees of motion occurs as the result of movement of the scapula on the thorax (Figure 2.53).

In the activities of daily living, the scapular muscles function primarily as stabilizers, but also are powerful muscles involved in upper extremity movements. Anatomical movements of the scapulae include elevation and depression, abduction (protraction) and adduction (retraction), and upward and downward rotation (Figure 2.54). Scapular muscles can be divided into two groups based on their location and function. Anterior shoulder girdle muscles connect the scapulae to the front of the trunk, while the posterior shoulder girdle muscles hold the scapulae to the back of the trunk.

The anatomical movements possible throughout the upper extremity are many. However, within the scope of this chapter, only the kinesiology of the scapulothoracic articulation and glenohumeral joint will be addressed.

Anterior Shoulder Girdle Muscles

The anterior shoulder girdle muscles, the pectoralis minor and serratus anterior, attach the scapula to the front of the thorax (Figure 2.55). Concentric and eccentric activity in these muscles results in scapular movement on the thorax; these muscles have no attachment to the humerus and thus do not directly cause glenohumeral motion. The pectoralis minor originates on the coracoid process of the scapula and inserts on the third, fourth, and fifth ribs. The pectoralis minor can have a positive or negative effect on posture, depending on the condition of the scapular adductors, specifically the middle trapezius and rhomboids. Concentric activity of the pectoralis minor results in abduction, depression, and downward rotation of the scapula. However, if the scapular adductors are weak, fatigued, or injured, the muscular tension created by the pectoralis minor will tilt the scapulae forward and down, worsening a rounded-shoulders posture (kyphosis).

The serratus anterior is a broad, knife-edged muscle that originates along the underside of the entire length of the medial border of the scapula and inserts onto the front parts of first through ninth ribs. The serratus anterior abducts the scapula and works as synergist with the upper trapezius to produce upward rotation of the scapula. A key function of the serratus is to hold the medial border of the scapula firmly against the rib cage, preventing "winging" of the scapula posteriorly away from the thorax. Concentric action of the serratus anterior enables powerful forward motion of the arm, as in the overhead throwing motion. Strengthening of the serratus can be done from a supine position with the shoulder flexed to 90 degrees, and the elbow extended, pushing a dumbbell or medicine ball held in the hand toward the ceiling in a "punching" motion without bending the elbow. The shoulder blade(s) should lift off the floor slightly when performing this exercise (Figure 2.56). Another effective method of working the serratus is to have clients perform push-ups with a "plus" — the addition of scapular abduction at the end of the upward phase of a regular push-up.

Posterior Shoulder Girdle Muscles

The posterior shoulder girdle muscles, the trapezius, the rhomboids, and levator scapulae, attach the scapula to the back of the thorax. Since these muscles have no attachment to the humerus, their action does not directly result in glenohumeral motion.

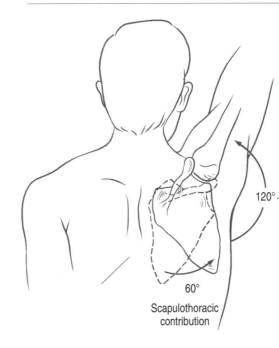

Figure 2.53
The movement of the arm is accompanied by movements of the shoulder girdle; the working relationship between the two is known as the scapulohumeral rhythm.

120° — Glenohumeral contribution

60°
Scapulothoracic contribution

Figure 2.54
Scapular movements
a. Elevation
b. Depression
c. Adduction (retraction)
d. Abduction (protraction)
e. Upward rotation
f. Downward rotation (return to anatomic position)

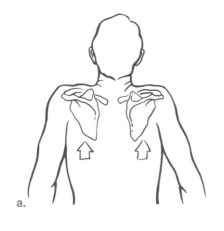

a.

b.

c.

d.

e.

f.

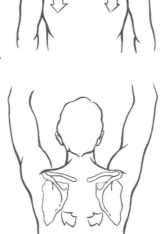

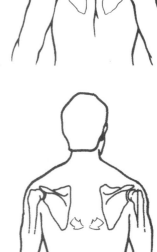

Figure 2.55
Anterior muscles of
the shoulder girdle

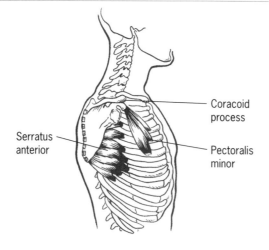

Coracoid
process

Serratus
anterior

Pectoralis
minor

The trapezius is the largest and most superficial of the posterior shoulder girdle muscles; it originates at the base of the skull and has attachments to the 19 vertebrae in the cervical and thoracic regions of the spine. Resembling the shape of a trapezoid, the muscle attaches laterally to the spine of the scapula and the lateral aspect of the clavicle. Recalling da Vinci's perspective of functional human anatomy as nothing more than "cords attached to skeletons," it is easy to understand the reason the trapezius has three different names. The trapezius is divided into three distinct units, upper, middle, and lower, because of the different directions that its fibers course and exert their pull. The fibers of the upper trapezius are upward and oblique, the fibers of the middle trapezius are purely horizontal in their direction and pull, and the fibers of the lower trapezius are angled obliquely downward. Therefore, if the upper fibers are activated concentrically they will produce elevation and adduction of the scapula. Stimulation of the fibers of the middle trapezius will cause pure adduction of the scapula, while concentric activity of the lower trapezius fibers will both depress and adduct the scapula.

The different fibers of the trapezius are alternately activated and relaxed in order to cause scapular rotation. If the arms are lifted in front (G/H flexion) or out to the side (G/H abduction), the shoulder blades rotate upward and away from the spine. This anatomical motion, upward rotation, occurs as the result of the upper and middle trapezius, rhomboids, and serratus anterior pulling on different aspects of the scapula. Concentric action of the lower

Figure 2.56
"Punches" to
strengthen the
serratus anterior
muscle

a. Starting position
b. Shoulder blades
   lifted off the floor
   slightly; do not
   bend elbows

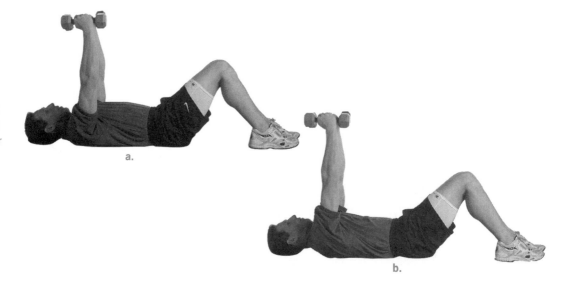

a.

b.

trapezius, together with eccentric activity in the rhomboids and levator scapulae return the shoulder blades to their original (anatomical) position.

To design effective exercises to strengthen each of the sections of the trapezius, consider the stresses and loads that the muscle encounters regularly. In typical sitting and standing postures, the upper trapezius acts isometrically to support the arms and head. The upper trapezius is also active when a heavy weight or object is held or carried at arm's length. This portion of the trapezius needs stretching and strengthening throughout the full range of motion and does not require long duration isometric resistance activities. The upper trapezius and the levator scapulae are strengthened in upright standing or sitting by performing shoulder shrugs with dumbbells or tubing with the arms extended behind (Figure 2.57).

The middle trapezius is commonly weak or fatigued in the client with a rounded-shoulders (kyphotic) sitting posture. Typically the middle trapezius does not need to be stretched but rather strengthened in an "antigravity" position; that is, the muscle must be used to lift some resistance against gravity. Simply adducting the scapulae in a standing position does not overload the middle trapezius because there is no resistance (other than gravity) to overcome. Examples of antigravity positions include a fully prone or a simulated-prone position (e.g., forward lunge, half-kneeling with the torso supported on the front thigh). Using dumbbells, the desired movement in the prone position is to "squeeze" the shoulder blades together causing the arms to lift in the direction opposite the pull of gravity (Figure 2.58a).

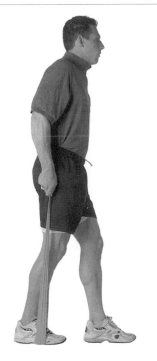

Figure 2.57
Exercise for the upper trapezius: hyperextend shoulders, then perform a shoulder shrug

To isolate the middle trapezius in a standing position, use elastic bands or surgical tubing to provide resistance. Instruct your clients to abduct their G/H joints to 90 degrees, maintain a neutral spine, and then "pull" their scapulae together with no movement at the elbows or wrists (Figure 2.58b).

The rhomboid major and rhomboid minor work as one functional unit, their fibers running upward and obliquely from the vertebral border of the scapulae to the spine. These muscles act primarily to adduct and elevate the scapulae and help with downward rotation of the scapulae. When the rhomboids are weak or over-stressed, the shoulder blades may tilt and pull away from the thorax due to the unopposed tension exerted by the serratus anterior and pectoralis minor. Bent-over rows with dumbbells or pulley machine weights or the use of a rowing ergometer are effective exercises to strengthen the rhomboids (Figure 2.59).

Figure 2.58

Exercises for the
middle trapezius
a. Maintain neutral
spine, pull scapulae
toward spine
keeping elbow
straight and arms
hanging down

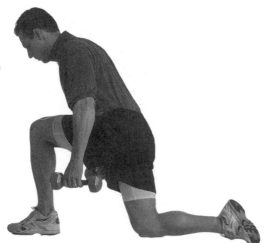

b. Maintain neutral spine;
pull scapulae together
with elbows slightly bent,
wrists neutral

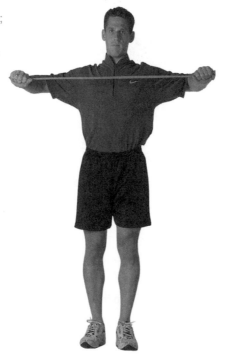

Glenohumeral Joint Muscles

The final group of muscles to be discussed are those that directly produce movement at the glenohumeral joint. These muscles include the pectoralis major, deltoid, rotator cuff, latissimus dorsi, and teres major (Figure 2.60). Due to the complexity of the anatomical functions of the major muscles acting at the G/H joint, they are not listed in groups as adductors, extensors, and so on.

The pectoralis major is a very large muscle that comprises the bulk of the muscle on the anterior chest wall. The pectoralis major is divided into two functional units based on the orientation of the muscle's fibers: a sternal portion and a clavicular portion. The clavicular portion of the pectoralis, located slightly superior to the G/H joint, acts concentrically as a flexor, while the angle of pull and inferior position relative to the shoulder joint make the sternal portion a powerful extensor. As a whole, the pectoralis major is a prime mover in glenohumeral adduction, internal rotation, and horizontal flexion. To strengthen the pectoralis major in a class using hand-held weights, have clients lie supine on a mat or on top of a step bench. From this position, a pectoral fly exercise involving horizontal flexion will overload the pectoralis major. The push-up is also an effective exercise for the pectorals. The pectoralis major, serratus anterior, and triceps brachii act eccentrically to slowly lower the body in the downward phase (same direction of movement as the force of gravity) of the push-up. These same muscles act concentrically during the upward phase of the push-up. As an added challenge for an advanced class, utilize a step-bench as the starting position for the hands to increase the level of difficulty of the push-up, or have clients place two benches close together, positioning one hand on each and performing the push-up between the benches. The increased height off the ground will permit a larger range of motion during the eccentric and concentric phases of the push-up, creating a greater overload of these muscles.

The deltoid has a configuration similar to the trapezius in that it has fibers running in three different directions and three names, according to location. As a whole, the deltoid muscle lies superior to the glenohumeral joint, and collectively functions as the primary abductor of the shoulder joint. The anterior deltoid is easily palpated in the front of the shoulder, attaching to the lateral one-third of the clavicle. Since the anterior deltoid crosses the shoulder joint anteriorly, it flexes, internally rotates, and horizontally flexes the arm at the shoulder. The most effective positions to strengthen the anterior deltoid are sitting and standing. Using free weights or elastic tubing, flex the arms forward from 0 degrees (anatomical position) to full flexion (180 degrees), in sets of eight to 12 repetitions.

The fibers of the middle deltoid are aligned perfectly with the frontal plane,

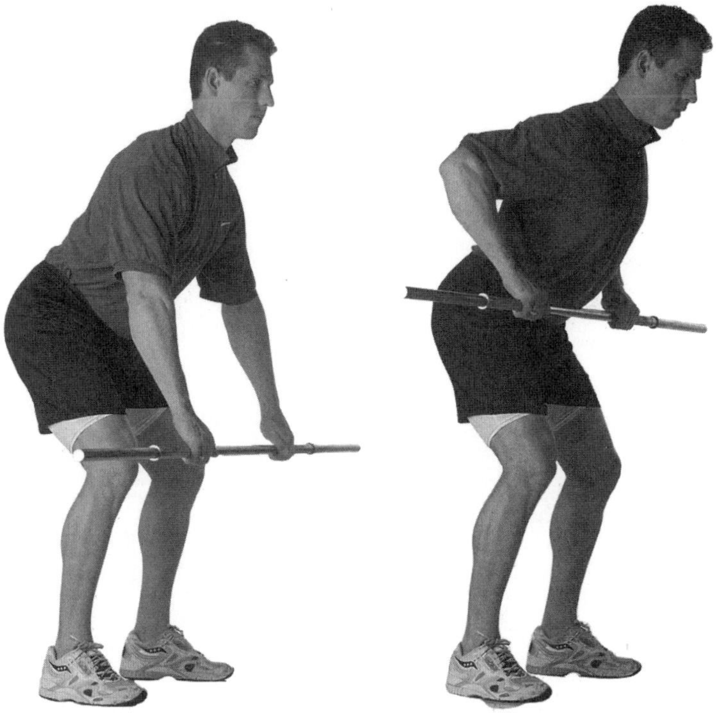

Figure 2.59

Bent-over row to strengthen scapular retractors (rhomboids and middle trapezius)

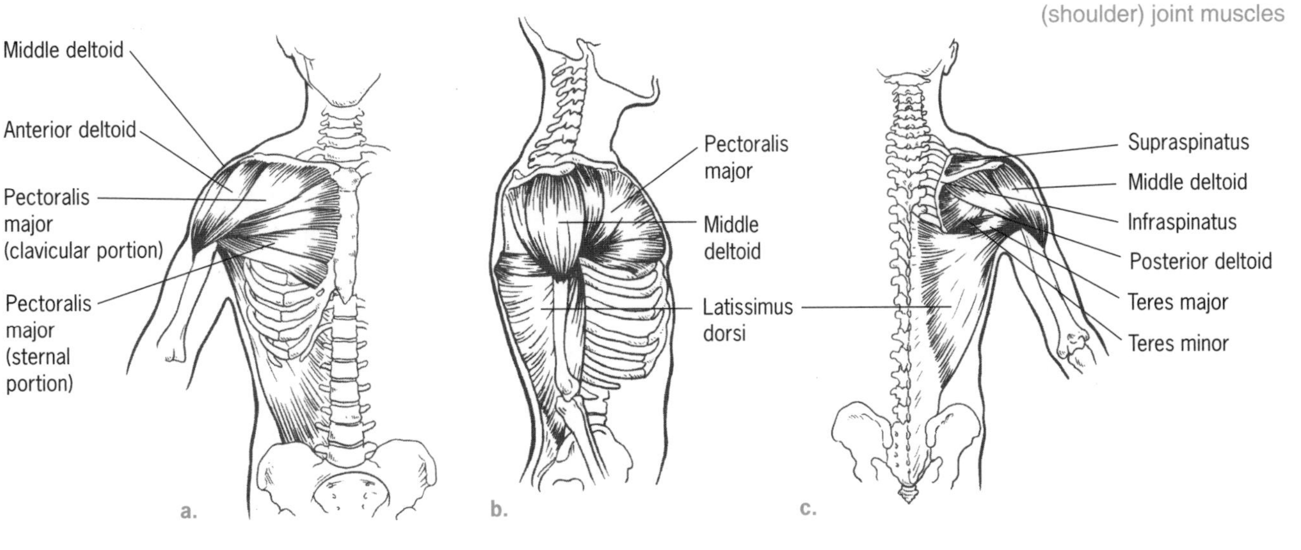

Figure 2.60

Superficial glenohumeral (shoulder) joint muscles

Middle deltoid
Anterior deltoid
Pectoralis major (clavicular portion)
Pectoralis major (sternal portion)

a.

Pectoralis major
Middle deltoid
Latissimus dorsi

b.

Supraspinatus
Middle deltoid
Infraspinatus
Posterior deltoid
Teres major
Teres minor

c.

a. Deltoid and pectoralis major

b. Latissimus dorsi, pectoralis major, and deltoid (lateral view)

c. Posterior muscles of the glenohumeral (shoulder) joint

and thus it is the prime mover in concentric abduction of the shoulder joint. When acting eccentrically, the middle deltoid controls adduction, as in the downward phase of a seated military press (Figure 2.61). When performing overhead weight lifting, such as a lateral raise, it is important to maintain the glenohumeral joint in neutral or external rotation. Abduction combined with internal rotation can ultimately irritate the rotator cuff muscles, impinging their tendons between the acromion process of the scapula and the head of the humerus (Figure 2.62).

The posterior deltoid fibers are located on the back of the G/H joint and act as an antagonist to the anterior deltoid. The posterior deltoid has the exact opposite functions as the anterior deltoid; it extends, externally rotates, and horizontally extends the arm at the shoulder. To

strengthen the posterior deltoid, have your clients stand in a forward lunge position with a neutral spine. Using hand weights, begin with the shoulder flexed, adducted, and internally rotated, and move into extension, abduction, and external rotation (Figure 2.63).

A group of four relatively small muscles comprise the rotator cuff group. These muscles act synergistically to pull the head of the humerus down and into the glenoid fossa, thus helping to stabilize the G/H joint against the constant downward pull of gravity acting to dislocate the joint. The rotator cuff muscles are sometimes referred to as the "compressor cuff" since they stabilize the humeral head in the joint. The tendons of these muscles cover the head of humerus, while the muscles themselves are mostly named for their location. The acronym SITS is used to recall the names of the muscle in this group. The supraspinatus, located as its name suggests superior to (above) the spine of the scapula, initiates abduction and is a prime mover through the early abduction range of motion. The infraspinatus, found inferior to (below) the spine of the scapula, and the teres minor, the smaller of the two "round" muscles, are synergists for external rotation of the G/H joint. The subscapularis, located on the anterior undersurface of the scapula, is not easily palpated and attaches to the anterior aspect of the joint. Since it is located anterior and medial, the subscapularis is an internal rotator.

Caution must be used when working the rotator cuff in isolation; the four tendons (primarily the supraspinatus) can become inflamed by performing many repetitions of movements that involve abduction, flex-

Figure 2.61

Seated military press for the deltoid muscle group

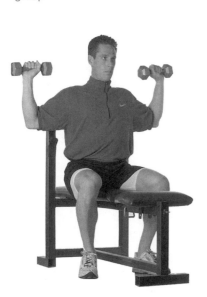
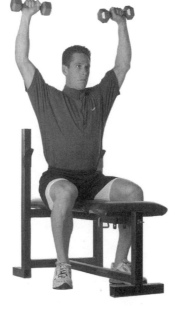

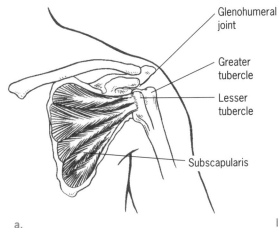

a.

Glenohumeral joint

Greater tubercle

Lesser tubercle

Subscapularis

Supraspinatus

Infraspinatus

Teres minor

b.

Figure 2.62
Rotator cuff muscles.
Avoid shoulder
abduction with
internal rotation to
prevent irritation of
the supraspinatus

a. Anterior view

b. Posterior view

ion, and rotation. For injury prevention, make sure that your clients' shoulders are in neutral or external rotation any time the arms are abducted or flexed.

The latissimus dorsi and the teres major are very similar muscles from a functional perspective (see Figure 2.30). Kinesiology instructors often nickname the teres major the "little lat" because its functions are identical to the much larger latissimus dorsi. The latissimus dorsi originates over a wide area in the lower thoracic and all of the lumbar regions of the spine, while the teres major arises from the inferior portion of the scapula. What makes these two muscles so functionally similar is the close proximity of their insertion sites on the medial aspect of the proximal humerus. Both muscles act concentrically to produce adduction, extension, and internal rotation of the glenohumeral joint. In the class setting, these muscles are strengthened with elastic cord resistance, starting with the arms overhead (elbows extended) and attempting to adduct and extend the G/H joint against the resistance provided by the tubing. Performing this same exercise with dumbbells will not involve the

Figure 2.63
Strengthening
exercise for the
posterior deltoid

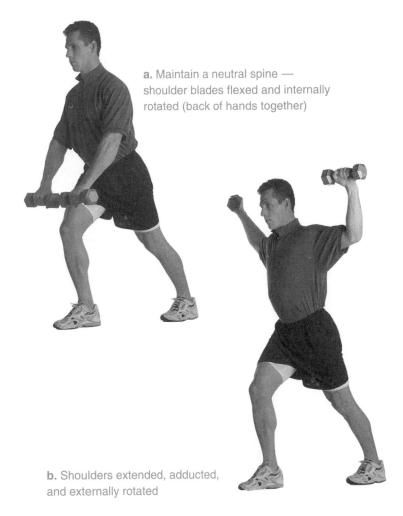

a. Maintain a neutral spine —
shoulder blades flexed and internally
rotated (back of hands together)

b. Shoulders extended, adducted,
and externally rotated

latissimus and teres major in adduction, but rather recruit the abductors (deltoids) eccentrically to lower the weights down. Regardless of the muscle targeted for strengthening, when working with hand-held weights be sure that the initial effort is in a direction opposite the pull of gravity.

Summary

Group fitness instructors are required to design programs that are safe and effective and that accomplish the desired fitness and/or personal goals of clients. Without a fundamental understanding of human anatomy and kinesiology, this task is nearly impossible. Anatomical terminology and the five major anatomical systems — cardiovascular, respiratory, nervous, skeletal, and muscular — were presented. A detailed region-by-region summary of the functional relationships of skeletal muscles was also presented. With this information, you have at your disposal sufficient information to identify specific exercises and physical activities that will safely and efficiently accomplish the fitness goals of your clients.

References

Maybury, M.C. & Waterfield, J. (1997). An investigation into the relation between step height and ground reaction forces in step exercise: A pilot study. *British Journal of Sports Medicine,* 31, 109.

Suggested Reading

Gardner, E., Gray, D. & O'Rahilly, R. (1975). *Anatomy: A Regional Study of Human Structure* (4th ed.). Philadelphia: W. B. Saunders.

Guyton, A. (1991). *Textbook of Medical Physiology* (8th ed.). Philadelphia: W. B. Saunders.

Hall, S.J. (1999). *Basic Biomechanics* (3rd ed.). Boston: WCB McGraw-Hill.

Hamill, J. & Knutzen, K.M. (1995). *Biomechanical Basis of Human Movement.* Baltimore: Williams & Wilkins.

Lephart, S.M., Pincivero, D.M., Giraldo, J.L., & Fu, F.H. (1997). Current concepts: The role of proprioception in the management and rehabilitation of athletic injuries. *American Journal of Sports Medicine,* 25, 130.

Luttgens, K. & Hamilton, N. (1997). *Kinesiology: Scientific Basis of Human Motion* (9th ed.). Boston: WCB McGraw-Hill.

Marieb, E.N. (1995). *Human Anatomy & Physiology,* (3rd ed.). Redwood City, Calif.: Benjamin-Cummings.

Pollock, M.L. & Evans, W.J. (1999). Symposium: Resistance training for health and disease. *Medicine & Science in Sports & Medicine,* 31, 10.

Smith, L.K., Weiss, E.L., & Lehmkuhl, L.D. (1996). *Brunnstrom's Clinical Kinesiology* (5th ed.). Philadelphia: F. A. Davis.

Snow-Harter, C. & Marcus, R. (1991). Exercise, bone mineral density, and osteoporosis. In Holloszy, J.O. (ed.) *Exercise & Sport Science Reviews,* 19, 351.

Thompson, C.W. & Floyd, R.T. (1998). *Manual of Structural Kinesiology* (13th ed.). Boston: WCB McGraw-Hill.

Chapter 3

In This Chapter:

Claudia S. Plaisted, M.S., R.D., L.D.N., is a clinical assistant professor and the director of Nutrition in Medicine Program® at the University of North Carolina at Chapel Hill. She graduated from Miami of Ohio with her bachelor's degree and earned her master's degree at Boston University. At UNC she teaches a graduate course in nutrition called Psychology of Eating, teaches in the UNC medical school, directs a program creating interactive CD-ROMs to teach nutrition to medical students, and teaches at the Duke Fuqua School of Business. Clinically she specializes in eating disorders/ disordered eating, weight cycling and obesity, and wellness.

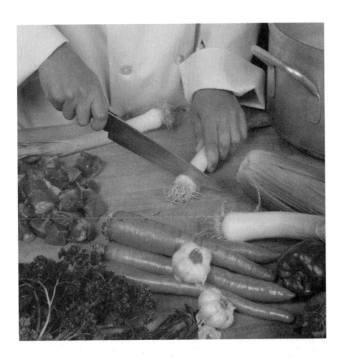

Introduction to
Nutrition

By Claudia S. Plaisted

As a group fitness instructor, you will be in a position to both teach and demonstrate healthy habits to your clients. This includes not only your fitness habits, but your nutritional habits as well. Since many of your clients will see you as an authority on basic issues of health, it is important that you can instruct them on appropriate nutritional guidelines, identify individuals at risk, and know when it is appropriate to make referrals.

As a group fitness instructor, your understanding of **nutrition** is fundamental to providing good guidance to your clients. There are four basic sets of dietary guidelines with which you should be very familiar: the USDA dietary guidelines, the American Heart Association Guidelines, The American Cancer Society Guidelines, and the Food Guide Pyramid (Table 3.1).

Table 3.1
National Nutrition Guidelines

UDSA Dietary Guidelines for Americans	The National Cancer Institute	The American Heart Association
• Balance the food you eat with physical activity — maintain or improve your weight. • Choose a diet with plenty of grain products, vegetables, and fruits. • Choose a diet low in fat, saturated fat, and cholesterol. • Eat a variety of foods. • Choose a diet moderate in salt and sodium. • Choose a diet moderate in sugars. • If you drink alcoholic beverages, do so in moderation.	• Americans should eat between 20 – 30 grams of fiber per day. For those who wish to consume more fiber, NCI recommends that individuals do not exceed 35 grams per day. • Fiber-rich foods, not fiber supplements, are the sources of fiber to choose unless your doctor advises otherwise. • Americans should consume a diet in which no more than 30% of calories come from fat. • Choose vegetables that are dark green and leafy or other green vegetables, the red, yellow, and orange vegetables and fruits, the citrus fruits and juices made from any of these • Other good vegetable choices include the cabbage family (cruciferous vegetables) which includes bok choy, broccoli, brussels sprouts, cabbage, cauliflower, collards, kale, kohlrabi, mustard greens, rutabagas, and turnips and their greens. • Eat a variety of vitamin-rich foods, rather than relying on vitamin supplements to help protect yourself from cancer.	• Dietary fat intake should be less than 30% of total calories. • Dietary carbohydrate intake should be 50% – 60% of total calories • Dietary protein intake should be 10% – 20% of total calories. • Cholesterol intake should be less than 300 mg/day. • Sodium intake should be less than 3000 mg/day. • AHA recommendations are also made for saturated, polyunsaturated, and monounsaturated fats: - Saturated fats should be less than 10% of total calories. - Polyunsaturated fats should be up to 10% of total calories. - Monounsaturated fats should be 10% – 15% of total calories.

The Food Guide
Pyramid

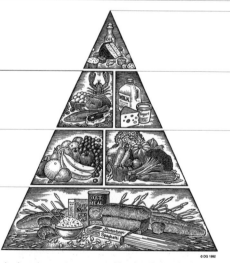

Fats, Oils and Sweets
Use sparingly

Meat, Poultry, Fish, Dry Beans,
Eggs and Nuts Group
2 – 3 Servings

Milk, Yogurt and Cheese Group
2 – 3 Servings

Fruit Group
2 – 4 Servings

Vegetable Group
3 – 5 Servings

Bread, Cereal, Rice
and Pasta Group
6 – 11 Servings

Use the Food Guide Pyramid to help you eat better every day ... the Dietary Guidelines way. Start with plenty of Breads, Cereals, Rice, and Pasta; Vegetables; and Fruits. Add two to three servings from the Milk group and two to three servings from the Meat group.

Each of these food groups provides some, but not all, of the nutrients you need. No one food group is more important than another — for good health you need them all. Go easy on fats, oils and sweets, the foods in the tip of the Pyramid.

Source: U.S. Department of Agriculture

This chapter is designed to provide you with the basics of nutrition so that you can serve as a guide in improving your client's health, based on these sets of public health guidelines. Some of your clients may have more complex health issues, such as chronic diseases or eating disorders. In these cases, it will be important for you to give sound nutritional guidance and to refer your client for the appropriate medical intervention, such as a medical doctor or a registered dietitian. Although you should have an understanding of basic nutrition after you master this chapter, it is not a substitute for a degree or a license in nutrition. In some states, nutrition assessment and prescription is a legally protected area of practice. Be aware of the laws governing the practice of nutrition in your state. Regardless of your home state's licensure laws, advanced training in nutrition (such as a bachelor's or master's degree in nutrition and passing a national competency exam) is required before one is competent to make assessments or give prescriptions. However, all allied health professionals should be able to give sound advice based on the four sets of guidelines mentioned above. Studying this chapter will help you to guide your clients to better health and answer some of their most common questions about nutrition.

The Human Body: An Energy System

Energy is a word with many meanings in common language, but when it comes to the human body, it refers exclusively to the capacity to do work. The ultimate source of **energy** is the sun, which plants turn into chemical energy through a process called **photosynthesis**. Animals, such as man, eat plants (and some animals eat other animals) to gain this energy. The energy in food is chemical energy. The human body can convert chemical energy from foods into mechanical energy (muscle activity), electrical activity (nerve conduction), and heat energy (metabolism). Energy is found in two forms: active (kinetic) energy and stored (potential) energy. Active energy is ready for the body's immediate use (for example "**ATP**" in muscles), while stored energy is in the body's reserve (body fat and **glycogen** stores).

Energy is measured in units called **kilocalories**, often written as "kcal," "Cal," or "**Calories**" (note the capital C). A kilocalorie is the amount of energy needed to raise 1 kilogram of **water** by 1°C. Although many people simply call these "**calories**," the correct scientific terminology is kilocalories. One kilocalorie equals 1,000 calories (note the lowercase c). The energy-burned units measured by exercise machines are actually in kilocalories, although they often read out as "calories."

The body requires energy — or calories — to function properly. **Total energy expenditure** is made up of basal metabolism, **physical activity**, and **dietary-induced thermogenesis**. Metabolism describes the chemical processes that happen in your body every day. Your **basal metabolic rate** (**BMR**) is the energy required to complete the sum total of these processes — including ion transport (about 40% of BMR), protein synthesis (about 20% of BMR), and daily functioning like breathing, circulation, and nutrient processing (also about 40% of BMR).

Physical activity requires energy as well. The amount of kilocalories needed depends on the duration and type of activity as well as the size of the object moving (larger people burn more calories). Energy expenditure

Figure 3.1
Breakdown of
energy expenditure

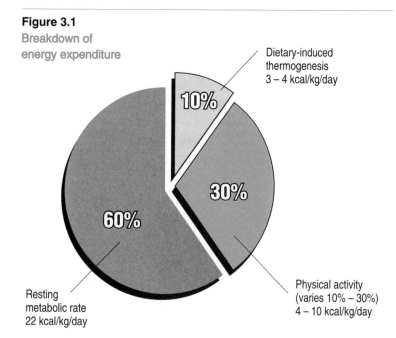

Dietary-induced
thermogenesis
3 – 4 kcal/kg/day

10%

30%

60%

Resting
metabolic rate
22 kcal/kg/day

Physical activity
(varies 10% – 30%)
4 – 10 kcal/kg/day

also increases after eating, which is called the "thermic (heat-producing) effect of food" or sometimes "dietary-induced thermogenesis." This energy is spent on digesting the carbohydrates, proteins, and fats into other substances and for some storage of energy in the form of body fat and glycogen. This body fat is called adipose tissue. Dietary-induced thermogenesis accounts for about 10% of daily energy expenditure (Figure 3.1).

How Much Energy?

Just how much energy does the human body need on a daily basis? General guidelines have been developed by the United States Department of Agriculture and the United States Department of Health and Human Services. For sedentary women and some older adults, 1600 kcal/day can provide sufficient energy intake. For most children, teenage girls, active women, and many sedentary men, 2200 kcal will be adequate. Teenage boys, many active men, and some active women will need closer to 2800 kcal/day. How this translates into food

choices is discussed later in this chapter. To get a general understanding of how much energy is needed by the human body, you can anticipate that about 10 kcal for every pound (.45 kg) of body weight will be used to supply body energy needs at rest, which include tissue growth and repair. For a 160-pound (72 kg) male, that means his resting energy expenditure will be about 1600 kcal/day. In addition, the body has energy needs for daily activities (general movement creates a need, often estimated at 300 – 500 kcal/day) and exercise, which varies with the individual. Growth, such as in children, pregnant women, and teenagers, requires extra energy. As you can see, energy needs can add up quickly in active individuals.

Since we generally eat several times a day rather than continuously, our bodies must store some of the energy we eat for later use, maybe minutes, hours, or even days away. The body ultimately converts all energy from food into ATP molecules — the energy currency of the body. Overall only about 25% of ATP energy ends up being used for work, and the other 75% is lost as heat. ATP is always present in small amounts in all body tissues. Its purpose is to deliver energy instantaneously. When you sprint for just a few seconds, you are drawing primarily on your muscular ATP stores and another compound called **phosphocreatine**, or **creatine phosphate** (**CP**). As you use up your immediate energy stores, you must continually provide more for your muscles to function.

Of course, many of us do activities for longer than just a few seconds, whether it is running, walking, or even standing. Food energy must be converted to meet these demands as well. This energy is directly related to the foods you eat: the type and the amount of **carbohydrates**, **proteins**, and fats. Not only does this food supply energy to the body, it also supplies the chemicals needed to process and use this energy. These chemicals are commonly called "vitamins" and "minerals." A diet high in carbohydrates helps the body to perform better on endurance activities, since a high-carbohydrate diet promotes glycogen storage. The other main energy source for the body is stored fat, called **fatty acids**, which are stored in adipose tissue in the form of **triglycerides**. Although a mix of fuel is consistently being used, during physical activity the body initially draws on ATP and CP, then primarily on glycogen, and eventually on fatty acids from fat stores. The well-trained athlete stores more glycogen, and can mobilize fat faster and more efficiently than the poorly trained individual.

All this chemistry and biology of health and physical fitness boils down to one major starting point: food. The energy to move, live, and grow comes from the foods we eat and the **nutrients** they contain. Helping your clients make healthy food choices is an important role you can play — a role that can have positive impacts not only on athletic performance, but also on life expectancy. In order to provide this guidance, you need to understand some of the basics of nutrition.

The Basics of Nutrition

The foods we eat supply energy. Energy only comes from four classes of nutrients: carbohydrates, protein, fat, and alcohol (Table 3.2). Fat is by far the most energy-dense of the substances we eat, with 9 kcal/g. Carbohydrate and pro-

tein both contain only 4 kcal/g, less than half of that found in fat. Alcohol is very energy-dense at 7 kcal/g but, unlike carbohydrate, protein, and fat, is very nutrient-poor. It contributes mostly calories to the diet with little to no nutritional benefit. Any energy eaten in excess of needs is converted to body fat for storage, thus no one category is more "fattening" than another.

Carbohydrate

Carbohydrate, protein, and fat are referred to as the **macronutrients,** while alcohol is not usually referred to as a macronutrient since it cannot be a large contributor to a healthy diet. These macronutrients are the "energy nutrients" since they provide the body with kilocalories. They also contain or carry vitamins, minerals, and other non-nutritive substances (dietary fiber, fluid, phytochemicals, etc.) that are critical for health.

**Table 3.2
Energy Content**

Carbohydrate	4 kcal/g
Protein	4 kcal/g
Fat	9 kcal/g
Alcohol	7 kcal/g

Carbohydrates are compounds of carbon, oxygen, and hydrogen atoms. They are consumed either as **simple carbohydrates** or as **complex carbohydrates** (Table 3.3). The simple carbohydrates are also called sugars, which fall into the category of **monosaccharides** ("single sugars") or **disaccharides** ("double sugars"). Regardless of the category into which they fall, all of these carbohydrates provide 4 kcal/g.

Table 3.3.
Carbohydrates (sugars)

Simple

Monosaccharides	Disaccharides
Glucose	Sucrose
Fructose	Lactose
Galactose	Maltose

Complex

Starch (polysaccharides)	Fibers (soluble, insoluble)

Simple carbohydrates contain naturally occurring sugars like those in fruit (fructose) and milk (lactose) and refined sugars (often sucrose or high-fructose corn syrup), such as table sugar, brown sugar, honey, and corn syrup. Since refined sugars provide little more than calories, excess consumption of foods high in refined sugars can cause health problems, particularly if sweetened, nutrient-poor foods replace more nutritious choices. The naturally occurring sugars in fruits and milk are found in combination with vitamins, minerals, proteins, and other non-nutritive but beneficial compounds (fiber, phytochemicals).

Complex carbohydrates are made up of longer chains of carbon atoms and have different tastes, textures, and health effects than their simple shorter-chain counterparts. Examples of complex carbohydrates are whole grain breads, cereals, legumes (beans and peas), and vegetables. Similar to the naturally occurring simple carbohydrates, the complex ones are good choices since they are packed with vitamins, minerals, some protein, and other non-nutritive but beneficial compounds.

Regardless of whether the carbohydrate eaten is in a simple or complex form, through the processes of digestion, absorption, and metabolism all carbohydrates are turned into **glucose**, the form of sugar in the blood and the main energy fuel for the body, brain, and central nervous system. Although muscle tissue can use fat as an energy source, the brain and central nervous system are dependent on glucose as their primary source of fuel. As one of the body's major energy sources, glucose is stored after eating to be used later. The muscles contain some glucose to meet their short-term energy needs while the liver stores up to approximately a 12-hour supply to meet the needs of the brain between meals or during an overnight fast (during sleep).

Many foods rich in carbohydrates actually contain a mix of simple and complex carbohydrates. There is some evidence that the body transforms this mix into blood glucose at slightly different rates. The speed of the relative rise in blood glucose is called the **glycemic index**. The blood glucose response of foods eaten is compared to either the response to glucose or white bread (set at a reference standard of 100). Foods with

Table 3.4
Recommended Healthy Intakes/Day for Carbohydrate, Protein, and Fat for Several Different Calorie Levels (grams and percent total calories)

Energy Intake (kcal)	Carbohydrate	Protein	Fat
	Goal % total kcal		
	50% – 60%	10% – 15%	25% – 30%
1600	200 – 240 g/day	40 – 60 g/day	44 – 53 g/day
2000	250 – 300 g/day	50 – 75 g/day	56 – 67 g/day
2200	275 – 330 g/day	55 – 83 g/day	61 – 73 g/day
2600	325 – 390 g/day	65 – 98 g/day	72 – 87 g/day
2800	250 – 420 g/day	70 – 105 g/day	78 – 93 g/day

higher glycemic index scores compared to glucose (for example, carrots at 92, instant rice at 91, corn flakes at 84, table sugar at 65, raisins at 64, potatoes at 62, orange juice at 57) raise blood glucose more quickly than those with lower scores (for example, bananas at 53, oranges at 43, apples at 36, chocolate milk at 34, yogurt at 33, skim milk at 32, whole milk at 27, and grapefruit at 25).

It is this type of provocative research that has shown that people with diabetes can have food containing sugar — or any other kind of carbohydrates — just like anybody else. Research into the glycemic index gives us evidence to say that we cannot classify foods into "good" or "bad" categories. It is important to remember that the glycemic index only applies when these foods are eaten alone — when they are eaten as part of a mixed meal the values change in complex and unpredictable ways. Carrots eaten by themselves as a snack do not react the same way as those in a salad, on a sandwich, or cooked. The glycemic index is sometimes used by people with a poor understanding of nutrition to label foods inappropriately, such as "provokes a strong insulin response," "promotes fat storage," "provokes high blood sugars," etc. The science just does not give evidence to draw those kinds of conclusions.

Guiding your clients to base their diet in complex carbohydrates and the naturally occurring simple ones can help them maximize their muscle glycogen stores, extend their endurance, and improve their athletic performance. However, even more importantly, it can help lower their risks for chronic diseases, such as cancer and heart disease, in part because of the **fiber**, **vitamins**, **minerals**, and **phytochemicals** they contain. The relationship between diet and disease will be discussed later in this chapter as

will the definition and role of dietary fiber. See Table 3.4 for recommended daily carbohydrate intakes in grams for several different calorie levels.

Protein

Proteins are large molecules that play a variety of roles in the body. They make up the major part of the body's structural components like muscles, skin, tendons, organs, and bones. They also work in the forms of enzymes to catalyze chemical reactions and they serve as neurotransmitters in the brain and are thus involved with thinking and emotions. Some hormones are made of protein and thus they transmit messages throughout the body. Proteins help balance fluid and electrolytes in the body compartments and help regulate acid-base balance. Also, they work as a veritable taxi service in the blood, serving as transport proteins for many nutrients, particularly fats. Proteins can provide energy too, but in light of all the other important functions they provide, it is best if carbohydrate and fat supply the majority of energy needs. In illness, severe injury, or poorly constructed diets (such as some fad diets), protein is sacrificed to meet energy demands instead of fulfilling its important biological roles.

How do proteins accomplish this incredible variety of vital tasks? They do this by taking on a virtually infinite variety of different shapes, most of them looking like long twisted chains or balls of string. In fact, that is exactly what they are: long chains of **amino acids**, the building blocks of proteins. There are approximately 20 amino acids, all but eight to 10 of which can be manufactured by the body if the basic metabolic parts are available. Those the body cannot make are called "essential amino acids" and must be provided in the diet. Complete proteins contain all the essential amino acids and are found in animal products like seafood, poultry, dairy products, and red meats. Although grains and legumes do not contain all the amino acids, they can be combined to provide complete protein sources. For example, serving black beans with rice, peanut butter on wheat bread, or tofu and stir-fried vegetables with brown rice will provide the complete array of essential amino acids.

Amino acid supplements are not necessary for either health or athletic performance. For most people living in westernized societies, protein deficiency is not a health issue. Most individuals in these societies eat too much protein, rather than too little. Instead, excess protein intake is quickly turned into fat and stored in the body.

Fat

Dietary fats, called **lipids**, are a group of organic compounds that are water-insoluble and include triglycerides, **cholesterol**, and **lecithin.** Of the fat you eat, 95% is in the form of triglycerides. This is also the major storage form of fat in the body's fat tissues, called **adipose tissues**. In the body, fat does more than store energy; it cushions vital organs, provides insulation, and is involved in basic functions, such as nerve conduction and tissue structure (for example, brain tissue). Fats are also important for the absorption and transport of **fat-soluble vitamins** and **essential fatty acids**.

Fat is the most efficient source of energy, since it contains 9 kcal/g. Even if 70 g sounds like a lot of fat (see Table 3.4), it is quite easy to consume that when eating the typical American diet. Consider that a popular fast-food hamburger contains 35 g of fat and a "bloomin' onion" (a popular breaded and deep fried onion) contains nearly 300 g of fat.

Fats, or triglycerides, are organized into two groups: saturated and unsaturated (you will also see these referred to as fatty acids). Regardless of the type of fat, all these fats contain 9 kcal/g. Like carbohydrates, fatty acids are made up of long chains of carbon molecules connected to hydrogen atoms. What determines whether a fat is saturated or unsaturated is how many carbons are bonded to each other (called a carbon-carbon double bond) and not just to hydrogen. **Saturated fats** have *no* double bonds, which makes them typically solid at room temperature. Examples include butter, stick margarine, hydrogenated vegetable shortening, lard, milk and meat fats, eggs, and tropical fats like coconut oil. Liquid oils that are turned into stick margarines or solid hydrogenated vegetable shortening undergo a process called **hydrogenation**, where the carbon-carbon double bonds are destroyed and replaced with more hydrogen atoms. This process creates a new type of fat, the **trans fatty acid**. Trans fatty acids are not commonly found in unprocessed foods. The health implications of saturated fats are addressed later in this chapter.

Unsaturated fats have at least one of these carbon-carbon double bonds. They also fall into two categories: **polyunsaturated** and **monounsaturated**. The polyunsaturated fats have more than one double bond and are liquid at room temperature. Examples include corn, sunflower, and safflower oils. The monounsaturated fatty acids have only one double bond and are also liquid at room temperature. Examples of these include olive, sesame, canola, avocado, and nut oils. Most naturally occurring fats in foods are actually a mix of all three types of fat: saturated, monounsaturated, and polyunsaturated. The category is determined by the proportion of the fatty acid types present. The health implications of these types of fats will be addressed later in this chapter.

Cholesterol is not actually a fat, but rather a waxy, fat-like substance. You cannot derive calories from cholesterol because your body cannot break it down; it is absorbed relatively intact. Cholesterol is commonly found in foods of animal origin rich in saturated fats (primarily meat and milk fats).

Cholesterol is made by the liver. In order for a food to contain cholesterol it must come from an animal-based food, such as beef, pork, dairy, poultry, etc. Organ meats are particularly rich in cholesterol and saturated fat and, therefore, should be consumed only in moderation. Some foods, such as peanut butter made with hydrogenated fat, are rich in saturated fat but contain no cholesterol. It is recommended to keep average daily intake of cholesterol to 300 mg or less.

Lecithin is a type of fat called a **phospholipid**, meaning it has a water-soluble and a fat-soluble portion. It is manufactured by the

Table 3.5
Vitamin RDA, Food Sources, and Functions

Vitamin	Adult RDA	Food Sources	Role in Health
Fat soluble			
Vitamin A	men: 1000RE women: 800RE or 4000–5000 IU	Dark green, leafy vegetables; yellow/orange vegetables and fruits; liver; fish liver oils; milk and milk products; margarine; eggs	Visual health; healthy skin and inside surfaces of mucous membranes, immune system; bone growth; cell membranes; red blood cells and nerve sheaths; thyroid hormone production
Vitamin D	5 µg; 400 IU	Fortified cow's milk; egg yolks; butter; liver; some fatty fish; fortified margarine (and sun exposure)	Regulates the metabolism of calcium and phosphorus; promotes growth of strong bones
Vitamin E	men: 10 mg; women: 8 mg α–tocopherol or 30 IU	Unprocessed grains; vegetables oils; margarine; salad dressing; shortening; nuts; seeds; poultry; fish; eggs	Antioxidant (prevent cell-membrane damage) scavenger for destructive substances that react against the unsaturated fats in the body (free radicals); tissue growth and repair
Vitamin K	65 – 80 µg	Green, leafy vegetables, milk, cabbage family vegetables, soybean oil, egg yolk, bacteria in the gut synthesizes vitamin K	Required for normal blood clotting
Water soluble			
Vitamin C	60 mg	Citrus fruits; broccoli; cauliflower; green pepper; strawberries	Maintaining and forming collagen; (part of connective tissue); bones and teeth; healing of skin and capillaries; blood vessel repair
B1 Thiamin	1.0 – 1.5 mg	Whole grains; legumes (beans and peas); seeds; pork; organ meats; brewer's yeast; breads made from enriched flours	Metabolizing food (carbohydrate) for use as energy

Table 3.5 (continued)

Vitamin	Adult RDA	Food Sources	Role in Health
B2 Riboflavin	1.2 – 1.7 mg	Dairy products; eggs; liver; whole grains; fortified cereals; baked goods made with enriched white wheat flour; green vegetables (broccoli, asparagus, turnip greens, spinach)	Metabolism of carbohydrates, proteins and fats; B6 and niacin functioning; red blood cells; building tissues; protection from skin and eye disorders
Niacin	13 – 19 mg	Protein rich foods such as meat, fish, poultry, breads made with enriched flour, fortified cereals, mushrooms, baked potatoes, peanuts	Metabolism of carbohydrates, protein and fat; protects skin, nervous tissues, and digestive tract from disorders
B6 Pyridoxine	1.6 – 2.0 mg	Chicken; fish; pork; eggs; liver; whole grains (unmilled rice, oats, whole wheat products); legumes (soybeans, peanuts); fruits; nuts; many vegetables (avocados and bananas especially)	Metabolism of protein; conversion of glycogen to glucose; amino acid building and conversion to hormones; red blood cell production; nerve tissue functioning
B12 Cyanocobalamin	2.0 µg	Meats; dairy products; eggs	Red blood cell manufacture; nerve fiber sheath development and protection; cell growth
Folic Acid, (folate, folacin)	400 – 600 µg	All leafy green vegetables; legumes; oranges; peanuts; sunflower seeds; whole grains	Essential for formation of DNA and RNA, bone marrow, red blood cells, and intestinal tract; synthesis and breakdown of amino acids; critical for fetal development
Pantothenic Acid	4 – 7 mg (safe & adequate range)	Whole grains; legumes; some vegetables and fruits; organ meats; yeast; egg yolk	Part of coenzyme A; widely involved in metabolism of carbohydrates; proteins and fat; formation of fatty acids, cholesterol, acetylcholine; and steroid hormones
Biotin	30 – 100 µg (safe & adequate)	Produced by intestinal bacteria; widely distributed in foods (liver, kidney, egg yolk, soy flour, cereals, yeast)	Carrier of carbon dioxide; coenzyme functions

These intake levels are meant for adult males and females between age 24 – 50 years. Ranges for adults 51+ years are very similar.
Vitamin A Note: RE=Retinol Equivalent, IU=International Units. IU is a cruder measure of Vitamin A activity and is less frequently used

body and does not contain calories. Although it is not needed as a supplement, it is sold in many health-food stores. The body can convert fatty acids to meet its needs for all fats except for **linoleic acid**, which is called an essential fatty acid. This fat is found in vegetable oils, nuts, seeds, wheat germ, and other foods that contain polyunsaturated fat. Supplements of essential fatty acids are not necessary since adequate amounts are supplied by even an extremely low fat intake.

Micronutrients

The body needs more than just carbohydrate, protein, and fat to function; it needs the special chemicals it cannot manufacture on its own. These chemicals, among a multitude of other tasks, help the body create tissues, release energy, regulate metabolic processes, and make DNA. Unlike the macronutrients, these special chemicals are needed only in minute amounts and are found widely in the foods you eat. You know these special chemicals as vitamins and minerals.

Vitamins are organic (carbon-containing) compounds that the body cannot manufacture on its own and, therefore, must be consumed. If a vitamin is not supplied in the diet, a deficiency symptom occurs. For example, lack of vitamin C causes scurvy, a condition particularly prevalent among sailors before the nineteenth century. By definition, when the vitamin is returned to the diet the deficiency symptoms go away. If lack of a substance does *not* cause deficiency symptoms, it cannot be a vitamin. Vitamins provide no calories and therefore they cannot be used as fuel. Some vitamins, such as the B-vitamins, help you liberate the energy from the foods you eat, but they do not themselves give you energy.

The 13 vitamins identified fall into two groups: water soluble and fat soluble. The **water-soluble vitamins** include the B-vitamins and vitamin C. These need to be supplied on a daily basis since the body has a limited ability to store them and excretes excesses in the urine daily. Vitamins A, D, E, and K are the fat-soluble vitamins. Unlike their water-soluble counterparts, they are stored in the body, particularly in the liver and body fat tissues. Table 3.5 lists the important vitamins, food sources, and how much

of the foods provide the necessary daily intake. It is challenging to meet all your nutrient needs when eating fewer than 1600 kcal/day. As an ACE-certified instructor, be aware that clients who are restricting their calorie intake might be depriving themselves of essential nutrition as well. They will need to make careful decisions about the foods they eat in order to protect their health. Later in this chapter we will address for whom supplements are appropriate.

Like vitamins, the minerals necessary for health are needed in tiny amounts. Minerals are inorganic compounds that enter the food chain as plants absorb them from soil and water. Humans eat either the plants or the animals that consumed the plants, and thus we get minerals in our diets. There are 15 minerals that have been recognized as essential (Table 3.6). Excess intake of minerals can be dangerous. Since such small amounts are required for health, it is important to keep mineral intake well balanced. Many minerals compete for absorption in the gut, such as iron, copper, and zinc. Supplementing with large doses of iron can cause a deficiency in copper or zinc, even if dietary intake meets the **recommended daily allowances (RDA)**. Similarly, the

Table 3.6
Mineral RDA, Food Sources, and Role in Health

Mineral	Adult RDA	Food Sources	Role in Health
Major Minerals			
Calcium	1000 mg	Milk, cheese, and other dairy products; dark green leafy vegetables; legumes; lime-processed corn tortillas; some brands of tofu; almonds	Bones; teeth; transmission of nerve impulses; proper muscle contraction; heart rhythm; function of several enzymes; absorption of B12
Phosphorus	800 – 1200 mg	Protein-rich foods and cereal grains; milk and milk products; meat	Formation of bones and teeth; part of DNA and RNA; new cell formation and growth; transport of nutrients through blood stream; used in many hormones

Table 3.6 (continued)

Mineral	Adult RDA	Food Sources	Role in Health
Magnesium	280 – 350 mg	Protein foods; unprocessed whole grains; legumes; nuts; seeds; chocolate; dark green vegetables; bananas	Bone and teeth formation and integrity (helps hold calcium in the bones and teeth); muscle relaxation; nerve impulse conduction; part of many enzymes
Potassium	2000 mg (safe & adequate)	Fresh fruits and vegetables; legumes	Fluid and electrolyte balance; cell integrity
Sodium	1100 – 3300 mg (safe & adequate)	Table salt; processed foods; soy sauce	Fluid balance; generating nerve impulses; acid-base balance; metabolism of carbohydrates and protein
Chloride	750 mg (safe & adequate)	Table salt; soy sauce; processed foods; moderate amounts in milk; meats and eggs	Normal fluid balance; hydrochloric acid in stomach; necessary for proper digestion

Trace Minerals

Mineral	Adult RDA	Food Sources	Role in Health
Iron	10 – 15 mg	Lean meats; fish; poultry; organ meats; legumes; nuts and seeds; whole grains; dark molasses; green leafy vegetables	Carries oxygen in the blood; helps accept, store, and release oxygen in the muscles
Copper	1.5 – 3.0 mg (safe & adequate range)	Legumes; seafood and shellfish; organ meats; whole grains; nuts; seeds; vegetables	Plays a key role in several enzymes; red blood cell formation; transportation of iron; healing wounds; nerve fiber sheath; bone formation; RNA synthesis; collagen formation
Zinc	10 – 15 mg	Protein foods; seafoods; meats; whole grains; legumes	Enzyme production; metabolism of protein, carbohydrates, fat, and alcohol; protein synthesis; DNA and RNA; immune functioning; growth and repair of tissues; function of hormone insulin
Iodine	150 µg	Iodized salt; some shellfish and seafoods	Constituent of thyroid hormones
Selenium	55 – 70 µg	Seafood; meats; eggs; whole grains; legumes; brazil nuts	Antioxidant functions; part of enzyme glutathione perioxidase
Fluoride	1.5 – 4.0 mg (safe & adequate range)	Drinking water; tea; seafood	Involved in formation of bones and teeth; resistance to tooth decay
Manganese	2.0 – 5.0 mg	Whole grains; cereal products; tea; some fruits and vegetables	Functions as a cofactor in many reactions; found in most of the body's organs and tissues
Chromium	50 – 200 µg (safe & adequate range)	Mushrooms; prunes; nuts; asparagus; wine; beer; meat; organ meat; whole grains; cheese	Metabolism of carbohydrates and lipids; helps the hormone insulin to function
Molybdenum	75 – 250 µg (safe & adequate range)	Legumes; cereals; organ meats	Metabolism of carbohydrates and lipids; helps the hormone insulin to function

These intake levels are meant for adult males and females age 24 – 50 years. Ranges for adults 51+ years are very similar.

proper balance between the minerals enhances their use. For example, magnesium and zinc affect how **calcium** is absorbed and used in the body.

The RDAs are set by a national panel of scientists for the Food and Nutrition Board and the National Academy of Science. Through evaluation of current research, this group of experts determines the amounts of selected nutrients considered to meet the known nutrient needs of practically all Americans. The RDA is set for energy, protein, vitamins A, D, E, K, thiamin (B1), riboflavin (B2), niacin, B6, folate, B12, calcium, phosphorous, magnesium, iron, zinc, iodine, and selenium. Estimated minimum requirements are set for sodium, potassium, and chloride. While nutritional needs vary somewhat from person to person, the RDAs are set to meet the needs of 98% of the population. The needs of most people will be met adequately if they make good food choices. For those individuals who wish to "hedge their nutritional bet," a general purpose multi-vitamin/mineral supplement should be sufficient. Under no circumstances should you ever suggest a client take a supplement with more than 100% to 150% of the RDA. While most nutrients are safe even in large doses, some, particularly the minerals and some fat soluble vitamins, can have toxic side effects at just a few-to-several times the RDA level.

When vitamins and minerals are obtained through foods, it is difficult to upset the proportional balances that nature intended. However, when an individual starts taking large doses (called **megadoses**) of the **micronutrients**, he or she risks imbalances that could affect long-term health outcomes, particularly for diseases such as osteoporosis (via an upset in calcium absorption or use) or blood sugar control (via aberrations in zinc or chromium absorption and use). Some minerals (and some vitamins) are toxic in large amounts, so megadoses should be avoided. Some minerals are referred to as major minerals, which indicates their relative quantity, not their importance. The major minerals include calcium and phosphorus (used in bones and teeth), sodium, potassium, chloride (found in body fluids), sulfur, and magnesium.

The **trace minerals**, found in much smaller quantities, include iron, zinc, copper, manganese, iodine, and selenium, among many others. Despite the fact the entire human body has less than 5 g in total of each of these minerals, they are far more likely to be consumed in nutritional supplements. Tables 3.5 and 3.6 provide you with an overview of these important vitamins and minerals: their function, how much you need each day, what foods contain these nutrients, and how much you need to eat to meet your health needs. Use these tables as references to steer your clients to healthy food choices and away from pills.

Other Important Dietary Components

There is more to the story of good nutrition than just macro- and micronutrients. There are substances important to health that are not nutritive at all. Non-nutritive substances include water, fiber, and phytochemicals.

As a fitness professional, you know the value of adequate **hydration**. Water is the most commonly overlooked endurance aid. It is literally the fluid in which all life processes occur in every cell. The body uses fluids to help regulate body temperature via sweat (to dissipate heat); to maintain blood pressure, thus influencing how substances move between the blood stream and the body cells; to deliver nutrients to cells; and to carry off waste products. You can survive without water for only a few days. Sudden **dehydration** from heat or excessive exercise can be life threatening.

Thirst and satiety guide most individual's water intake. The changes in the mouth, hypothalamus (a gland in the brain), and the nerves help signal the need for increased fluid intake. Although your thirst may drive you to seek water, it lags behind your body's fluid needs. A fluid deficiency that develops quickly, such as during strenuous exercise, may not alert the body's fluid sensors in time to prevent dehydration. The adult body must excrete a minimum of about 500 milliliters per day (almost 17 oz) of urine to carry away the waste products generated by the day's metabolic activities. Your kidneys can adjust to high fluid intake to keep you in a normal fluid balance. How much fluid does a person need in a day? You've probably heard the recommendation to consume eight 8-oz glasses of water, but the true amount varies with age, gender, activity, and environment. In general a person consuming about 2000 kcal/day needs about 2 – 3 liters (7 to 11 cups).

Table 3.7
Tips for Increasing Dietary Fiber

- Increase intake of whole grain breads and cereals
- Choose foods with as little processing as possible (whole wheat breads and flours, brown rice)
- Include several servings of fresh fruits and vegetables daily
- Include legumes (beans and peas) in your diet on a regular basis
- Consume moderate amounts of meat

Estimating Fiber Intake

Fresh, whole, and dried fruits — ~ 2 g/serving
 (fruit juice contains very little fiber)
Whole grain breads — ~ 2 g/slice
Whole grain cereals — between 3 to 12 g/serving
Vegetables — ~1 – 4 g/serving

Not all fluid intake must be in the form of water; fluid comes from other beverages as well as foods. Although fluid needs are best met by water, particularly in an exercising adult, lowfat milk and juice are excellent choices to round out the day's liquid intake since they contain the minerals involved in fluid balance: potassium, sodium, chloride, and, to some extent, calcium. Poor choices for rehydration include alcohol and caffeine-containing beverages (sodas, coffees, and teas), since both these substances act as diuretics.

Fiber

Another important non-nutritive substance is fiber. **Dietary fiber** is basically carbohydrate chains that the body cannot break down, thus they pass through the entire gastrointestinal tract intact. As they move through the gut these fibers serve two central functions, depending on their type. **Soluble fibers** form a gel with fluids in the gut and bowel. They delay the emptying of the stomach, delay glucose (sugar) absorption, and help lower blood cholesterol. These fibers help keep the stool soft and easy to pass, thus aiding in the relief of constipation. These fibers are found primarily in fruits, oats, barley, and legumes. The names for these fibers, which you might see added on ingredient lists, are gums, pectins, hemicelluloses, and mucilages.

Insoluble fibers, in contrast to soluble fibers, do not tend to bind water, fluids, or cholesterol. They accelerate the passage of foods through the gut, make the stool larger, and slow the digestive processes. These fibers, found in wheat bran, whole-grain breads and cereals, and vegetables, are called cellulose, hemicellulose, and lignins. You can think of these fibers as scraping the sides of the bowel, thus helping to remove old gut tissue cells. Both types of dietary fiber are thought to play a role in preventing colon cancer.

The average American does not eat enough dietary fiber. Recommendations for health suggest an intake of 25 – 35 g a day as a healthy goal, but the average American consumes only about 15 g per day. If there is a health benefit to dietary fiber, such as lowering cholesterol or reducing the risks for colon cancer, individuals need to consume it in sufficient amounts. Table 3.7 provides a list of suggestions you can use with your clients to help them include good sources of dietary fiber. Although fiber supplements are available, it is best to consume fiber with foods and with plenty of fluids. If a client requests advice for problems with constipation that do not respond to increased dietary fiber and fluid intake, refer him or her to their physician.

Phytochemicals

You have probably been told that fruits and vegetables are good for you. You should know (and tell your clients) that whole grain breads and cereals, fruits, and vegetables contain more than just vitamins, minerals, and fiber. Recent research has uncovered exciting news about those garden-fresh foods mothers have been pushing for centuries. Vitamins and minerals are extremely important to our health, but these foods also contain other non-nutritive substances that seem to play amazing roles in protecting our health. These special compounds are called phytochemicals. Phytochemicals are the biologically active compounds in plants that give them their color, flavor, and natural disease resistance. This exciting new research has shown that many of these phytochemicals have benefits for humans as well since they are potent cancer-fighters, blocking one or more of the steps in the process that leads to cancer. Some help fight the process of heart disease by working as **antioxidants**. The chemistry of phytochemicals makes the biochemistry of vitamins and minerals look easy; there are just a few vitamins and minerals but there are literally thousands and thousands of phytochemicals. Supplements of these compounds are available in health food stores, but they are not recommended. While most phytochemicals protect our health, some encourage the cancer process. Keeping your dietary intake in a natural balance is the best way to reap the benefits of phytochemicals without upsetting the natural balance

Table 3.8
Phytochemicals from Food

Food	Phytochemical	Action
Broccoli	Sulforaphane	Helps remove carcinogens from cells
Citrus fruits and berries	Flavonoids	Blocks the cancer-promotion process
Soybeans	Genistein	Works against tumors by preventing the formation of capillaries needed to nourish them
Cruciferous vegetables (broccoli, cabbage, brussels sprouts, and cauliflower)	Indoles	Increase immunity and make it easier for the body to excrete toxins
Tomatoes	Lycopene	May fight lung cancer
Cherries, citrus fruits, strawberries, blueberries	Monoterpenes (polyphenols)	May inhibit growth of early cancers

between them. Similar to vitamins and minerals, while it is hard to over-consume these from foods, it is easy to get too much from a pill. The research is just too recent to be sure about safety and efficacy. Instead, encourage your clients to fill their shopping baskets with phytochemical-packed fruits, vegetables, and whole grains every time they shop. See Table 3.8 for some examples of phyto-chemical-rich foods.

Putting Together a Healthy Diet

Now you have a basic understanding of macro- and micronutrients, but how do you guide your clients in making healthy food choices? The **Food Guide Pyramid** is your best tool to translate all this complex nutrition information into simple-to-follow, healthy eating guidelines (Tables 3.4 and 3.9).

When you use the Food Guide Pyramid as a teaching tool, remember that it represents the variety, moderation, and proportions of foods that make up a healthy diet. The base of the pyramid is the largest section — and represents where the majority of calorie and food intake should come from

Table 3.9
Sample Diets for a Day at Three Calorie Levels

| | Servings from Food Group | | |
	1600 kcal	2200 kcal	2800 kcal
Bread/grains	6	6	11
Vegetables	3	4	5
Fruits	2	3	4
Milk and dairy	2 – 3	3	4
Protein (oz)	5	6	7
Total added sugars	6 tsp	12 tsp	18 tsp

Source: *How to Make the Pyramid Work for You.*
U.S. Department of Agriculture/U.S. Department
of Health and Human Services.

Table 3.10
Daily Intake Patterns with Increased Nutritional Risk

Food Group	Servings/day	Deficiency
Dairy	<3 to 5 servings	Calcium
Protein	<2 servings	Protein and iron
Vegetables	<5 servings	Vitamin, mineral, fat
Fruit fiber, vitamins	<4 servings	Energy, mineral,
Bread & whole grains	<4 servings	Energy, mineral, fiber, vitamins

in a healthy diet. Whole grains, breads, and cereals are the foundation of a healthy eating strategy. The next level contains fruits and vegetables, indicating that they should be the next most abundant choices for a healthy intake. Dairy and meats appear next, having a less prominent role since only a few servings are needed to obtain the valuable nutrients found in these foods. At the very top and in the smallest portion of the pyramid are the fats and sugars, indicating that they should be used sparingly. To some extent, fats and sugars are spread throughout all the levels of the pyramid, particularly in processed foods. That is another reason why added fats and sugars should be considered carefully as part of the daily food choices.

To help Americans use the Food Guide Pyramid, the United States Department of Agriculture and the United States Department of Health and Human Services have developed a healthy eating guideline for individuals needing 1600 kcal/day, 2200 kcal/day, and 2800 kcal/day. You can use the information in Table 3.9 as an example of recommended dietary patterns.

When individuals do not consume adequate servings from a food group, or miss it entirely, they are at risk of getting inadequate nutrients as well. Over time, this can have devastating consequences on one's health. Table 3.10 illustrates the nutritional components at risk when daily patterns do not meet the recommended guidelines. In the next section we will discuss the health implications of eating an unbalanced diet.

There are no perfect teaching tools, and the Food Guide Pyramid is no exception. It may not provide enough information for people who already know a lot about nutrition, and one still must be aware of fats. For example, ice cream and milk appear in the same food group, as do french fries and broccoli. Obviously, ice cream and milk are not nutritionally equivalent. And no matter how much we might wish it were so, french fries are just not as good for your body as broccoli. Thus, fat gram counting is a good tool for you and your clients as well. See Table 3.4 for information on reasonable fat gram intakes. There are many fat gram guides available to help your clients track their fat intake. Be careful, however. Just as you can get too much of a good thing, you can get too little as well. In general, most people need a minimum of 20 g of fat, and 50 g is a reasonable intake for many adults. Being too restrictive on fat intake can lead to dissatisfaction with the diet, feelings of hunger, and "throwing in the towel" on making dietary changes. Moderation is the key, even when it comes to limiting fat.

Diet and Disease

O f course, eating well on a day-to-day basis will help you feel your best, have energy, and think clearly. However, eating well on a month-to-month and year-to-year basis can save or prolong

your life. There is a strong relationship between diet and disease. Four of the 10 leading causes of death are diet related, which means they are preventable to a large extent. As a fitness professional, you will have the opportunity to affect peoples' health in a profound way, both by the information you give and the by the example you set.

The relationship between diet and disease is a complex medical association. Fortunately, the nutritional guidance is simple. The principles you can employ via the Food Guide Pyramid, the Dietary Guidelines, and an awareness of fat intake (such as using fat gram counting) can help lower the risks for many chronic diseases. Of all the nutrients, fat is most related to chronic disease.

Cardiovascular Disease

Cardiovascular disease, more commonly known as heart disease or "CVD," is the most common killer of adults in the United States. The types and quantity of the foods chosen in the diet have a strong influence on the risk of developing CVD. The nutrient of most concern is of course fat. A high total dietary fat intake is associated with increased rates of CVD in all ages. One of the early and major biological indicators of CVD is elevated blood cholesterol, called "serum cholesterol." When total serum cholesterol is above 200 mg/dL, the risks of developing CVD are increased. Measuring your serum cholesterol is usually referred to as measuring "**serum lipids**." Lipids are fats in the blood — there is more than just cholesterol to think about. **Low-density lipoprotein**, or **LDL**, **cholesterol** is the type known as "bad" cholesterol. It is very much involved in the artery-blocking process. Risk of heart disease is elevated when LDL cholesterol is >130 mg/dL.

High-density lipoprotein, or **HDL**, is often called "good cholesterol" since it helps move body lipids from places of storage to places of use. Athletes often have very high HDL levels since they have trained their bodies to be efficient fat-burning machines and to produce more HDL cholesterol. It is desirable for HDL levels to be >35 mg/dL. Triglycerides are another type of blood fat, often elevated right after eating. It is desirable for triglyceride levels to be <200 mg/dL after an overnight fast.

Where do all these types of cholesterol come from? Cholesterol is made in the livers of animals. For the most part, the cholesterol in your blood is the cholesterol that you manufactured yourself, not the cholesterol in what you may have eaten. Although there is some relationship between eating a high-cholesterol diet and having high serum cholesterol, the much stronger relationship is with saturated fat. Saturated fat is solid at room temperature, except for some tropical oils, and is found in animal and plant foods. Saturated fat biochemically signals the liver to increase its cholesterol production. In individuals with a strong genetic predisposition to heart disease, this effect may be particu-

larly potent. Therefore, for all individuals, it is recommended that saturated fat be kept to less than 10% of total caloric intake.

Some of the saturated fats are made from plant sources, such as stick margarine or solid shortening. These fats, used in food preparation or at the table, are made by blowing hydrogen gas through the liquid vegetable oil. During this process, a type of fat known as transfatty acid is created. Some research indicates that trans fatty acids may be even more heart disease-provoking than saturated fats of animal origin.

Since tracking saturated fat grams in addition to total fat grams can be too confusing for many individuals, you can safely recommend the tips listed in Table 3.11 for lowering both total and saturated fat intake.

The unsaturated fats consist of polyunsaturated and monounsaturated fats. Polyunsaturated fats can help lower LDL cholesterol, but the monounsaturated fats have little to no independent effect. Why then are monounsaturated fats touted as being so healthful? Because while the polyunsaturated fats can help lower cholesterol, they lower *all* cholesterol: HDL and LDL. Remember, you want HDL to be as high as possible. In

---

Table 3.11
Tips for Lowering Both Total and Saturated Fat Intake

- Read food labels to track total fat gram intake, keeping intake within reasonable limits.

- Choose lowfat (1% or less) dairy products.

- If you choose margarine, choose one with "liquid vegetable oil" as the first ingredient; try jam or jelly on breads instead of butter or margarine.

- In cooking, use moderate amounts of canola or olive oils. You can usually cut about 1/2 the fat out of recipes without changing their quality.

- Use cooking methods that do not use fat (bake, broil, steam, roast, poach) or that use very little (stir fry).

- Eat meats in moderation, choosing the leanest selections; trim all visible fat and remove any skin.

- Keep protein portions to about 6 oz/day (the size of two decks of cards).

- Choose red meats once or twice a week at most; choose seafoods or poultry for the majority of your meals with meat.

- Limit egg yolks to fewer than three per week.

- Consume several meatless meals per week for lunches and dinners.

- Avoid organ meats and processed meat products, such as bacon, sausage, hot dogs etc., or choose the non-fat, very low fat, or meatless alternatives

---

contrast, some research shows that mono-unsaturated fats help *raise* HDL cholesterol, thus improving lipid profiles and lowering CVD risk. Overall, total fat should be kept to <30% of total caloric intake, with <10% coming from saturated fats, and up to 10% coming from each of the unsaturated fats.

There is one more type of fat worth mentioning: **omega-3 fatty acids.** These are the fats found in cold water fish, including salmon, mackerel, menhaden, sardines, herring, and tuna. Research has shown that diets rich in these marine oils can lower blood cholesterol. Further, these oils can help prevent blood clots (the instigators of heart attacks and strokes) and may also lower high blood pressure. Some research has shown that consumption of cold water fish just once a week cut rates of heart disease by 50%. Supplements have not been shown to have these protective benefits and can have some side effects. Therefore it is not advisable to take these oils as a supplement. It *is* advisable to consume deep-sea cold water fish regularly.

Antioxidants protect membranes, lipid-rich organelles, and **lipoproteins**, like HDL, from being attacked by destructive agents known as free radicals. Vitamins E, C, and A, selenium, and omega-3 fatty acids all function as antioxidants in the body. They are interdependent and perform complementary functions, which in part explains why supplements seem to be less effective in preventing heart disease than eating foods rich in these nutrients.

Elevated **homocysteine** is now being recognized as a risk factor for heart disease, much in the same way as cholesterol. Although high homocysteine levels are in part due to genetics, diets poor in folate and vitamins B6 and B12 can also play a role. Use the information in Tables 3.5 and 3.6 to help guide your clients to healthy food selections.

Obesity

Diets high in fat can also lead to **obesity**, which is a complex and poorly understood disease that has several contributing factors. Certainly diet is one, but so are physical inactivity and genetic predisposition, among a host of others. One pound (.45 kg) of excess body fat stores about 3500 kcal of energy. In order to lose this fat, the stored energy must be burned. This is called creating an "**energy deficit**." To lose 2 pounds (.9 kg) a week, one must burn 1000 calories a day more than one takes in. To lose 1 pound (.45 kg) a week, a 500-kcal deficit must be created each day (500 kcal/day x 7 days = 3500 kcal).

The rate of weight loss should average no greater than 2 lb/week (.9 kg/week) after the first week (a greater amount of fluid is lost initially accounting for larger weight losses typically seen in the first week of a weight loss attempt). Losing weight faster than this rate can be harmful to some individuals and it has not been shown to be associated with successful long-term weight loss.

Small changes in lifestyle that are sustainable are more likely to result in the permanent changes your clients are seeking. Therefore, discourage your clients from engaging in starvation or low-calorie diets when they attempt to lose weight. Instead, encourage a 500-kcal deficit from the energy intake needed to maintain body weight — half this deficit created by decreasing food intake and half created by increasing physical activity. For most people, cutting out 250 – 300 kcal of food is easy; almost everyone has some higher-fat, less-nutritious food choices they could substitute with fruits, vegetables, and whole grains. Similarly, for most people needing to lose weight, there are opportunities for increasing energy output, even without planned exercise. Planned or structured exercise sessions can make obese individuals uncomfortable or nervous due to physical discomfort on exertion, shortness of breath, joint pain, or other somatic complaints. Physical activity can be increased by simple walking, parking the car farther away, taking the stairs instead of the elevator, and limiting television watching. All obese individuals should be cleared by their physician before starting an exercise program.

In general, most obese or overweight individuals do not need severe caloric restriction. Many will be able to improve their health dramatically by following the principles of a healthy lifestyle, which apply to everyone. Overweight or obese individuals are no different from healthy individuals, in that they should consume only 25% – 30% of their total calories as fat, choose a wide variety of fruits, vegetables, and whole grains, consume protein foods in moderation (~ 6 oz/day [170 g/day]), and include low-fat dairy products. Weight loss is not easy, however, as the body seems to store energy more easily than it mobilizes it from storage. But with patience, persistence, and an eye toward overall health improvements (not just weight on a scale), the overweight or obese individual has great power to improve his or her health.

Hypertension

One disease common in obese people and older adults is **hypertension,** or high blood pressure. Hypertension can damage the eyes, kidneys, liver, and the nervous system, and increases the risk for heart attacks and strokes. It is particularly common in people of African-American descent and is more prevalent in African-American women than

men. Although genetic predisposition plays a big role in whether or not someone has hypertension, so do many lifestyle factors: obesity, high-salt diets, alcohol consumption, and smoking. It is estimated that with weight loss, 80% of people with hypertension will have lower blood pressures. A recent study called the Dietary Approaches to Stop Hypertension trial (DASH) also showed that diet can lower blood pressure even without weight loss. Diets low in total and saturated fat and rich in fruits, vegetables, and low-fat dairy products had as strong an effect on blood pressure as some drugs (Apfel, 1998). Diets like these are rich in calcium, potassium, and magnesium, and when cold water fish is chosen as a protein source, they are rich in omega-3 fatty acids as well.

A high intake of sodium in the diet can aggravate blood pressure in about 40% of hypertensive individuals. Sodium is most commonly found in table salt and in many processed foods, canned soups, and cured meats and cheeses. Although not all individuals are sodium sensitive, you should recommend that your clients avoid adding salt at the table or during cooking, and to limit the number of highly processed foods they choose. Some hypertensive individuals are sensitive to alcohol as well. They can greatly reduce their blood pressure by limiting or eliminating alcohol. Caffeine has been found in some studies to raise blood pressure mildly throughout the day.

By far the most effective way to lower blood pressure in overweight or obese individuals is through weight loss. For many individuals, achieving and maintaining a healthy body weight can mean being able to discontinue medications. Hypertension should never be ignored; it should be managed by the client working with their physician, using strategies like healthy nutrition, exercise, smoking cessation, and medications as needed.

Diabetes Mellitus

As body weight increases, **diabetes mellitus** may also develop, particularly in those individuals with abdominal or upper-body obesity. Earlier we discussed how all carbohydrates eaten are transformed into blood sugar, called glucose. In diabetes, the body cannot control the blood glucose level, which can have serious short- and long-term consequences, including impaired vision, numbness in the extremities, non-healing ulcers and wounds, heart disease, and death. Diabetes is a very serious condition if left untreated and half of all individuals with diabetes do not know they even have the disease since they have never been tested. Most of these individuals suffer from the obesity-related condition called Type 2 diabetes. (Type 1 diabetes usually strikes children and is not related to being overweight.) Helping your clients to achieve and maintain a healthy body weight can help prevent them from developing Type 2 diabetes. A commitment to exercise and a healthy eating plan is vital to managing diabetes once an individual has been diagnosed. The dietary guidelines are appropriate for individuals with diabetes. However these people should be monitored by their physician and a registered dietitian (R.D.) or certified diabetes educator (C.D.E.).

Cancer

Diet is one of the many factors that influence the development of **cancer**. Cigarette smoking is one of the strongest cancer promoters for lung and oral cancers. Diet is more closely related to cancers of the esophagus, stomach, colon, rectum, breast, lung, liver, pancreas, endometrium, ovaries, bladder, and prostate. Although not all of these associations are clearly understood and some of the data are still debated, experts do agree that the way you eat affects your risk of developing cancer. In countries where the typical diet is similar to our Dietary Guidelines, the incidence of cancer is about half that in the United States (Woteki & Thomas, 1992). The components of food that are particularly important are fats, folic acid, vitamins A, C, and E, selenium, zinc, fiber, and the phytochemicals discussed previously. Fruits, vegetables, and whole grains are low in fats and rich in these food components.

Some foods can raise your risk of developing cancer. For example, salt-cured, smoked, and nitrate- or nitrite-containing foods should be avoided or consumed only in limited amounts. Foods preserved with **nitrates** and **nitrites,** like lunch meats, hams, and hot dogs, can increase the risk for stomach cancers since they can be converted to **nitrosamines,** which are carcinogenic. Charbroiling or grilling foods generates a broad spectrum of compounds that increase cancer risk, such as **polycyclic aromatic hydrocarbons** and **heterocyclic amines**. Enzymes in the liver (called Phase I enzymes) activate these compounds, which form **DNA adducts** (attach themselves to DNA) and may cause mutations. Although char-broiling adds attractive flavors, it is recommended these foods be consumed in moderation. Some of the phytochemicals in fruits and vegetables enhance the liver's Phase II enzymes, which helps the body deactivate polycyclic aromatic hydrocarbons and heterocyclic amines. Alcohol intake has also been associated with increased risks for cancers of the mouth, esophagus, stomach, liver, and breast.

Some food components are often blamed for increasing cancer risk, but the data do not support those assertions. Artificial sweeteners are safe when consumed in moderate amounts. Food additives other than nitrates and nitrites are generally regarded as safe since no studies have shown any added risk of cancer. Irradiation of foods kills harmful organisms and increases the shelf life of foods. It does not increase cancer risk. While pesticides and herbicides are toxic in high doses, there is no current evidence linking them with an increase in cancer rates. However, it is good advice to thoroughly wash all produce before consuming it to remove dirt and any pesticide residue. While organic foods may be a personal preference, they are not thought to reduce one's risk for cancer to any greater extent than consuming non-organic fruits and vegetables.

Physical activity may play a role in cancer development as well. Statistically, sedentary women are three times as likely to develop breast cancers as active women (McArdle, 1987). The risk of developing colon cancers in men may also decrease as physical activity increases. More scientific work needs to be done before a direct link between physical activity and cancer prevention can be made; it may be that people who exercise regularly are more likely to have better overall health habits, thus lowering their risk. Regardless, regular exercise is fundamental to achieving optimal health.

Osteoporosis

Osteoporosis is yet another important chronic disease related to nutrition and exercise. It affects more than 25 million people in the United States alone, most of these women. In osteoporosis, the bones become soft and later brittle, making them very prone to breaking at the spine, wrist, and hip area, sometimes even spontaneously (without a causative event or accident). Once osteoporosis has set in, it is almost too late to make significant improvements in bone mass, although research is advancing in this area. Peak bone mass is achieved by about age 25. It is important to optimize the amounts of hard mineral deposited into bone by providing sufficient calcium and vitamin D intake during the growing years. After age 30, calcium intake and exercise are still important to maintain bone mass density. Adult women need 1000 – 1300 mg of calcium per day, depending on their age and condition (i.e., post-menopausal, pregnancy, lactating mothers). One cup of milk, yogurt, or calcium-fortified orange juice provides about 300 mg of calcium. An ounce of cheese can contain from 70 (parmesan) to 270 (swiss) mg of calcium. Some green leafy vegetables, like collards (179 mg per 1/2 cup) or turnip greens (138 mg per 1/2 cup), are also good sources of calcium. Without sufficient dietary calcium, the bones cannot grow strong and maintain their integrity.

There are some other nutritional factors that play a role in bone development. Vitamin D is integral to the process of forming hard bones. Vitamin D is found in fortified milk and your body can synthesize it during sun exposure. About 30 minutes of sun on the face and hands can meet the daily needs for vitamin D. Weight-bearing exercise (walking, aerobic dance, weight lifting, tennis, stair climbing) also promotes good bone density, but nonweightbearing exercises (swimming, cycling) do not. A high-protein or a high-sodium diet can increase calcium loss in the urine, which lowers the amount of calcium available to your bones. Excessive alcohol intake impairs calcium absorption as well.

Teas, cocoa, spinach, asparagus, beet greens, and swiss chard are all high in chemicals called **oxylates.** Legumes and cereals high in bran are rich in **phytates**. Oxylates and phytates bind with calcium in your intestines, thus interfering with absorption. These foods should not be eliminated from the diet, since they contain many other beneficial components, but it is a good strategy not to rely on the calcium contained in them as it might not be absorbed. It is not thought that the oxylates and phytates interfere with other sources of calcium eaten at the same time. Smoking also contributes to bone loss. See Table 3.12 for a listing of tips to increase calcium intake.

Anemia

Iron-deficiency anemia is the most common nutritional deficiency in the United States, affecting about 40% of women between the ages of 20 and 50 (Aftergood & Alfin-Slater, 1982). Iron is a part of hemoglobin synthesis; hemoglobin carries the oxygen to your cells, allowing them to function. A lack of hemoglobin or poorly formed red blood cells is called **anemia**. Anemia is diagnosed when laboratory red blood cell counts fall below 12 mg/dL for women and below 14 mg/dL for men. Individuals with anemia often feel tired and listless, their endurance capacity is diminished, and their immune system is weakened, making them less resistant to colds or infections.

Most cases of anemia are due to poor iron intake, although poor intake of either folate or vitamin B12 can also result in this condition. Another cause is blood loss, either naturally (e.g., menstrual losses) or through injury or infection (e.g., gastrointestinal bleeding). The RDA for iron is 10 mg/day for adult males and postmenopausal women and 15 mg/day for premenopausal women. The average woman, in consuming only 10 mg/day does not meet this guideline. Table 3.13 presents tips for increasing iron intake and absorption. Because of the difficulty of obtaining sufficient dietary iron, individuals

---

Table 3.12
Tips for Increasing Calcium Intake

- Add nonfat milk powder to milk, soups, shakes or smoothies, meat loaf, baked goods, and mashed potatoes.
- Use milk or evaporated skim milk in cream soups, sauces, cocoa, and casseroles instead of cream.
- Top angel food cake, fruit, or gelatin with nonfat yogurt.
- Choose calcium-rich desserts such as frozen yogurt, puddings and custards.
- Freeze milk in ice cube trays to use in shakes or smoothies.
- Substitute nonfat plain yogurt for sour cream or mayonnaise in dips, salad dressings, or as a baked potato topping.
- Sprinkle lowfat cheese on vegetables, salads, soups, or popcorn or choose lowfat cheeses instead of meats.
- Use calcium-fortified products (orange juice, breakfast bars, etc.).
- Use tofu in meals (a 4 oz [113 gram] serving has 150 mg of calcium).

Table 3.13
Tips for Increasing Iron Intake and Absorption

- Because acids enhance iron absorption, you should eat foods rich in vitamin C (particularly citrus foods) with each meal. Orange juice with breakfast can increase iron absorption by nearly 300%.
- Avoid coffee and tea with meals; they contain tannins, which inhibit iron absorption.
- Use cast iron cookware, as elemental iron will transfer to the foods, particularly when those foods are acidic.For example, the iron content of 1/2 cup of spaghetti sauce increases from 3 mg to 88 mg when simmered in a cast iron pot for 3 hours.
- Red meats and the dark meats of poultry are excellent sources of iron.
- Choose iron-rich fruits and vegetables, such as raisins, dried apricots, prunes, strawberries, dark green leafy vegetables, and legumes.
- Combine vegetable sources of iron with animal sources of iron (meat and vegetable or bean burritos, meat and bean soups and stews, etc.).

might be tempted to take an iron supplement. If one chooses to do so, it is best to take small amounts, such as that contained in a general-purpose daily multivitamin/mineral supplement.

Iron supplementation will not improve endurance or performance in an individual with normal iron stores. Clients should be warned that feelings of fatigue can have many causes and may be completely unrelated to iron status. Iron overload is also a possibility and a serious medical concern.

Long-term high iron intake may even be related to heart disease (Monsen, 1992). Excessive iron supplementation can also result in deficiencies of copper and zinc. Individuals concerned about anemia should be tested by their physician and referred to a registered dietitian for assessment and dietary counseling.

There are different nutritional concerns at each stage of the lifecycle. See Table 3.14 for a listing of what you should be aware of for your clients at these different stages.

Table 3.14
Nutritional Concerns of Different Age Groups

Age Group	Nutrition-Related Risk	Related Nutritional Component
Children	Anemia	Inadequate iron, folate, vitamin B12
	Obesity	Excess caloric consumption, fat intake
	Eating disorders	Inadequate total intake
Young adults	Anemia	Inadequate iron, folate, vitamin B12 intake
	Obesity	Excess caloric consumption, fat intake
	Neural tube defects in offspring during pregnancy	Folate and vitamin B12 deficiency during the first 28 days of pregnancy
Middle-aged adults	Obesity	Excess caloric consumption, fat intake
	Hypertension	Excess body fat; inadequate calcium, magnesium, or potassium
	Diabetes	Excess body fat; possible other components
	Cancer	Excess body fat and dietary fat; poor intake of vitamins and minerals (for antioxidant nutrients), fiber, and phytochemicals
Older adults	Cardiovascular disease	Excess body fat and dietary fat, poor intake of vitamins and minerals (for antioxidant nutrients), fiber, and phytochemical
	Hypertension	Excess body fat; inadequate calcium, magnesium, or potassium
	Diabetes	Excess body fat; possible other components (eg., diet, inactivity)
	Cancer	Excess body fat and dietary fat; poor intake of vitamins and minerals (for antioxidant nutrients), fiber, and phytochemicals
	Osteoporosis	Inadequate calcium and vitamin D intake

Special Topics of Concern

Caffeine

Caffeine is a naturally occurring substance found in about 63 different species of plants, most notably coffee beans, cocoa beans, cola nuts, and tea leaves. Unless a food is processed for its removal, caffeine is present in any products made from those foods, such as coffee, tea, chocolate, and some soft drinks. Caffeine simulates the central nervous system, making some people feel more awake and giving others the "jitters." Although it is relatively harmless, caffeine's side effects can include headache, nausea, muscle tremors, anxiety, nervousness, irritability, and insomnia. Though caffeine was once thought to be an "energy-enhancing" or **ergogenic aid**, research has not continued to support that idea. Caffeine is one of the substances banned by the United States Olympic Committee. This chemical acts in the body as a diuretic and will contribute to fluid loss unless habitually used. Since the body quickly develops a tolerance for caffeine the diuretic effect is not notable in regular caffeine users. It can also contribute to elevated blood pressure.

Nutrition for Athletic Performance

Many active individuals want to eat to fuel their bodies, using nutrition to enhance athletic performance. Adequate nutritional status is an important part of a training program, just as it is an important part of general health. However, there is no secret to healthy nutrition for the athlete. Supplements, special diets, and food fads have not been shown to significantly impact endurance or strength. The guidelines for healthy eating can benefit all physically active individuals, from the merely active to the elite athlete. In fact, people who exercise regularly will need more food to meet their energy needs. They are more likely to actually consume *more* nutrients as they consume a greater amount and a wider variety of foods. The current recommendation on nutrition for fitness is to consume a diet rich in carbohydrates, particularly complex carbohydrates, and moderate in protein and fat. Following the dietary guidelines and pattern outlined in Tables 3.4 and 3.9 will more than adequately meet the needs for protein and should meet the needs for the vitamins and minerals and other nutrients as long as the individual makes reasonable food choices (i.e., the french fry/broccoli example given earlier).

Consuming a high carbohydrate diet also promotes glycogen storage. As discussed previously, glycogen is the storage form of carbohydrate in the muscles and used for energy during physical activity. Adequate glycogen stores promote better endurance.

Even for individuals who are working to add lean body mass and build their muscles, excess protein is not necessary. A healthy diet can provide more than the needed amino acids, which are the building blocks of body protein. Protein powders and supplements are not cost-effective and excess protein intake is converted either to glucose for the brain, burned for energy, or stored as body fat.

Eating Disorders

The alarming increase in the incidence of **eating disorders** is of great concern to every health and fitness professional today. An eating disorder is a disturbance in eating behavior that jeopardizes a person's physical or psychological health. They affect both men and women, although they are more common in women. These problems stem in part from unrealistic standards for body weight and body proportions. Dancers, wrestlers, gymnasts, and other athletes who strive for low body fat are the most vulnerable, although these disorders have also been noted in swimmers and cyclists. **Anorexia nervosa**, **bulimia nervosa**, and **binge eating disorder** are the three types of eating disorders currently recognized by the medical community.

Anorexia nervosa is usually characterized by an extremely low body weight and a denial of both hunger and thinness. To individuals suffering from this disorder, eating normally feels "out of control" and a normal body shape and size often "feels fat." Anorexics are obsessed with resisting food and often engage in vigorous exercise as a way to control both their eating and their body weight. Anorexia nervosa can be fatal. Eating disorders have the highest mortality rate of all the psychiatric illnesses.

Bulimia nervosa is characterized by a cycle of binging and purging. Typically, huge amounts of food is consumed prior to purging, which could include vomiting, fasting, and diuretic or laxative use. Like the anorexic, the bulimic is trapped by an obsession with thinness and a preoccupation with food.

Binge eating disorder (sometimes called compulsive overeating) is the least understood of the eating disorders. In this disorder, individuals usually consume large amounts of food without purging, yet they feel the same degree of guilt and emotional trauma as individuals with anorexia or bulimia. Although these individuals are quite often overweight or obese, not all overweight/obese individuals have a compulsive eating disorder.

On the surface, it may not be easy to tell the difference between a participant's healthy concern for body composition and athletic performance and an obsessive, destructive concern for being thin. An instructor cannot treat a person with an eating disorder; he or she should be seen by a medical team specializing in this field. By providing sound nutritional guidance, supporting realistic weight goals, and acknowledging that bodies come in many shapes and sizes, you might be able to help prevent someone from developing an eating disorder.

Summary

People who are interested in fitness are often interested in their nutritional health as well. This interest makes them susceptible to many of the diet, supplement, and food fads constantly promoted in today's media and marketplace. As an ACE-certified group fitness instructor, you can provide accurate information about the basics of nutrition, which can save your clients time and money as well as improve their health.

Decades of research have found that there is no "quick fix" to improved health or athletic performance. If you could "fix" your health, weight, or athletic performance overnight, you could just as easily put it in jeopardy. The human body is far more resilient than that. In a healthy diet, there is room for all foods in moderation, just as there is room for some sedentary activities, like watching a movie, in an active lifestyle.

Unfortunately, many people do not practice moderation when it comes to nutrition or exercise. Instead, they live an unbalanced lifestyle consuming nutrient-poor, high-calorie foods and engaging in little physical activity. While dietary fat intake is above recommended guidelines, fruit, vegetable, and whole grain consumption are far too low in the population in general, resulting in low dietary fiber intakes. All of these nutritional issues can create significant health problems over just a few decades of life. Balance is the key to avoiding chronic health conditions such as obesity, heart disease, and diabetes on the excess side, and eating disorders such as anorexia nervosa on the other.

Help your patients set realistic and achievable goals by making lifestyle changes they can truly live with. As an ACE-certified group fitness instructor, you can use your knowledge of nutrition to help your clients achieve balance in their lives, help prevent or manage chronic disease, and improve their quality of life.

References

Appel, L.J., Moore, T.J., Obarzanek, E., Vollmer, W.M., Svetkey, L.P., Sacks, F.M., Bray, G.A., Vogt, T.M., Cutler, J.A., Windhauser, M.M., Lin, P.H., & Karanja, N., for the DASH Collaborative Research Group. (1997). A clinical trial of the effects of dietary patterns on blood pressure. *New England Journal of Medicine*, 336, 1117 – 1124.

Aftergood, L. & Alfin-Slater, P. (1980). Women and Nutrition. *Contemporary Nutrition* (General Mills, Inc.).

Albertson, A.M., Tobelmann, R.C. & Marquart, L. (1997). Estimated dietary calcium intake and food sources for adolescent females: 1980-92. *Journal of Adolescent Health*, 20, 20 – 26.

American Diabetes Association. (1981). *The Exchange Lists for Meal Planning.*

American Heart Association. (1982). Report of AHA Nutrition Committee: Rationale of the diet-heart statement of the American Heart Association. *Arteriosclerosis*, 2, 177 – 191.

Drezner, M.K. & Hoben, K.P. (1996). *Eating Well, Living Well with Osteoporosis.* New York: Viking Press.

Foster-Powell, K. & Miller, J.B. (1995). International tables of glycemic index. *American Journal of Clinical Nutrition*, 62, 871S – 893S.

Guthrie, H.A., Picciano, M.F., & Scott, A. (1995). *Human Nutrition,* 1st ed. Boston: McGraw-Hill.

Hands, E.S. (1995). *Food Finder, Food Sources of Vitamins and Minerals.* 4th ed. Salem, Oregon: ESHA Research.

McArdle, W. (1987). *Building Endurance.* New York: Time Life Books.

McGinnes, J.M. & Foege, W.H. (1993). Actual causes of death in the United States. *Journal of the American Medical Association*, 270, 2207 – 2212.

Monsen, E. (1992). Iron and serum lipids in the pathogenesis of heart disease. *Journal of the American Dietetic Association*, 92,12, 1502.

National Research Council (U.S.) Subcommittee on the Tenth Edition of the RDAs. (1989). *Recommended Dietary Allowances,* 10th ed. National Academy of Sciences. Washington, DC.

Schleicher, E. & Nerlich, A. (1996). The role of hyperglycemia in the development of diabetic complications. *Hormone and Metabolic Research*, 28, 367 – 373.

Wardlaw, G.M. (1999). *Perspectives in Nutrition.* 4th ed. Boston: McGraw-Hill.

Whitney, E.N. & Rolfes, S.R. (1996). *Understanding Nutrition.* 7th ed. St. Paul, Minn.: West Publishing Company.

Woteki, C. & Thomas, P. (1992). *Eat for Life.* Washington, D.C.: National Academy Press.

U.S. Department of Agriculture. (1980). *Dietary Guidelines for Americans.* Washington, D.C.

Suggested Reading

Dalton, S. (1997). *Overweight and Weight Management: the health professionals guide to understanding and practice.* Gaithersburg, Md.: Aspen Publishers.

Sifton, D.W., ed. (1995). *PDR Family Guide to Nutrition and Health.* Montvale, N.J.: Medical Economics.

Credible Sources for Nutrition Information

National Center for Nutrition and Dietetics (NCND) - the education center of The American Dietetic Association — www.eatright.org

Federal Trade Commission — www.ftc.gov

US Department of Health and Human Services — www.dhhs.gov

Food and Drug Administration — www.fda.gov

US Department of Agriculture — www.usda.gov

National Institutes of Health — www.nih.gov

National Cancer Institute — www.nci.nih.gov

National Heart, Lung and Blood Institute — www.nhlbi.nih.gov/nhilbi/nhlbi.htm

Scientific and Professional Organizations Offering Credible Nutrition Information

The American Dietetic Association — www.eatright.com

American Academy of Pediatrics — www.aap.org

American Society for Clinical Nutrition — www.faseb.org/ascn

American Medical Association — www.ama-assn.org

American Cancer Society — www.ca.cancer.org

American Diabetes Association — www.diabetes.org

American Heart Association — www.americanheart.org

Reputable Consumer Organizations

Better Business Bureau — www.bbb.org

Consumer Union — www.consumerreports.org

National Council Against Health Fraud — www.ncahf.org

Industry Groups that Provide Reputable Nutrition Information to the Public

National Live Stock and Meat Board — www.foodsafety.org

Food Marketing Institute — www.fmi.org

National Dairy Council — www.nationaldairycouncil.org

Chapter 4

David C. Nieman, Dr. P. H., F.A.C.S.M., is a professor of Health and Exercise Science and director of the Human Performance Laboratory at Appalachian State University in Boone, North Carolina. He is the author of eight books and more than 130 articles in research journals and books.

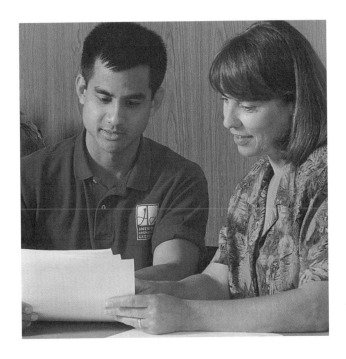

Health
Screening

By David C. Nieman

The modern-day fitness movement is more than 30 years old. It started in 1968, when Kenneth Cooper, at that time a physician for the Air Force, published his book Aerobics (Cooper, 1968). In this book, Cooper challenged Americans to take personal charge of their lifestyles and counter the epidemics of heart disease, obesity, and rising healthcare costs through regular exercise. Millions took up the "aerobic challenge" and began running, cycling, walking, and swimming their way to better health.

Much has been learned about exercise and health during these 30-plus years. In general, exercise has been found to be both safe and beneficial for most people (Nieman, 1999). However, there are some individuals that can suffer ill health from exercise. There is probably not a single fitness enthusiast in America who has not read the reports of famous athletes dying on basketball courts, runners found dead with their running shoes on, executives discovered slumped over their treadmills, or middle-aged men suffering heart attacks while shoveling snow.

Whether exercise is beneficial or hazardous to the heart depends on who the person is. For most people, regular exercise reduces the risk of heart disease by about one-half compared to those who are physically inactive (USDHHS, 1996). However, for those who are at high risk for heart disease to begin with, vigorous exercise bouts can trigger fatal heart attacks. About 75,000 Americans suffer heart attacks during or after exercise each year (ACSM, 1995). Studies show that these victims tended to be men who were sedentary, over age 35, already had heart disease or were at high risk for it, and then exercised too hard for their fitness levels. And for patients with heart disease, the incidence of a heart attack or death during exercise is 10 times that of otherwise healthy individuals (ACSM/AHA, 1998).

Also of concern is **congenital** cardiovascular disease, now the major cause of athletic death in high school and college. In one study of 158 athletes who died young (average age 17) and in their prime, 134 of them had heart or blood vessel defects that were present at birth (Maron et al., 1996). Most common was **hypertrophic cardiomyopathy**, a thickening of the heart's main pumping muscle. In other words, when a young athlete dies during or shortly after exercise, it is most often due to a birth defect of the cardiovascular system (AHA, 1996; Cantwell, 1998).

Health screening is a vital process in first identifying individuals at high risk for exercise-induced heart problems, and then referring them to appropriate medical care (ACSM/AHA, 1998). According to the American College of Sports Medicine, "the incidence of cardiovascular problems during physical activity is reduced by nearly 50 percent when individuals are first screened and those identified with **risk factors** or disease are diverted to other professionally established activity programs" (ACSM, 1995). Despite the proven benefits of screening, efforts to screen new members at enrollment into health/fitness facilities are limited and inconsistent (ACSM/AHA, 1998).

Several agencies and organizations recommend that every person participate in at least moderate-intensity physical activity for 30 minutes or more on most days of the week (USDHHS, 1996). Efforts to promote physical activity will result in increasing numbers of individuals with and without risk of heart disease joining health/fitness facilities and community exercise programs. Surveys reveal that 50% of health/ fitness facility members are older than 35 years, and the fastest growing segments are middle-aged and elderly participants (ACSM/ AHA, 1998). According to the American Heart Association, more than one-fourth of all Americans have some form of **cardiovascular disease** (including high blood pressure), and prevalence rises with age (AHA, 1998). To ensure safe exercise participation, it is essential that people with underlying cardiovascular disease be identified before they initiate exercise programs (Fletcher et al., 1995; Gibbons et al., 1997).

This chapter focuses on procedures group fitness instructors can implement to help protect participants when initiating exercise or athletic programs and emphasizes several key issues:

1. Always obtain a medical history or pre-exercise health-risk appraisal on each participant.
2. Stratify individuals according to their disease risk.

3. Refer high-risk individuals to a health-care provider for medical evaluation and a **graded exercise test**.

The Pre-exercise Health Appraisal Questionnaire

All facilities offering exercise equipment or services should conduct a cardiovascular screening of all new members and/or prospective users, regardless of age (ACSM/AHA, 1998; Tharrett & Peterson, 1997). The screening procedure should be simple, easy to perform, and not so intensive that it discourages participation. The screening questionnaires should be interpreted and documented by qualified staff to limit the number of unnecessary medical referrals and avoid barriers to participation.

The health appraisal questionnaire is useful in classifying a potential exercise participant according to disease risk, and in facilitating the exercise prescription process. In general, the background information obtained from the questionnaire improves the instructor's ability to meet individual needs.

There are many questionnaires available for pre-exercise screening. A comprehensive questionnaire should include the following (ACSM, 1995):

- Medical diagnoses
- Previous physical examination findings
- History of symptoms
- Recent illness, hospitalization, or surgical procedures
- Orthopedic problems
- Medication use and drug allergies
- Lifestyle habits
- Exercise history
- Work history
- Family history of disease

When testing large numbers of individuals in a short period of time, or in most health/fitness facility settings, a short, simple medical/health questionnaire is used. A brief, self-administered medical questionnaire called the **Physical Activity Readiness Questionnaire (PAR-Q)** has been used very successfully (Figure 4.1) (Shephard et al., 1991). The PAR-Q was designed in the 1970s by Canadian researchers, and used in conjunction with the Canadian fitness testing program. After years of successful use and a revision in 1994, the PAR-Q is now recognized by experts as a safe pre-exercise screening measure for low-to-moderate (but not vigorous) exercise training (Canadian Society for Exercise Physiology, 1996). Participants are directed to contact their personal physician if they answer "yes" to one or more questions.

In 1998, the American College of Sports Medicine and the American Heart Association published a slightly more complex questionnaire than the PAR-Q (Figure 4.2) (ACSM/AHA, 1998). The ACSM/AHA questionnaire uses history, symptoms, and risk factors to direct individuals to either initiate an exercise program or contact their physician. Persons at higher risk are directed to seek facilities providing appropriate levels of staff supervision. The questionnaire takes only a few minutes to complete, identifies high-risk participants, documents the results of screening, educates the consumer, and encourages and fosters appropriate use of the healthcare system.

Disease Risk Stratification

The American College of Sports Medicine and the American Heart Association have jointly published guidelines for classifying individuals according to

Figure 4.1

The Physical Activity Readiness Questionnaire -
PAR-Q (revised 1994)

PAR Q & YOU (A Questionnaire for People Age 15 to 69)

Regular physical activity is fun and healthy, and increasingly more people are starting to become more active every day. Being more active is very safe for most people. However, some people should check with their doctor before they start becoming much more physically active.

If you are planning to become much more physically active than you are now, start by answering the seven questions in the box below. If you are between the ages of 15 and 69, the PAR-Q will tell you if you should check with your doctor before you start. If you are over 69 years of age, and you are not used to being very active, check with your doctor.

Common sense is your best guide when you answer these questions. Please read the questions carefully and answer each one honestly: check YES or NO.

YES	NO	
☐	☐	1. Has your doctor ever said that you have a heart condition and that you should only do physical activity recommended by a doctor?
☐	☐	2. Do you feel pain in your chest when you do physical activity?
☐	☐	3. In the past month, have you had chest pain when you were not doing physical activity?
☐	☐	4. Do you lose your balance because of dizziness or do you ever lose consciousness?
☐	☐	5. Do you have a bone or joint problem that could be made worse by a change in your physical activity?
☐	☐	6. Is your doctor currently prescribing drugs (for example, water pills) for your blood pressure or heart condition?
☐	☐	7. Do you know of any other reason why you should not do physical activity?

If you answered Yes to one or more questions:

✔ Talk with your doctor by phone or in person BEFORE you start becoming much more physically active or BEFORE you have a fitness appraisal. Tell your doctor about the PAR-Q and which questions you answered YES.

✔ You may be able to do any activity you want — as long as you start slowly and build up gradually. Or, you may need to restrict your activities to those that are safe for you. Talk with your doctor about the kinds of activities you wish to participate in and follow his/her advice.

✔ Find out which community programs are safe and helpful for you.

If you answered NO honestly to all PAR-Q questions, you can be reasonably sure that you can:

✔ Start becoming much more physically active — begin slowly and build up gradually. This is the safest and easiest way to go.

✔ Take part in a fitness appraisal — this is an excellent way to determine your basic fitness so that you can plan the best way for you to live actively.

continued on next page

DELAY BECOMING MUCH MORE ACTIVE:

✔ If you are not feeling well because of a temporary illness such as a cold or a fever — wait until you feel better; or

✔ If you are or may be pregnant — talk to your doctor before you start becoming more active.

Please note: If your health changes so that you then answer YES to any of the above questions, tell your fitness or health professional. Ask whether you should change your physical activity plan.

Informed Use of the PAR-Q: The Canadian Society for Exercise Physiology, Health Canada, and their agents assume no liability for persons who undertake physical activity and, if in doubt after completing this questionnaire, consult your doctor prior to physical activity.

You are encouraged to copy the PAR-Q, but only if you use the entire form.

Note: If the PAR-Q is being given to a person before he or she participates in a physical activity program or a fitness appraisal, this section may be used for legal or administrative purposes.

I have read, understood and completed this questionnaire. Any questions I had were answered to my full satisfaction.

_____

Name

_____

Signature   Date

_____

Signature of Parent   Witness
or Guardian (for participants under the age of majority)

© Canadian Society for Exercise Physiology   Supported by: Health   Santé
Societe canadienne de physiologie de l'exercice   Canada   Canada

Figure 4.2
ACSM/AHA participation screening questionnaire
(ACSM/AHA, 1998)

Assess your health needs by marking all true statements

History

You have had:

☐ a heart attack
☐ heart surgery
☐ cardiac catheterization
☐ coronary angioplasty (PTCA)
☐ pacemaker/implantable cardiac
☐ defibrillator/rhythm disturbance
☐ heart valve disease
☐ heart failure
☐ heart transplantation
☐ congenital heart disease

Other health issues:

☐ You have musculoskeletal problems.
☐ You have concerns about the safety of exercise
☐ You take prescription medication(s).
☐ You are pregnant.

Symptoms

☐ You experience chest discomfort with exertion.
☐ You experience unreasonable breathlessness.
☐ You experience dizziness, fainting, blackouts.
☐ You take heart medications.

Recommendations

If you marked any of the statements in this section, consult your healthcare provider before engaging in exercise. You may need to use a facility with a medically qualified staff.

Cardiovascular risk factors

☐ You are a man older than 45 years.
☐ You are a woman older than 55 years or you have had a hysterectomy or you are postmenopausal.
☐ You smoke.
☐ Your blood pressure is greater than 140/90 mm Hg.
☐ You don't know your blood pressure.
☐ You take blood pressure medication.
☐ Your blood cholesterol level is >240 mg/dl.
☐ You don't know your cholesterol level.
☐ You have a blood relative who had a heart attack before age 55 (father/brother) or 65 (mother/sister).
☐ You are diabetic or take medicine to control your blood sugar.
☐ You are physically inactive (i.e., you get less than 30 minutes of physical activity on at least 3 d/wk).
☐ You are more than 20 pounds (9 kg) overweight.

If you marked two or more of the statements in this section, you should consult your healthcare provider before engaging in exercise. You might benefit by using a facility with a professionally qualified exercise staff to guide your exercise program.

☐ None of the above is true.

You should be able to exercise safely without consulting your healthcare provider in almost any facility that meets your exercise program needs.

disease risk (ACSM/AHA, 1998). Stratification according to disease risk is important for several reasons:

- To identify those in need of referral to a healthcare provider for more extensive medical evaluation.
- To ensure the safety of exercise testing and participation.
- To determine the appropriate type of exercise test or program.

ACSM/AHA recommends that participants be classified into one of three risk strata: **apparently healthy** (class A-1), persons at increased risk (classes A-2 and A-3), or persons with known cardiovascular disease (classes B, C, and D):

■ Class A — Apparently healthy

A-1 (younger): Children, adolescents, men ≤45 years, women ≤55 years, no symptoms of disease, apparently healthy with no known disease, no cardiovascular risk factors.

A-2 (older): Men >45 years, women >55 years, no symptoms of disease, apparently healthy with no known disease, no cardiovascular risk factors.

A-3 (risk factors): Men >45 years, women >55 years, no symptoms of disease, apparently healthy with no known disease, ≥2 cardiovascular risk factors.

■ Class B — Cardiovascular disease patient at low risk

Presence of known, stable cardiovascular disease with low risk for vigorous exercise, but slightly greater than for apparently healthy persons.

■ Class C — Cardiovascular disease patient at moderate- to high-risk

Those at moderate-to-high risk for cardiac complications during exercise and/or who are unable to self-regulate activity or understand the recommended activity level.

■ Class D — Cardiovascular disease patient at high risk

Patients with unstable cardiovascular conditions; in this population, no physical activity is recommended for conditioning purposes.

The Medical/Physical Examination

The depth of the medical or physical examination for any individual considering an exercise program depends on the disease **risk stratification**. When a medical evaluation or recommendation is advised or required, written and active communication by the exercise staff with the individual's personal physician is strongly recommended. The form in Figure 4.3 can be used for this referral (ACSM/AHA, 1998).

Apparently healthy individuals, young or old (classes A-1 and A-2), can begin moderate exercise programs such as brisk walking without the need for exercise testing or medical examination. Moderate intensity is defined as 45% – 59% $\dot{V}O_2$ max or heart rate reserve, or 11 – 12 on the rating of perceived exertion (RPE) scale (6 – 20 version) (ACSM/AHA, 1998). Even apparently healthy individuals who have two or more cardiovascular disease risk factors but no history of disease symptoms (class A-3) can safely

Figure 4.3a

Sample physician referral form

Dear Dr. _____

Your patient _____ would like to begin a program of exercise and/or sports

activity at _____.
                  [Name of health/fitness facility]

After reviewing his/her responses to our cardiovascular screening questionnaire, we would appreciate your medical opinion and recommendations concerning his/her participation in exercise/sports activity. Please provide the following information and return this form to:

_____
                [Name]

_____
                [Address]

_____
                [Telephone, fax]

1. Are there specific concerns or conditions our staff should be aware of before this individual engages in exercise/sports activity at our facility? Yes/No. If yes, please specify:

_____

_____

_____

2. If this Individual has completed an exercise test, please provide the following:

    a. Date of test: _____

    b. A copy of the final exercise test report and interpretation.

    c. Your specific recommendations for exercise training, including heart rate limits during exercise:

    _____

3. Please provide the following information so that we may contact you if we have any further questions:

_____   I AGREE to the participation of this individual in exercise/sports activity at your health/fitness facility.

_____   I DO NOT AGREE that this individual is a candidate to exercise at your health/fitness facility because

_____

Physician's signature _____

Physician's name _____

Address _____

Telephone/Fax _____

Thank you for your help.

Must be accompanied by a medical release form.

Figure 4.3b

Sample authorization for release of medical information

1. I hereby authorize_____to release the following information from the medical record of:

_____
(Patients name)

_____
(Address)

_____   _____
(Telephone)   (Date of birth)

2. Information to be released *(If specific treatment dates are not indicated, information from the most recent visit will be released)*:

_____ Exercise test

_____ Most recent history and physical exam

_____ Most recent clinic visit

_____ Consultations

_____ Laboratory results *(specify)* _____

_____ Other *(specify)*_____

3. Information to be released to:

Name of person/organization _____

Address _____

Telephone _____

4. Purpose of disclosure information _____

5. I do not give permission for disclosure or redisclosure of this information other than that specified above.

6. I request that this consent become invalid 90 days from the date I sign it or _____

I understand that this consent can be revoked at any time except to the extent that disclosure made in good faith has already occurred in reliance of this consent.

7. Patient's signature _____   Date _____

Witness _____
(Please print)

Signature _____

initiate moderate-exercise programs without medical examination. This is especially true when the moderate-exercise program proceeds gradually and the individual is alert to the development of disease signs and symptoms.

Apparently healthy younger persons (class A-1) may participate in vigorous exercise without first undergoing medical examination. Prior to starting a vigorous, high intensity exercise program (i.e., $\dot{V}O_2$ max $\geq 60\%$, or an RPE ≥ 13), older apparently healthy men (above age 45) or women (above age 55) (class A-2), and apparently healthy persons with cardiovascular disease risk factors (class A-3) should have a medical examination and a diagnostic graded exercise test under the supervision of a physician. The contrast between moderate and vigorous exercise is an important issue, and group fitness instructors should carefully monitor intensity through RPE or heart-rate methods (Figure 4.4).

All other persons (classes B and C) should undergo a medical examination and exercise testing before participating in any type of exercise program unless exercise should be avoided altogether (class D). For any individual (young or old, apparently healthy or at increased risk), the information garnered from a maximal, graded exercise test is useful in establishing an effective and safe exercise prescription.

In general, most individuals, except for those with known serious disease, can begin a moderate-exercise program such as walking without a medical evaluation or graded exercise test. Whenever people are in doubt about their own personal health and safety while exercising, a medical evaluation is recommended. Diagnostic exercise testing is not recommended as a routine screening procedure in adults who have no evidence of heart disease. As emphasized earlier in this chapter, risk of serious medical complications during exercise is low unless an individual is at high risk for cardiovascular disease. Exercise physiologist Dr. Per Olaf Åstrand, has emphasized that "anyone who is in doubt about the condition of his health should consult his physician. But as a general rule, moderate activity is less harmful to the health than inactivity. You could also put it this way: A medical examination is more urgent for those who plan to remain inactive than for those who intend to get into good physical shape" (Sharkey, 1979).

Figure 4.4

The Borg Ratings of Perceived Exertion (RPE) Scale (Borg, 1985). The RPE scale is a reliable method to evaluate an individual's level of exertion while exercising. Individuals are asked to select a number that corresponds to their overall, general feeling of exertion. The rating should be based on total body feelings and not on leg fatigue or other localized sensations. For individuals beginning to exercise, an appropriate level of exertion is between 11 and 15 — if the RPE is greater than that, the individual should lower the exercise intensity.

Perceived Exertion Scale	
6	**Light Exercise** *Some health benefits, but minimal fitness improvement*
7 Very, very light	
8	
9 Very light	
10	
11 Fairly light	
12	**Moderate Exercise** *Both health and fitness benefits with minimal risk*
13 Somewhat hard	
14	
15 Hard	**Intense Exercise** *For those who desire high fitness. Can precipitate heart attack in high risk*
16	
17 Very hard	
18	
19 Very, very hard	
20 Maximal exertion	

Cardiovascular Screening
of Competitive Athletes

An average of 12 to 20 athletes, most of them high school students, die suddenly each year from congenital heart defects that aren't detected during normal physical examinations (AHA, 1996; Maron et al., 1996). About a third of the cases of sudden cardiac death are caused by a congenital heart defect called hypertrophic cardiomyopathy (thickened heart muscle), with the next most frequent cause being congenital coronary anomalies (AHA, 1996).

In the United States there are nearly six million scholastic athletes. Although most states require a regular physical once a year or once every 2 years for these athletes, the cost for the more sensitive tests (e.g., two-dimensional **echocardiography**) that would detect heart defects ranges from $400 to $2,000 a screening. However, even with echocardiography, some athletes are incorrectly classified (e.g., false-positive or false-negative) (AHA, 1996).

The sudden death of a young athlete is tragic, but the financial, ethical, medical, and legal issues involved in **preparticipation screening** have created huge barriers (Cantwell, 1998; Corrado et al., 1998). In 1996, the American Heart Association published a consensus statement on this issue from a panel of experts (AHA, 1996). The group fitness instructor should support all efforts to encourage preparticipation screening of athletes. Here are the key recommendations from the American Heart Association (AHA, 1996):

■ Some form of preparticipation cardiovascular screening for high school and collegiate athletes is justifiable and compelling, based on ethical, legal, and medical grounds.

■ A complete and careful personal and family history and physical examination designed to identify cardiovascular problems known to cause sudden death or disease progression in young athletes is the best available and most practical approach to screening populations of competitive sports participants, regardless of age. Such cardiovascular screening is an obtainable objective and should be mandatory for all athletes.

■ Both a history and a physical examination should be performed before participation in organized high school (grades 9 through 12) and collegiate sports. Screening should then be repeated every 2 years. In intervening years an interim history should be obtained.

■ The athletic screening should be performed by a healthcare worker with the requisite training, medical skills, and background to reliably obtain a detailed cardiovascular history, perform a physical examination, and recognize heart disease.

Summary

■ For those who are at high risk for heart disease to begin with, vigorous exercise bouts can trigger fatal heart attacks. These victims tend to be men who were sedentary, over 35 years old, already had heart disease or were at high risk for it, and then exercised too hard for their fitness levels.

■ Health screening is a vital process in first identifying individuals at high risk for exercise-induced heart problems, and then referring them to appropriate medical care.

■ All facilities offering exercise equipment or services should conduct a health and cardiovascular screening of all new members and/or prospective users, regardless of age.

■ Several types of health appraisal questionnaires are available including the *Physical Activity Readiness Questionnaire* (PAR-Q) and the 1998 ACSM/AHA questionnaire.

■ When a medical evaluation or recommendation is advised or required, written and active communication by the exercise staff with the individual's personal physician is strongly recommended.

■ ACSM/AHA recommends that participants be classified into one of three risk strata: apparently healthy (class A-1), persons at increased risk (classes A-2 and A-3), or persons with known cardiovascular disease (classes B, C, and D).

■ The depth of the medical or physical examination for any individual considering an exercise program depends on the disease risk stratification. Apparently healthy individuals (classes A-1, A-2, A-3) can begin moderate-exercise programs such as brisk walking without the need for exercise testing or medical examination.

■ Prior to starting a vigorous exercise program, older, apparently healthy persons (class A-2), and apparently healthy persons with cardiovascular disease risk factors (class A-3) should have a medical examination and a diagnostic graded exercise test under the supervision of a physician.

■ All other persons (classes B and C) should undergo a medical examination and exercise testing before participating in any type of exercise program or exercise should be avoided altogether (class D).

■ Some form of preparticipation cardiovascular screening for high school and collegiate athletes is justifiable and

compelling, based on ethical, legal, and medical grounds.

■ Appendix C details the general effects of several categories of medications on heart-rate response. This table should *not* serve as a substitute for consultation with a participant's physician.

References

American College of Sports Medicine. (1995). *ACSM's Guidelines for Graded Exercise Testing and Prescription,* 5th ed. Baltimore: Williams & Wilkins.

American College of Sports Medicine and American Heart Association. (1998). Recommendations for cardiovascular screening, staffing, and emergency policies at health/fitness facilities. *Medicine & Science in Sports & Exercise,* 30, 1009 – 1018.

American Heart Association. (1996). Cardiovascular preparticipation screening of competitive athletes. *Circulation,* 94, 850 – 856.

American Heart Association. (1998). 1999 Heart and Stroke Statistical Update. *Heart and Stroke Facts.* Dallas.

Canadian Society for Exercise Physiology. (1996). *The Canadian Physical Activity, Fitness & Lifestyle Appraisal.* Ottawa, Ontario.

Cantwell, J.D. (1998). Preparticipation physical evaluation: getting to the heart of the matter. *Medicine & Science in Sports & Exercise,* 30 (suppl), S341 – S344.

Cooper, K.H. (1968). *Aerobics.* New York: Bantam Books, Inc.

Corrado, D., Basso, C., Schiavon, M., & Thiene, G. (1998). Screening for hypertrophic cardiomyopathy in young athletes. *New England Journal of Medicine,* 339, 364 – 369.

Fletcher, G.F., Balady, G., Froelicher, V.F., Hartley, L.H., Haskell, W.L., & Pollock, M.L. (1995). Exercise standards: A statement for healthcare professionals from the American Heart Association. *Circulation,* 91, 580 – 615.

Gibbons, R.J., Balady, G.J., & Beasley, J.W. (1997). ACC/AHA guidelines for exercise testing: Executive summary. A report of the American College of Cardiology/American Heart Association Task Force on Practice Guidelines

(Committee on Exercise Testing). *Circulation,* 96, 345 – 354.

Maron, B.J., Shirani, J., Poliac, L.C., Mathenge, R., Roberts, W.C., & Mueller, F.O. (1996). Sudden death in young competitive athletes: Clinical, demographic, and pathological profiles. *Journal of the American Medical Association,* 276, 199 – 204.

Nieman, D.C. (1999). *Exercise Testing and Prescription: A Health-Related Approach.* Mountain View: Mayfield Publishing.

Sharkey, B.J. (1979). *Physiology of Fitness.* Champaign, Ill.: Human Kinetics.

Shephard, R.J., Thomas, S., & Weller, I. (1991). The Canadian Home Fitness Test: 1991 update. *Sports Medicine,* 11, 358 – 366.

Tharrett, S.J. & Peterson, J.A. (1997). *ACSM's Health/Fitness Facility Standards and Guidelines* 2nd ed. Champaign, Ill.: Human Kinetics.

U.S. Department of Health and Human Services. (1996). *Physical Activity and Health: A Report of the Surgeon General.* Atlanta, GA: U.S. Department of Health and Human Services, Centers for Disease Control and Prevention, National Center for Chronic Disease Prevention and Health Promotion.

Suggested Reading

American College of Sports Medicine. (1995). *ACSM's Guidelines for Graded Exercise Testing and Prescription,* 5th ed. Baltimore: Williams & Wilkins.

American College of Sports Medicine and American Heart Association. (1998). Recommendations for cardiovascular screening, staffing, and emergency policies at health/fitness facilities. *Medicine & Science in Sports & Exercise,* 30, 1009 – 1018.

McInnis, K.J. & Balady, G.J. (1999). Higher cardiovascular risk clients in health clubs. *ACSM's Health & Fitness Journal,* 3, 19 – 24.

Nieman, D.C. (1999). *Exercise Testing and Prescription: A Health-Related Approach.* Mountain View: Mayfield Publishing.

Tharrett, S.J. & Peterson, J.A. (1997). *ACSM's Health/Fitness Facility Standards and Guidelines,* 2nd ed. Champaign, Ill.: Human Kinetics.

Chapter 5

In This Chapter:

Carol Kennedy, M.S., is the program director for Fitness/Wellness at Indiana University. She has created and taught exercise leadership classes at three major universities. Kennedy has also instructed group exercise sessions for more than 20 years and currently oversees a comprehensive fitness/wellness program at Indiana University – Bloomington that offers group exercise, personal training, and strength and conditioning fitness programming.

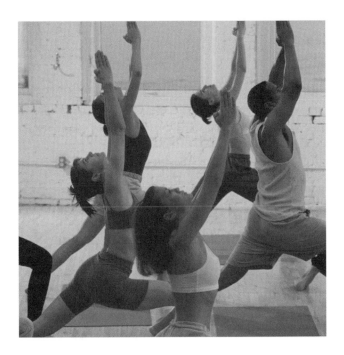

Group Exercise
Program Design

Carol Kennedy

The underlying purpose of a group exercise class is to enhance all health-related components of fitness. These include a participant's cardiorespiratory endurance, muscular strength and endurance, flexibility, and body composition. Group exercise has grown to include traditional hi/lo impact classes, step, indoor cycling, boxing, sports conditioning, water exercise, use of strength and conditioning equipment for group exercise, mind/body classes such as yoga and tai chi, stretching-only classes, and more.

As these different types of group exercise workouts continue to be created and studied, the American College of Sports Medicine (ACSM) Position Stand on Fitness for Healthy Adults continues to be updated as well (ACSM, 1998). See Table 5.1 for a summation of the 1998 ACSM position stand on fitness for healthy adults. The biggest change in the standards from the 1990 position stand that impacts group exercise is the change in duration to 20 – 60 continuous minutes or discontinuous 10-minute bouts that add up to 20 – 60 minutes total. Many group exercise class formats are set to be 1 hour long, with the cardiorespiratory segment being 20 – 40 minutes of continuous exercise to meet the old ACSM guidelines. Rethinking class schedules and offering a variety of times and activities are important for all successful fitness programs. Many facilities offering group exercise are finding success with 30-minute or shorter classes to help accommodate the busy schedules of participants. The 1998 ACSM position stand validates what group exercise has offered all along, which is a balanced workout that contains cardiorespiratory training, muscular strength and endurance training, and flexibility training. Finally, it is important also to consider the Surgeon General's Report on Physical Activity and Health (Pate et al., 1995). This report focuses on the importance of physical activity in daily life, such as walking the dog or taking the stairs. It states, "Every U.S. adult should accumulate 30 minutes or more of moderate-intensity physical activity on most, preferably all, days of the week." It cannot be assumed that people are generally active. Guidelines for structured exercise as well as the activities of daily life need to be stressed. The challenge is to apply the information in this manual, current research, and information from the ACSM Position Stand and The Surgeon General's Report into safe, effective, and highly motivating workouts in order to make a difference in the health and wellness of participants.

Group Exercise Professionalism/Attitude

Combining current research with participant needs and designing a safe and effective class begins with the attitude and atmosphere established by the instructor. A comfortable environment can be influenced by a wide range of factors, whether it be the quality of your communication or attire. Each helps establish a professional and caring attitude. As a group fitness instructor, you need to be a motivator and an educator (Kennedy, 1992).

Student-centered Instructor

The motivational/inspirational aspect of instructing includes having new moves, new music, and state-of-the-art equipment. The educational part of instructing includes having the knowledge of why certain moves are selected, making sure current research and knowledge are incorporated into the group exercise session, and making educated choices and decisions about the information given to participants. According to Westcott (1991), the most important characteristic of fitness instructors, as rated and ranked by participants, was knowledge of physical fitness. Let's compare and contrast a teacher-centered instructor with a student-centered instructor. The teacher-centered instructor can often foster depen-

Table 5.1
1998 ACSM Position Stand on Fitness for Healthy Adults

Frequency:	3 – 5 days per week
Intensity:	60% – 90% of max heart rate(HR) and 50% – 85% of VO_2 max
Duration:	20 – 60 continuous minutes or 10-minute bouts accumulated throughout the day to equal 20 – 60 minutes.
Mode:	Walk, run, row, stairs, cycle, aerobics
Resistance training:	One set of 8 – 12 reps < 50 years old and 10 – 15 reps > 50 years old for a minimum of 2 times per week, 8 – 10 major muscle groups worked.
Flexibility:	Recommended – three times per week

dence, intimidation, unattainable goals, and quick fixes (Table 5.2). The student-centered instructor, on the other hand, strives to establish an atmosphere of independence, encouragement, attainable goals, and realism (Table 5.3). Learning to take responsibility for the health and well-being of participants starts with understanding the importance of establishing a positive attitude and atmosphere.

Table 5.2
Teacher-centered Instructor

1. *Dependence:* I know the way – do what I do and you'll look like me!
2. *Intimidation:* This is an easy exercise: come on, do 10 more! No wimps in my class!
3. *Unattainable goals:* One more week and you'll start to see some changes.
4. *Quick fixes:* 20 more crunches will flatten those abdominals.

Table 5.3
Student-centered Instructor

1. *Independence:* Remember to work at your own pace. I will be teaching an intermediate class but will show modifications. It will be your responsibility to monitor your intensity level accordingly. Here's how to do that …
2. *Encouragement:* You're doing great! Keep up the good work. Remember if there is pain, there will be little gain. Stay with it, you'll achieve your goals.
3. *Attainable goals:* Learning to exercise regularly is a process that will take time. Adding extra activity outside of class, like taking the stairs or mowing your yard, will help you reach your goals faster.
4. *Reality:* Abdominal exercises will strengthen your abdominal muscles, but you will not be able to spot-reduce.

Creating a Healthy Emotional Environment

Another major factor in creating a comfortable environment for participants is establishing a healthy emotional environment. Education and motivation alone are not what keep participants coming back to group exercise. It is necessary to tap into the feelings and emotions of participants in order to impact adherence. One study (Bain et al., 1989) concerning overweight women's perceptions of an exercise class revealed that the most powerful influences affecting their exercise behavior were concerns about embarrassment and judgment by others. Instructors spend many hours preparing music, organizing the class flow, and selecting equipment, when, in fact, working on establishing a comfortable atmosphere can be just as important to participants. You might try greeting participants as they enter the class, learning their names and talking to everyone, not just to the participants in the front. If mirrors are utilized during the workout, it is important to face the participants when possible throughout the class so that direct eye contact is made. Looking at people through a mirror does not promote true interaction.

Instructors also need to realize that what they do and say has an impact on the class atmosphere. According to Goleman (1998), having "emotional intelligence" in any group setting dictates the success of the group experience. Goleman believes that "the emotional economy is the sum total of the exchanges of feeling among us. In subtle (or not so subtle) ways, we all make each other feel a bit better (or a lot worse) as part of any contact we have; every encounter can be weighted along a scale from emotionally toxic to nourishing." A specific example of this within a group exercise setting would be announcing before class how great it feels to be in a group exercise class to improve overall health and well-being. Contrast this with telling an overeating indulgence story and stating specific intentions to "work it off" during the class. The first statement leaves participants with a health-related sense of purpose for the workout. The second statement can send a message that punishment through exercise is recommended after over-indulging. Sending positive health messages throughout the group exercise experience is important for establishing the "emotional atmosphere" of the workout and utilizing the role-model aspect of teaching in a positive way.

Feeling comfortable in an environment where instructors present a "body beautiful" can also be rather intimidating. Crawford and Eklund (1994) compared similar video exercise routines, with the instructor wearing a thong in one and the same instructor wearing shorts and a T-shirt in another. "High physique-anxious" participants rated the thong video more unfavorably than the shorts and T-shirt video. Instructors can help participants become more comfortable with their own bodies and keep them exercising by wearing a variety of exercise clothing to help facilitate this process. A study (Nardini et al., 1999) of 148 female fitness instructors at an instructor conference found that 64% of instructors perceived an ideal body as one that was thinner than their current body. The average percent fat of the instructors was 20.5%; the national average for this age group is 23.1%. Instructors' body image perceptions are just that, perceptions. Perceptions can be changed, and this begins with the exercise instructor's self-awareness (Evans & Kennedy, 1993). If instructors are to make an impact on the health and well-being of participants it will be important to address this issue on a personal level.

Role of Fitness Assessment

Keying into the needs of participants through basic fitness assessments to educate and set goals is an option for the group exercise instructor. In many cases the role of the group exercise instructor in fitness assessment is minimal. Most group exercise classes do not include fitness assessments because assessments are usually performed one-on-one in a private setting. Should the group fitness instructor, then, not be concerned at all about performing fitness assessment? Not necessarily. Group fitness instructors are often asked to give advice on fitness assessment results. Therefore, having an understanding of the various assessment tests is important, as is learning some basic **field tests** applicable to the group exercise setting.

Establishing a positive attitude and atmosphere in group exercise involves letting participants know the physiological health benefits of coming to class. Performing basic group assessments allows participants to perform measurements on themselves, thus teaching them to take responsibility for their own health. Often, in a one-on-one setting, the clinician, clinical exercise physiologist, or personal trainer will perform measurements on the participants. The role of the group fitness instructor has a preventive healthcare aspect; it is important to encourage participants, who are apparently healthy people, to take personal responsibility for their health. This message can be sent quite clearly by allowing participants to learn and perform self-assessments, which is often the main objective of "field tests" such as waist-to-hip circumference measurements to assess body composition. Your role as a group fitness instructor in doing assessments, then, can be to help participants take more personal responsibility for their health by performing basic assessments. Although it's difficult to incorporate fitness assessment activities into a group class, this can be accomplished with field tests.

In addition to encouraging participants to take personal responsibility for their health, another goal when performing a field test assessment with a group is to educate participants about their health.

An overview of a sample field test for each of the health-related components of fitness (body composition, cardiorespiratory endurance, muscular strength and endurance, and flexibility) is presented later in this chapter. Other information on options available in a one-on-one setting are included in this chapter. Since there is little time in a group exercise setting to individualize participant results, it will be important to focus on educating participants as well as setting goals. Keep in mind that it is suggested to use field tests with an apparently healthy population. Participants with increased risk (two or more major health risk factors, according to ACSM) are to be referred to a clinical setting. Taking appropriate health-history information can help you discover who needs a one-on-one assessment. Field tests are not the "most accurate" type of test, but if performed in exactly the same way as both pre- and post-tests, results can be compared. Also, the tests are much less expensive and more convenient than one-on-one testing. Performing group fitness assessments is certainly not a requirement of a group exercise class. This portion is presented only as an option for the purpose of establishing a positive attitude and atmosphere and allowing the instructor to goal-set and educate participants.

Fitness Assessment/Health-related Components of Fitness

Outlined below are sample fitness-assessment tests utilized in a one-on-one setting. It is important to note that proper training is required to perform one-on-one assessments. This training is beyond the scope of this book and beyond the scope of practice of most group fitness instructors. However, being able to answer questions about these tests is important.

Body Composition

Hydrostatic weighing, also known as underwater weighing, is considered the "gold standard" of body-composition assessment. Body density is calculated from the relationship of normal body weight to underwater weight with percent fat being calculated from body density. Though hydrostatic weighing is more precise and the choice of many researchers, it is often impractical in terms of expense, time, and equipment.

Bioelectrical impedance is another popular method for determining body composition. It is based on the principle that the conductivity of an electrical impulse is greater through lean tissue than through fatty tissue. Reliability using this method is problematic because environmental issues, such as hydration state, temperature, and humidity, can have an impact on the results and are hard to standardize. Assessing body composition via bioelectrical impedance requires minimal technical training with the analyzers, which range in price from $300 to $5,000.

Near-infrared (NIR) light interactance is another method of assessing body composition. The FUTREX 5000 is the most popular commercial NIR analyzer available. It emits near-infrared light at two frequencies into the biceps area of the dominant arm. At these frequencies, body fat absorbs the light while lean body mass reflects the light. Although convenient and easy to use, researchers (McLean et al., 1992) have reported some problems with prediction errors.

Anthropometric assessments for measuring body composition include circumference measurements using a tape measure, waist-to-hip circumference ratio, and skinfold caliper measurements. Skinfold caliper measurements require special training and are not practical for a group setting. They are therefore recommended for use in a one-on-one setting. It is important to keep in mind that there is a margin of error (plus or minus 3% – 4%) with each skinfold test, and all tests must be compared to identical tests performed by the same tester under identical testing situations for optimum results. General body-fat percentage categories are listed in Table 5.4. Field tests for measuring body composition within a group exercise setting are discussed later in this chapter. These tests include waist-to-hip circumference and body mass index.

Table 5.4
General Body – fat Percentage Categories

Classification	Women (% fat)	Men (% fat)
Essential fat	10 – 12	2 – 4
Athletes	14 – 20	6 – 13
Fitness	21 – 24	14 – 17
Acceptable	25 – 31	18 – 25
Obese	32 and higher	25 and higher

Cardiorespiratory Endurance

There are many different tests available for measuring cardiorespiratory endurance. The measurement of $\dot{V}O_2$ max looks at the body's ability to take in oxygen from the atmosphere via the pulmonary system, transport it via the cardiovascular system, and utilize it via the muscular system. Field tests and sub-maximal tests such as the Rockport walking test or 12-minute walk/ run test estimate maximum **oxygen uptake** indirectly. Tests may vary in complexity from the relatively simple, such as **step tests**, walking tests, or running tests, which estimate maximum oxygen uptake ($\dot{V}O_2$ max), to those that use gas analyzers to measure oxygen uptake directly. Sub-maximal bicycle ergometer tests are a popular clinical alternative. These tests use heart-rate response to a given work intensity to predict $\dot{V}O_2$ max. The direct measurement of $\dot{V}O_2$ max using gas exchange can provide the most accurate results and is considered the gold standard. Direct $\dot{V}O_2$ max tests may be prohibitive in cost and are generally not practical for instructors. $\dot{V}O_2$ max norms for men and women are shown in Tables 5.5 and 5.6.

Acquiring $\dot{V}O_2$ max, whether it be from an indirect or direct method, is useful for being able to quantify percentage of work load by utilizing the metabolic equivalent (METs) system. Many cardiovascular machines

Table 5.5
Norms for Relative Maximal Oxygen Uptake (Men) (mL/kg)^2

Relative Maximal O₂ Uptake	Age (years)					
	18 – 25	26 – 35	36 – 45	46 – 55	56 – 65	65+
Excellent	> 60	> 60	> 55	> 49	> 43	> 38
Good	52 – 60	49 – 60	44 – 55	40 – 49	36 – 43	32 – 38
Above average	47 – 51	43 – 48	39 – 43	36 – 39	33 – 35	29 – 31
Average	43 – 46	39 – 42	36 – 38	32 – 35	30 – 32	26 – 28
Below average	37 – 42	34 – 38	31 – 35	29 – 31	26 – 29	23 – 25
Poor	30 – 36	30 – 33	27 – 30	25 – 28	22 – 25	20 – 22
Very poor	< 30	< 30	< 27	< 25	< 22	< 20

Source: Adapted from YMCA, 2000.

Table 5.6
Norms for Relative Maximal Oxygen Uptake (Women) (mL/kg)[2]

Relative Maximal O$_2$ Uptake	Age (years)					
	18 – 25	26 – 35	36 – 45	46 – 55	56 – 65	65+
Excellent	> 59	> 58	> 50	> 45	> 40	> 34
Good	49 – 59	47 – 57	42 – 50	36 – 45	33 – 40	29 – 34
Above average	43 – 48	42 – 46	37 – 41	32 – 35	30 – 32	26 – 28
Average	39 – 42	37 – 41	33 – 36	29 – 31	26 – 29	23 – 25
Below average	34 – 38	33 – 36	29 – 32	26 – 28	23 – 25	20 – 22
Poor	30 – 33	28 – 32	25 – 28	22 – 25	19 – 22	17 – 19
Very poor	< 30	< 28	< 25	< 22	< 19	< 17

Source: Adapted from YMCA, 2000.

(treadmills, upright steppers, etc.) list METs on their display boards. With group exercise sessions gravitating to this environment, it will be important to have a basic understanding of the use of METs. METs is a simplified system for classifying physical activities in which one MET is equal to resting oxygen consumption, which is approximately 3.5 milliliters of oxygen per kilogram of body weight per minute (3.5 mL/kg/min). $\dot{V}O_2$ max is measured in mL/kg/min. Therefore if $\dot{V}O_2$ max was estimated to be 42 mL/kg/min, this number could be divided by 3.5 to obtain maximum METs or 12 METs. Working at 50% of 12 METs would be 6 METs. A cardiovascular machine could then be set at 6 METs to accomplish this work load. This is one practical example of why cardiovascular testing can be useful for training. This would be a good group test to administer to educate group exercise participants about their cardiorespiratory fitness level.

Muscular Strength and Endurance

Muscular strength and muscular endurance are two components of muscular fitness testing. Muscular strength is the amount of force a muscle can produce in a single maximal effort. Muscular endurance is a muscle's ability to exert a force repeatedly over time.

Tests to measure muscular strength include the one-repetition maximum (1 RM) test using weight equipment to overload, and isometric strength tests, which are usually done in a one-on-one setting. The grip strength test using a hand dynamometer is also used to measure strength. The pull-up and the flexed arm hang are two muscular endurance tests used by the President's Council on Physical Fitness. The YMCA also has a bench press test for muscular endurance. Muscular endurance tests more commonly used by group fitness instructors are the push-up and bent knee curl-up test. It would be appropriate to administer these tests in a group setting in order to educate participants about the importance of muscular strength and endurance and to compare results over time to assess improvement.

Flexibility

Flexibility is defined as the range of motion around a joint or set of joints. Flexibility affects both health and fitness. Inflexibility increases the risk for joint and muscle injury, and excessive flexibility also can lead to joint instability. There is no one flexibility test that predicts range of motion for all other joints of the body. Therefore, each joint must be assessed individually. This is usually performed in a one-on-one setting using a goniometer to measure degrees of flexibility. These flexibility tests are often performed on an athletic training bench. Included below are descriptions of the following flexibility field tests: trunk extension, shoulder flexibility, and hamstring flexibility. These field tests work well within a group exercise setting. Including field test assessments within a group exercise setting is one way to establish an atmosphere of care and concern for the participants as well as help them identify the health benefits of group exercise.

Fitness Testing

Field Tests for Group Exercise Instructors

Waist-to-hip Circumference

Waist-to-hip measurements are an easy way to teach participants about the risks associated with poor body-fat distribution. Provide a basic tape measure (these cost around 99 cents at a local fabric store) and instruct students how to perform a waist to hip measurement appropriately. Waist measurement is the smallest waist circumference below the rib cage and above the umbilicus, measured while standing with abdominal muscles relaxed (not pulled in). If there appears

to be no smallest area around the waist, the measurement should be made at the level of the navel. Hip circumference is defined as the largest circumference of the buttocks – hip area taken while the person is standing. The waist-to-hip ratio is quick, easy, and focuses students on where they carry their body fat and whether this is a risk factor for diseases of the heart, diabetes, and some types of cancer. (Figures 5.1 and 5.2 and Table 5.7)

Body mass index (BMI) is another way to estimate body composition that is quick, easy, and does not require equipment or training. Of course, strictly speaking, BMI does not estimate body composition. It attempts to determine whether an individual is obese and how much their health risks are increased with increasing obesity. It is calculated as follows:

BMI= Weight in kilograms divided by height squared in meters

See Tables 5.8 and 5.9 for an example and reference chart. This test is a good one to include in a newsletter or handout for group exercise participants to do at home. Caution should be used whenever using total body weight instead of taking into account fat and lean body weight. More muscular, athletic types may be calculated as overweight when

Figure 5.1
Abdominal circumference

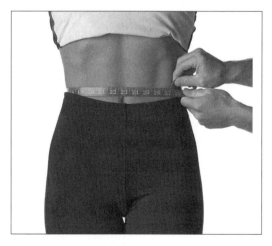

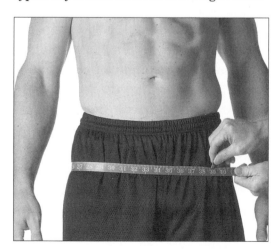

Figure 5.2
Hip circumference

Table 5.7
Waist-to-hip Ratios and
Associated Level of Health Risks

Classification	Men	Women
High risk	> 1.0	> 0.85
Moderately high risk	0.90 – 1.0	0.80 – 0.85
Lower risk	< 0.90	< 0.80

Adapted from Van Itallie (1988).

in fact they simply have a lot of lean body weight. This is the limitation of BMI testing.

Step Test

A practical field test appropriate for a group exercise setting is the YMCA Sub-maximal step test. This type of test is easy to administer in a group setting. A disadvantage of this test is that it does not result in an estimation of maximal oxygen consumption ($\dot{V}O_2$ max). An advantage is that participants can perform this test on their own without any assistance, once they know the protocol. The comparison to established norms is based on recovery HR. How quickly the heart recovers from work is one way to measure cardiorespiratory fitness.

The following equipment is needed to administer the test:

- A 12-inch step bench (bench and four risers)
- A cassette tape with a music tempo of 96 beats per minute
- A timer for timing the 3-minute test and 1-minute recovery time
- Forms on which to record the data

Utilize the following test administration procedures:

- Start stepping to a four beat cycle — up, up, down, down — either alternating feet or keeping the same lead foot. Make sure both feet touch the floor during the down portion and both feet touch the top of the bench on the up portion.

Table 5.8
Body Mass Index Example

$$BMI = \frac{Weight\ (kg)}{Height^2\ (m)}$$

Convert weight from pounds (lbs) to kilograms by dividing weight in lbs by 2.2

Weight = 140 lbs $\quad \frac{140}{2.2} = 63.6\ kg$

Convert height from inches to centimeters, and then to meters, by multiplying weight in inches by 2.54 and then dividing by 100:

Height = 58 inches
$\quad\quad$ 58 x 2.54 = 147.3 cm $\quad\quad \frac{147.3}{100} = 1.47\ m$

$$BMI = \frac{63.6}{1.47^2} = 29.4$$

- Have participants step for 3 minutes then sit on the bench for 1 minute and count their recovery HR for 1 minute. Remind participants to press lightly if using the carotid arteries as their HR location. (See *Methods of Monitoring Cardiorespiratory Intensity,* on page 163, for how to take a pulse rate)

Utilize the 1-minute postexercise HR to score the test and compare to the norms in Tables 5.10 and 5.11.

Push-up and Bent Knee Curl-up

The purpose of the push-up test is to evaluate the muscular strength and endurance of the upper body, specifically the triceps, anterior deltoid, and pectoralis

Table 5.9
Body Mass Index Reference Chart

Weight Category	BMI Range	Percent Above Normal Weight
Normal weight	19 to 25	————
Overweight	26 to 30	20 to 40 percent
Obese	31 to 35	41 to 100 percent
Seriously obese	Over 35	> 100 percent

Table 5.10
Norms for 3-Minute Step Test (Men) (bpm)

Fitness Category	Age (years)					
	18 – 25	26 – 35	36 – 45	46 – 55	56 – 65	65+
Excellent	< 79	< 81	< 83	< 87	< 86	< 88
Good	79 – 89	81 – 89	83 – 96	87 – 97	86 – 97	88 – 96
Above average	90 – 99	90 – 99	97 – 103	98 – 105	98 – 103	97 – 103
Average	100 – 105	100 – 107	104 – 112	106 – 116	104 – 112	104 – 113
Below average	106 – 116	108 – 117	113 – 119	117 – 122	113 – 120	114 – 120
Poor	117 – 128	118 – 128	120 – 130	123 – 132	121 – 129	121 – 130
Very poor	>128	>128	>130	>132	>129	>130

Source: Adapted from Golding et al. (1986). Reprinted with permission of the YMCA of the USA.

muscles. This test can be included in the muscular strength and conditioning segment of a group exercise class.

The participants can be allowed to keep their own count in order to promote independence and self-responsibility. Protocol for the norm charts listed in Table 5.12 are based on men performing full push-ups and women performing bent knee push-ups. The following tips are offered for making the test effective:

- Have participants partner up or allow individuals to count their repetitions on their own.

- Make sure hands are shoulder-width apart.
- The push-up is complete when the chest touches the fist of a partner and returns to the start position with arms fully extended.
- Rest is allowed in the up position only.
- Count the total number of push-ups completed before reaching the point of exhaustion.

The purpose of the bent knee curl-up test is to evaluate abdominal muscle strength and endurance. Procedures for administering the test are as follows:

Table 5.11
Norms for 3-Minute Step Test (Women) (bpm)

Fitness Category	Age (years)					
	18 – 25	26 – 35	36 – 45	46 – 55	56 – 65	65+
Excellent	<85	<88	<90	<94	<95	<90
Good	85 – 98	88 – 99	90 – 102	94 – 104	95 – 104	90 – 102
Above average	99 – 108	100 – 111	103 – 111	105 – 115	105 – 112	103 – 115
Average	109 – 117	112 – 119	111 – 118	116 – 120	113 – 118	116 – 122
Below average	118 – 126	120 – 126	119 – 128	121 – 126	119 – 128	123 – 128
Poor	127 – 140	127 – 138	129 – 140	127 – 135	129 – 139	129 – 134
Very poor	>140	>138	>140	>135	>139	>134

Source: Adapted from Golding et al. (1986). Reprinted with permission of the YMCA of the USA.

Table 5.12
Push-up Norms for Men and Women by Age Groups Using Number Completed

Age (Years)	(15-19)		(20-29)		(30-39)		(40-49)		(50-59)		(60-69)	
Gender	M	F	M	F	M	F	M	F	M	F	M	F
Excellent	>39	>33	>36	>30	>30	>27	>22	>24	>21	>21	>18	>17
Above average	29-38	25-32	29-35	21-29	22-29	20-26	17-21	15-23	13-20	11-20	11-17	12-16
Average	23-28	18-24	22-28	15-20	17-21	13-19	13-16	11-14	10-12	7-10	8-10	5-11
Below average	18-22	12-17	17-21	10-14	12-16	8-12	10-12	5-10	7-9	2-6	5-7	1-4
Poor	<17	<11	<16	<9	<11	<7	<9	<4	<6	<1	<4	<1

Source: CSTF Operations Manual. (3rd ed.) *Ottawa, Fitness and Amateur Sport*, 1986.
The Canadian Standardized Test of Fitness was developed by, and is reproduced with the permission of, Fitness Canada, Government of Canada.

- Place two strips of tape parallel to each other and 8 cm apart.
- Have participants lie on a mat with feet flat on the floor and knees bent at about 90 degrees. They should place their hands palms-down at their sides, with fingertips touching the first strip of tape.
- Begin the cadence at 40 bpm, which is equal to 3 seconds per curl-up or 20 curl-ups per minute, and make sure the fingertips touch the second strip with each curl-up.
- Participants should perform as many curl-ups as possible without stopping, up to a maximum of 75 or until the test is terminated if the cadence is broken.

Because push-ups and curl-ups are often selected to work muscle groups within the group exercise setting, it would be efficient to do a testing session occasionally to allow the participants the chance to compare their results. Have the participants keep a log of these results and keep them on file at the exercise class.

Trunk Extension, Shoulder Flexibility, and Hamstring Flexibility

The trunk extension test evaluates the amount of backward bend (extension) available to the lumbar spine. As flexibility in the lumbar spine is lost, the risk for low-back pain and injury increases significantly. Pro-

Table 5.13
Evaluation of Trunk Extension

Extension	Characteristics
Good	The hips remain in contact with the floor while the arms are fully extended.
Fair	The hips rise from the ground up to 2 inches.
Poor	The hips rise from the ground 2 inches or more.

Source: Adapted from Krepton, D. & Chu, D. (1984). *Everybody's Aerobics Book*. Oakland: Star Rover House. Reprinted with permission.

cedures for instruction on a self-test for the trunk extension are:
- Lie face down as if in the beginning stages of a push-up.
- Push the upper body up, relax the lower back, and keep the hip bones on the ground while working to fully extend the arms. See norms in Table 5.13.

The shoulder flexibility test is a good test for a group exercise setting. Procedures for testing are as follows:
- Have participants sit or stand with one arm straight up.
- Let the elbow bend so the hand comes to rest, palm down between the shoulder blades.
- Have participants reach back with the other hand palm up.
- Have participants attempt to touch hands with the fingers. See norms in Table 5.14.

Table 5.14
Evaluation of Shoulder Flexibility

Flexibility	Characteristics
Good	The fingers can touch.
Fair	The fingertips are not touching, but are less than 2 inches apart.
Poor	The fingertips are more than 2 inches apart.

Source: Adapted from Krepton, D. & Chu, D. (1984). *Everybody's Aerobics Book*. Oakland: Star Rover House. Reprinted with permission.

The hamstring flexibility test is another good test for a group exercise setting. Procedures for testing are as follows:

- Warm up slightly with some gentle stretching before performing the test.
- Place a yardstick on the floor and put a piece of tape at least 12 inches long at a right angle to the stick, between the legs, with the zero mark toward the body.
- Participants feet should be 12 inches apart and their heels aligned with the tape at the 15-inch mark on the yardstick (Figure 5.3).
- Have participants put one hand on top of the other with the tips of the fingers aligned.
- Participants should exhale slowly and lean forward by dropping the head

Figure 5.3
Hamstring
flexibility test

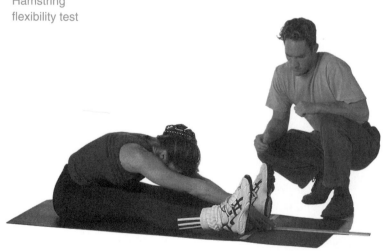

toward or between the arms. The fingers should maintain contact with the yard-stick while keeping the knees straight.
- The score is the farthest point reached after three trials. Scores can be compared to norms in Tables 5.15 and 5.16.

Class Format

Taking the positive attitude and atmosphere concept into the development of the overall class format is the next challenge. There is no single class format that is appropriate for every type of group exercise class. In a step class it is very appropriate to warm up using the steps; however, in a boxing class it may not be appropriate to use a bench but rather to practice boxing moves during the warm-up segment. In a water exercise session thermoregulation is important, so performing static stretches to enhance flexibility at the end of the workout may not be appropriate. It may be appropriate to perform some static stretching in the warm-up/stretching segment of a low-impact class for seniors. A 15-minute abdominal class may not even contain any stretching since the purpose of the session is confined to abdominal strengthening. These are just a few examples of why the same class format may not be appropriate for all group exercise classes.

A closer look will be taken at the general principles involved in each segment of group exercise from the pre-class preparation to the warm-up, cardiorespiratory, muscular strength and endurance, and flexibility/cooldown segments. These general principles apply to all types of group exercise from hi/lo impact, step, water exercise, indoor cycling, to sports conditioning, etc. Typically, most group exercise classes begin with **pre-class**

Table 5.15
Norms for Trunk Flexibility Test (Men) (inches)

Flexibility	Age (years)					
	18-25	26-35	36-45	46-55	56-65	65+
Excellent	>20	>20	>19	>19	>17	>17
Good	18-20	18-19	17-19	16-17	14-17	13-16
Above average	17-18	16-17	15-17	14-15	12-14	11-13
Average	15-16	15-16	13-15	12-13	10-12	9-11
Below average	13-14	12-14	11-13	10-11	8-10	8-9
Poor	10-12	10-12	9-11	7-9	5-8	5-7
Very poor	<10	<10	<8	<7	<5	<5

Source: Adapted from Golding, et al. (1986). Reprinted with permission of the YMCA of the USA.

preparation followed by a warm-up, which includes using specific movement to prepare for the cardiorespiratory activity. These movements are performed at a low-to-moderate speed and range of motion. They are also designed to specifically warm up for the activity to follow and to increase blood flow to the muscles. A **cardiorespiratory segment** follows the warm-up that is aimed at improving cardiorespiratory endurance and body composition and keeping the HR elevated for 10 – 30 minutes. Following the cardiorespiratory workout a gradual cooldown reduces the HR toward resting levels and prevents excessive pooling of blood in the lower extremities. A muscular strength

and endurance segment can also be included either before or after the cardiorespiratory segment, depending on the activity. The class then ends with a flexibility/cool-down component that includes stretching and relaxation exercises designed to further lower HR, help prevent muscle soreness, and enhance overall flexibility.

Offering Options

Notice how the four components — warm-up, cardiorespiratory endurance, muscular strength and endurance, and flexibility — common to most group fitness classes are also similar to the health-related components of fitness. It is important to note that

Table 5.16
Norms for Trunk Flexibility Test (Women) (inches)

Flexibility	Age (years)					
	18-25	26-35	36-45	46-55	56-65	65+
Excellent	>24	>23	>22	>21	>20	>20
Good	21-23	20-22	19-21	18-20	18-19	18-19
Above average	20-21	19-20	17-19	17-18	16-17	16-17
Average	18-19	18	16-17	15-16	15	14-15
Below average	17-18	16-17	14-15	14-15	13-14	12-13
Poor	14-16	14-15	11-13	11-13	10-12	9-11
Very poor	<13	<13	<10	<10	<9	<8

Source: Adapted from Golding et al. (1986). Reprinted with permission of the YMCA of the USA.

the emphasis given to each will vary depending on the objective of the class as well as the fitness level, age, health, and physical skill of its participants. It is difficult to schedule a specific type of group exercise class to meet everyone's needs. Putting beginners in with advanced participants can be challenging for instructors. Therefore, leveling the sessions by using names like "Fresh Start" for classes to appeal to beginners will be helpful. These classes should be shorter in duration and less intense, and the skills needed to perform the cardiorespiratory segment also need to be basic. Using names like "Plus" or "Extra" to describe longer-duration sessions that contain more skills for the cardiorespiratory segment would help the advanced exerciser locate the class that is right for them. Offering some shorter 20 – 30 minute classes of stretching or muscular strength and endurance only will also help prepare some of the more sedentary participants for the longer classes, which contain all components of fitness. Keep in mind that participants may walk to work in the morning and only need a flexibility or muscular strength and conditioning class. Offering different options and not staying with the typical hour-long format that encompasses all components will help meet more people's health goals.

Pre-class Preparation

There are a few common principles in the pre-class preparation for any group exercise class. They are listed below and will be reviewed in this segment. The instructor:

- Knows participants' health histories and surveys for new participants (see the chapter on health history)

- Is available before class/orients new participants
- Discusses/models appropriate attire/footwear
- Has music cued up and equipment ready before class begins
- Acknowledges class and introduces self
- Previews class format and individual responsibilities
- Brings, and encourages participants to bring, water to classes

Know Your Participants

Chapter 4 provides an in-depth review on acquiring health information and discussed waivers. What is important to note is that the information gathered from these sources needs to be transferred into making a safe and effective class. For example, if two participants say they have occasional lower-back pain, incorporating abdominal and low-back strengthening as well as hamstring stretching into the class format on a regular basis would help their conditions. Make sure participants are aware that the time they took to fill out the health information is useful time by asking participants' questions and also letting them know about the modifications. Of course some modifications will need to be explained directly to an individual participant if it is not appropriate to address the issue to the entire class.

Orient New Participants

A professional student-centered group fitness instructor takes the time to meet and orient new participants as well as be available if any participants have questions. Participants tend to respond more sincerely to questions such as "who has been to a step class three times or less" rather than "who has never been to step?" This is such an important part of customer service to participants, and it is also a time when instructors get the most amount of feedback about the class in general. Instructors need to learn to be open to input and also to take the time to get to know new participants. This is a part of continuing to establish a positive, comfortable class environment and is also essential to the adherence of the participant.

Choose Appropriate Attire

As mentioned earlier under "Creating a Healthy Emotional Environment," it is important that attire be appropriate for the specific group exercise class. For example, when teaching a senior class it would not be appropriate to wear a midriff spandex outfit, as it might be intimidating. Observe what the participants wear to class and try to match their attire so they will feel more comfortable. Ask what attire they prefer. However, as a fitness professional, try to balance the comfort level of the class with functional wear. Correct spinal alignment and form should be visible with each movement you demonstrate. Make sure to notice and discuss appropriate footwear for the various group exercise classes. For example, some indoor cycles have special clipless pedals that require that appropriate cycling shoes be worn for the workout. Encouraging use of cross-training shoes with adequate cushioning for a participant's first step class will make them more comfortable than if they wear running shoes that catch on the tracked platform. Finally, in water exercise it is important to note that a regular swimming suit often does not give the "support" needed to perform water exercise effectively. Have information available at all times on where to locate shoes and attire for the new participant.

Equipment Preparation

With all the different "toys" available for group exercise (i.e., physioballs, hand-held weights, bands, weighted bars, stretching devices, yoga blocks, etc.), it's important to be prepared ahead of time and inform participants about what toys will be used. Posting a note close to where the participants enter the facility to inform them which equipment will be used also works well. Consider playing welcoming music before the beginning of class and always make sure to have tapes cued and ready to go. It is also important to use good quality tapes and plan for minimal changes in order to have a better class flow. Prior preparation can make the actual class run much more professionally.

Acknowledge Class Participants

Creating a positive attitude and atmosphere begins with an instructor making sure to welcome people before class begins and introducing himself/herself, especially when teaching in a facility where different people come to class every week and there is no set class list.

This concept may sound minor, but it establishes an attitude of "we're in this together." Also, if participants are aware of your name they will be more likely to come up and ask questions afterward. New people coming to a group exercise class are often afraid of asking questions or feeling out of place. Understanding this and asking for feedback will create a more open, safe environment for all participants, not just the regular participants.

Preview Class Format

An overview of what the specific class format is should accompany the instructor introduction. With so many different classes being offered, people often find themselves in the wrong class. They do not always realize this until halfway through. Therefore, always make sure to introduce the class format before each class begins. A good example is, "This is a 30-minute stretching class. There will not be an aerobic component to it." After previewing the class format, it is also important that participants understand their individual responsibilities. There is nothing worse than having a participant come up after class and say, "That was not a hard enough workout." Intensity is the responsibility of the participant, not the instructor. It is your responsibility to make sure that modifications are given for various intensities in order to allow participants to make a choice.

Warm-up

There are a few common principles in the warm-up for any group exercise class. They are listed below and will be reviewed in this segment.

- The beginning segment is designed to "break a sweat."
- The warm-up focuses on rehearsal moves as a large part of the movement selection.
- Stretches, if appropriate, are done after "breaking a sweat" and performing rehearsal movements.
- Verbal directions should be clear and volume and tempo of music and atmosphere created appropriate.
- The instructor demonstrates proper form and observes participants' form and suggests adaptations for injuries and special needs.

"Break a Sweat"

The purpose of the warm-up is to prepare the body for the more rigorous demands of the cardiorespiratory and/or muscular strength and conditioning segments by raising the internal temperature. For each degree of temperature elevation, the metabolic rate of cells increases by about 13% (Astrand & Rodahl, 1977). In addition, at higher body temperatures, blood flow to the working muscles increases, as does the release of oxygen to the muscles. Because these effects allow more efficient energy production to fuel muscle contraction, the goal of an effective warm-up should be to elevate internal temperatures 1 or 2° Fahrenheit, so that sweating occurs.

Increasing body temperature has other effects that are beneficial for exercisers as well. The potential physiological benefits of warm-up include:

- increased metabolic rate
- higher rate of oxygen exchange between blood and muscles
- more oxygen released within muscles
- faster nerve impulse transmission
- gradual redistribution of blood flow to working muscles
- decreased muscle relaxation time following contraction
- increased speed and force of muscle contraction
- increased muscle elasticity
- increased flexibility of tendons and ligaments
- gradual increase in energy production, which limits lactic acid buildup
- reduced risk of abnormal **electrocardiogram**

Many of these physiological effects may reduce the risk of injury because they have the potential to increase neuromuscular coordination, delay fatigue, and make the tissues less susceptible to damage (Shellock, 1983; Alter, 1996). Therefore, the overall focus in the warm-up period should be on movements that increase core body temperature. "Breaking a sweat" is a way to measure if you are successfully increasing core temperature.

Rehearsal Moves - in warm up

Blahnik (1996) defines rehearsal moves as "movements that are identical to, but less intense than, the movements your students will execute during the workout phase." Examples of these would be utilizing the bench to warm up during a step class, teaching participants how to hill climb briefly in an indoor cycling class, performing one water interval segment to prepare for the cardiorespiratory water interval-training segment, or utilizing light weights to prepare for a muscle-conditioning class. The whole concept of rehearsal moves relates to the principle of specificity of training. This principle states that the body adapts specifically to whatever demands are placed on it. Durstine and Davis (ACSM, 1998) believe that specificity applies not only to energy systems and muscle groups, but also to movement patterns. Since motor units used during training demonstrate the majority of physiological alterations, movement patterns must also be specifically trained. In a group exercise session, one of the main reasons participants become frustrated is that they are not able to perform the movements effectively. Introducing these movement patterns in the warm-up will assist with waking up associated motor units.

Utilizing rehearsal moves in the warm-up not only specifically warms up the body for the movement ahead, but also can serve as a time to set down some neuromuscular patterns by introducing new skills not yet used. For example, in a hi/lo class where a grapevine half-turn movement is used, utilize the warm-up to break down the move,

identify the directional landmarks in the room, and name the specific move. This way, when a grapevine half-turn is referred to in the cardiorespiratory segment, the class participants will know what to do. The same idea applies to a complex choreography movement in a step class. Practice this movement slowly in the warm-up when maintaining a higher level of intensity is not the main focus. When this movement comes up in the routine it will have been "rehearsed," and this will make it easier for participants to maintain their cardiorespiratory intensity level. Rehearsal moves, therefore, ought to make up a large part of the warm-up.

Stretches, if Appropriate

To stretch or not to stretch during the warm-up is a much-debated issue. This issue is one on which the literature has not come to complete agreement. Taylor et al. (1990) found that gains in flexibility were most significant when a stretch was held for 12 to 18 seconds and repeated four times per muscle group. Another study (Walter et al., 1995) found that stretching the hamstrings for 30 seconds produced significantly greater flexibility than stretching for 10 seconds. If these two studies were the complete story, we would probably recommend not stretching in a group exercise warm-up, since it is impossible to stretch a muscle group four times and hold it for 30 seconds and still accomplish the goal of Another study (Girouard, 1995) looking at strength and flexibility training in older adults found that stretching before and after strength training did not increase flexibility when resistance training was involved. Finally, the 1998 ACSM position stand on exercise now includes flexibility for the first time. This position stand states, "The inclusion of recommendations for flexibility exercise in this position stand is based on growing evidence of its multiple benefits including: improving joint range of motion and function and in enhancing muscular performance." It is generally agreed that flexibility exercises are good for health, but we are not quite sure where to put them in the class format for group exercise.

Most prominent exercise leadership books (Neiman, 1999; Howley, 1997; McArdle et al., 1996) and stretching books (Alter, 1996) recommend an active warm-up with rehearsal moves followed by brief stretching with a focus on the warm-up and not on enhancing flexibility until the cool-down portion of the workout. However, these books are written with the individual and, often, the athlete in mind, not necessarily with an emphasis on how to work with a group. Generally, though, they do not leave out stretching within the warm-up, but they all advocate that a warm-up precede any stretching. There is no conclusive evidence showing any inherent benefit to stretching during the warm-up, but also no study shows that it is dangerous. With this in mind, the warm-up should contain mostly warm-up movements.

In terms of organizing a group exercise class format for the warm-up segment, perform several rehearsal movements and, if static stretches are included, try to focus on active movement as well. For example, while performing a standing hamstring stretch, keep the upper body moving with triceps extensions to stay warm. In a cycling class keep the legs pedaling and perform some upper-body stretches. When teaching a 30-minute session, it might be better to save the stretching for the end when it will be most beneficial in terms of enhancing flexi-

bility. In this situation, it might not be appropriate to do static stretching. When teaching an hour class, in which there is more time for the warm-up segment, actively contract the hamstrings and then stretch them briefly for optimum effectiveness. When teaching a group of seniors, warming up and then performing several minutes of static stretching might be their preference. For seniors, balance is also an issue. After they have warmed up they can hold a stretch for increased flexibility. By the end of the class, fatigue may keep them from being able to perform static stretches appropriately.

Only instructors know their clientele and what's best for them. The decision on how to go about warming up and stretching is an individual one. What definitively is known is that flexibility is a health-related component of fitness and needs to be included in the workout. Whether it is at the end of the workout, in the middle, or during the warm-up should be a choice made by the instructor based on feedback from the participants until we have more definite research on the topic. We do know that optimum flexibility is achieved at the end of the workout, and it is suggested that warming up and breaking a sweat be performed before any static stretching in the warm-up.

Use of Music

Many group exercise classes utilize music as a way to motivate participants and create more overall enjoyment in the experience. Several research studies (Gfeller, 1988; Boutcher, 1990) have validated the idea that music is beneficial from a motivational standpoint. In terms of utilizing music to create a beat to follow, research (Staum, 1983) has found that external auditory cues, such as rhythmic music and percussion pulses, favorably affect coordinated walking and proprioceptive control. Moving to the beat of the music is not always necessary in a group exercise setting. In fact, some yoga, tai chi, sports conditioning, or even outdoor group exercise sessions do not use music at all. However, while using the beat is important in most step and hi/lo classes, music is often used in cycling, boxing/sports conditioning, and water exercise as background sound to help motivate or set a mood. Keep in mind that even in a "beat-driven" step class, participants may benefit by sing along, less beat-driven music in part of the strength or stretching portion. Also, in an indoor cycling class the warm-up music might be something to sing along with that does not contain a lot of hard drums or fast-paced tempos. The mood the music establishes helps to create and control the individual segments of the class.

It is important to balance music and verbal cueing. If the music is so loud that the verbal cueing is not heard, that can be a problem for the participants. Seniors especially need to be asked about the volume of the music, as they often have the most opinions and feedback about volume. IDEA (1997) published an opinion statement on the volume of music based on standards established by the United States Occupational Safety and Health Administration (OSHA). It stated that music intensity during group exercise classes should measure no more than 90 decibels (dB) and, since the instructor's voice needs to be about 10 dB louder than the music in order to be heard, the instructor's voice should measure no more than 100 dB. A decibel meter measuring device can be purchased at a local electronics store for less than $50. It is worth the investment since music volume is often a common source of complaints for partici-

pants. To protect the voice of instructors it is also important to have a microphone system available.

Instructor's Responsibilities

Instructors are often selected because excellent form is something they naturally have. For example, potential hi/lo instructors are often picked from among the front row participants who regularly attend class. Cyclists often instruct indoor cycling classes. It is important to note that having the skill and "teaching" the skill are two different things. Instructors who have good form may need instruction on teaching good cueing for the skills they naturally have, whereas those who need instruction on good form may learn more readily how to explain what good form looks like. As an instructor, it is essential to have good alignment in all exercises demonstrated, especially for the benefit of the visual learners in the class.

One of the most important differences between the teacher-centered instructor and the student-centered instructor is that the student-centered instructor can and will help participants with individual needs to make exercise safe and less painful or problematic. To facilitate this, you must know the problems and limitations of participants and *observe* what the participants are doing (Figure 5.4). For example, if a participant has tight hamstrings and occasionally talks of back pain, they may deviate from the demonstrated exercise as in Figure 5.4. Verbalizing a modification involving putting the hands back to support the back and then slowly inching the hands forward demonstrates properly observing participants' form and suggesting adaptations for special needs.

The point of this example is to encourage all group exercise instructors to get out on the floor and observe and assist, not just during the warm-up stretch segment but during the entire workout. Demonstrate a move, perform a few repetitions, and then get up and begin watching participants or occasionally move around the room while demonstrating. Staying in one place only gives one frame of reference to participants. Plus, being a coach is a large part of the group exercise experience. It is a known fact that when the instructor is nearby and observing, listening and practicing of skills are improved by the participants. The skill of being a coach applies to all segments of the class format and needs to be evaluated throughout the class. It is important to allow participants to see that you have empathy.

Cardiorespiratory Segment

There are a few common principles in the cardiorespiratory segment of most group exercise classes. They are listed below and will be reviewed in this segment.

As a group fitness instructor, you should:
- Promote independence/self-responsibility
- Gradually increase intensity
- Gives impact and/or intensity options
- Build sequences logically and progressively
- Utilize a variety of muscle groups
- Use music to create a motivational atmosphere
- Monitor intensity through HR and/or rate of perceived exertion (RPE) checks
- Incorporate a post-cardio cool-down/stretch segment

Promote Self-responsibility

Whether leading a hi/lo class or teaching a treadmill class or a circuit/cardio class, it is impossible to be everywhere or help everyone simultaneously. Each participant is working at a different fitness level and has different goals. Ideally it would be nice if all classes could be organized according to intensity and duration levels. The reality is that many participants come to a class because its time is convenient, not necessarily because the class length or intensity level is suitable. If participants try to exercise at the instructors' level or another participant's level, they may work too hard and sustain an injury or they may not work hard enough to meet their goals. A few ways to help promote independence and self-responsibility are to encourage participants to work at their own pace, utilize HR monitoring or RPE checks, and inform them how they should feel through common examples. For example,

Figure 5.4
Sit and reach hamstring stretch

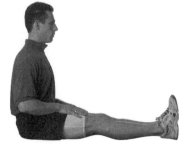

Demonstrated exercise

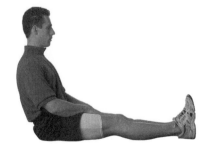

Deviation

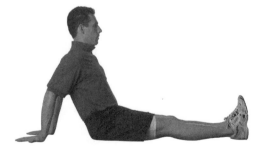

Modification — stretch hamstrings by walking hands toward torso

during the peak portion of the cardiorespiratory segment let them know they should feel out of breath. During the post-cardio cool-down tell them they should feel their HRs slowing down. Be as descriptive as possible of perceived exertion throughout the workout. Also, it is important to demonstrate high-, medium-, and low-intensity options in order to teach the class at various levels. Help participants achieve the level of effort they need to reach and continually remind them it is their responsibility. The instructor cannot be responsible for participants' exercise intensity. Pointing out participants who work at higher or lower levels can also help. It is recommended that you maintain a medium intensity most of the time, but that you also present other options and intensities as the need arises. Mastering this concept is the true "art" of group exercise and the reason why group exercise is more difficult than one-on-one instruction.

Gradually Increase Intensity

Even though the human body adapts to exercise very efficiently, gradually increasing intensity is necessary for the following physiological reasons:

1. It allows blood flow to be redistributed from internal organs to the working muscles.
2. It allows the heart muscle time to adapt to the change from a resting to a working level. The hardest and most dangerous time for changes in the heart's rhythm is in the transition from resting to high-intensity work or from high-intensity activity back to resting levels. At rest, the cardio-vascular system circulates about 5 liters of blood per minute. Imagine the contents of 2 ½ 2-liter soda pop containers circulating through the body every minute. At maximal strenuous exercise, the increase in workload requires as much as 25 liters per minute to accommodate working muscles — that's 12 ½ pop containers per minute!

3. It allows for an increase in respiratory rate. Remember that the diaphragm, the major muscle involved in breathing, is like any other muscle and needs time to shift gears. A rapid increase in breathing without time to warm up properly results in side aches and hyperventilation (rapid, shallow breathing). Some hyperventilation is a part of beginning exercise, but sudden increases in breathing mean that the transition into the cardiorespiratory segment was not gradual enough.

For example, to gradually increase intensity within a group exercise setting, exaggerate moves less in hi/lo in the first few minutes, and travel less. Make sure to keep moves less intense by not using propulsion-type moves in a step class. In a water exercise class, use moves that have a smaller range of motion or shorter lever length. Finally, in an indoor cycling class keep the flywheel tension set at a lower resistance for the first few minutes.

Impact and/or Intensity Options

In most group exercise classes, movement selection can increase impact and/or intensity. It is your job to make sure that this increase is balanced and appropriate for the participants. For example, in a boxing or sports-conditioning class you may elect to jump with both feet back and forth over lines on the floor. This is a high-impact movement. The next movement selection might then be a more moderate-impact movement like a brisk walk around the room. Impact is not as much an issue in an indoor cycling class where intensity options become more important. For example, a hill climb out of the saddle at a high resistance that lasts longer than three minutes is considered a higher-intensity option. This might be followed by a lower-resistance seated movement. All group exercise sessions have movements that can vary impact and intensity. Taking this into consideration when choosing movement combinations and segments is important.

Building Sequences

In a hi/lo class an example of building sequences logically would be teaching a group a grapevine move for the first time by breaking down the movement. Perform two step touches to the right followed by two step touches to the left. Then perform the same step touches, only this time step behind to make a grapevine move. In a complex choreography step class, this might mean teaching a complex series by breaking it down into segments of eight counts and then adding on until a series of four counts of eight is completed. Progressing properly in a water exercise class would mean marking a specific move by performing it, then increasing the speed of movement, traveling with the move, and then resisting the movement. If sequences are logically and progressively put together, there is a certain "flow" to the class that makes the participants want to come back. Participants know when the flow is not there — they usually end up standing and watching, feel confused while doing the movement, or execute it improperly.

Target a Variety of Muscle Groups

Instructors often have base moves (a series of movements that appear over and over again in their routine) within the car-

diorespiratory segment. These base moves often involve the use of the quadriceps and hip flexor muscle groups. Examples include the basic march in place, walk around the room, and the basic step. Some participants use these muscle groups exclusively in daily living activities; therefore, continuing to use the quadriceps and hip flexors repeatedly during exercise is unnecessary. Striving to balance daily flexion with other movements is important. Although it is impossible to individualize within a group exercise setting, understanding how the body functions in daily movement can help instructors determine which muscles are stronger and which muscles need to be focused on within group exercise. For example, walking forward works the hip flexors. Focusing on movement selection that utilizes the hamstrings (the opposing muscle group to the hip flexors) would help with muscle balance. The abductors are important stabilizer muscles for posture. Incorporating some abductor moves within the cardiorespiratory segment is recommended. In water exercise, muscle balance is automatically achieved since there is no gravity. If we flex the hip in water, the iliopsoas and rectus femoris perform the work. When the hip is extended in the water the hamstrings perform the work. On land, this movement would be an eccentric contraction of the quadriceps. With the exception of water exercise, it is important to analyze what movements work which muscle group and vary the selection to promote overall muscle balance.

Music

Most group exercise classes that contain a cardiorespiratory segment utilize music to motivate and inspire participants. Always ask participants about their preference for music. Just as many personal trainers will often give "their" workout to potential clients, group fitness instructors choose music that is motivating to them. Although it is important that music motivate the instructor, it is imperative that it motivate the participants. With the wide array of commercial tapes available, it is easy to find a variety of music. Take formal and informal surveys often of participants' preferences in order to get feedback on music. Probably one of the most time-consuming parts of teaching group exercise is finding good music. However, it is worth the time, since music can make or break the experience for the participants. It is recommended that you use pre-made fitness-specific workout tapes for group exercise classes.

Methods of Monitoring Cardiorespiratory Intensity

Monitoring exercise intensity within the cardiorespiratory segment is important. Participants need to be given instruction regarding the purpose of monitoring HR during exercise and information on how to obtain a pulse rate. Proper instruction on how to take an HR is the first step to monitoring intensity effectively. The following are a few recommended sites for taking heart rate:

Carotid pulse site. This pulse is taken from the carotid artery just to the side of the larynx using light pressure from the fingertips of the first two fingers, not the thumb. Remember, never palpate both carotid arteries at the same time and always press lightly.

Radial pulse site. This pulse is taken from the radial artery at the wrist, in line with the thumb, using the fingertips of the first two fingers.

Apical pulse site. This pulse is taken at the apex of the heart and can sometimes be felt very clearly by placing the heel of the hand over the left side of the chest.

Temporal pulse site. This pulse can sometimes be obtained from the left or right temple with light pressure from the fingertips of the first two fingers (Figure 5.5).

Understanding the use of HR, RPE, dyspnea scale, and **talk test** is the next step in monitoring exercise intensity effectively. One method is not advocated over another, as all have applications depending on the type of activities participants will be performing during the group exercise class. However, research (Parker et al., 1989) on group exercise has determined that HRs taken in hi/lo group exercise represent a lower relative exercise intensity ($\dot{V}O_2$ max) than that of running. Other research (Roach, 1994) on different forms of group exercise (step, interval hi/lo, and progressive treadmill training) concluded that HR may not be an appropriate predictor of exercise intensity and that RPE is the preferred method. Finally, there is research (Frangolias, 1995) suggesting that utilizing HRs in water exercise when the chest is submerged is not an appropriate technique. There is no one test that works for all different group exercise sessions or participants. It may be appropriate to utilize HR training for beginners or advanced participants, but use RPE more on a day-to-day basis. Many group exercise instructors have stopped using manual HR monitoring since it disrupts the flow of the class. Utilizing HR monitors is always an option as well. There are no hard and fast rules for monitoring intensity other than that it is an important responsibility of the group fitness instructor. Not monitoring intensity or giving constant intensity monitoring gauges does not show empathy for the participants. A summary of how to utilize

Figure 5.5a

Carotid heart rate monitoring

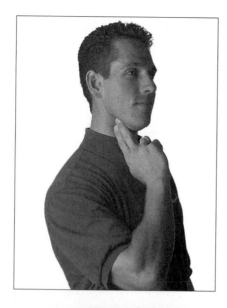

Figure 5.5b

Radial heart rate monitoring

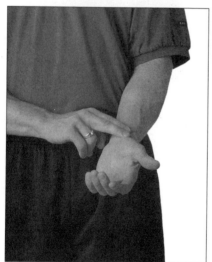

Figure 5.5c

Temporal heart rate monitoring

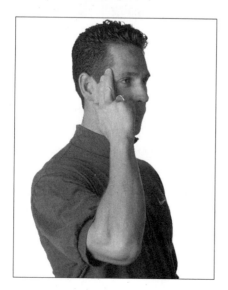

target HRs, RPE, dyspnea scale, and the talk test is given below.

Percentage of Maximal HR

One very common and easy-to-calculate way of determining target HR method is the percentage of maximal HR method. To use this method, HRmax must first be determined from either a maximal stress test or the age-adjusted **maximal HR formula**:

Estimated Maximal HR = 220 – Age in Years

The accuracy of **target heart rate** (THR) is slightly compromised when using the age-adjusted maximal HR rather than a measured maximal HR. Also, if a participant is taking medication that alters HR (e.g., beta blockers), then measured maximal HR must be used. THR is calculated by taking a percentage of HRmax and adjusting it by about 15% to better reflect aerobic capacity or maximal oxygen uptake. The formula is:

THR = (HRmax x percent intensity desired) x 1.15
(Table 5.17)

Percent of HR Reserve

Another method to determine THR range is to use a percentage of HR reserve, commonly known as the Karvonen formula. The recommended percent of HR reserve (50% – 85%) corresponds to a similar percent of maximal oxygen uptake (50% – 85%). This method differs from the HRmax method in that the **resting heart rate** is taken into account when determining THR. As in the HRmax method, measured **maximal heart rate** must be used in this method when the participant is taking prescribed medications that alter HR.

The key to this method is to take a percentage of the difference between maximal HR and resting HR, then add the resting HR to

Table 5.17
Using Percentage of Maximal HR to
Determine Target HR Range

Example: 38 year old participant who wants to exercise at 60% – 90% of HRmax:

$$\text{Maximal HR} = 220 - \text{age}$$

$$220 - 38 = 182 \text{ maximal HR} \times 0.60 \text{ to } 0.90 = \text{Target HR range}$$

$$
\begin{array}{cc}
182 & 182 \\
\underline{\times\,0.60} & \underline{\times\,0.90} \\
109 & 163.8 = 164
\end{array}
$$

Target heart rate range = 109 – 164

identify the THR. The reserve capacity of the heart reflects its ability to increase the rate of beating and cardiac output above resting level to maximal intensity (Table 5.18).

Rate of Perceived Exertion (RPE)

Using RPE is another common method of determining exercise intensity. Based on subjective perceptions of intensity, clients rate the level of steady-state work, using the 6 – 20 RPE scale or 0 – 10 RPE scale developed by Borg (1982). Interestingly, RPE is both valid and reliable (Dunbar et al., 1992; Robertson et al., 1990) and is closely associated with increases in most cardiorespiratory parameters, including work, maximal

Table 5.18
Using HR Reserve (Karvonen's formula)
to Determine Target HR Range

220 – 38 years old=182		
Maximal heart rate (220-age)	182	182
minus resting heart rate (RHR)	−70 (RHR)	−70 (RHR)
	112	112
x 0.50 to 0.85	x .50	x .85
	56	95.2
+ RHR	+ 70 (RHR)	+70 (RHR)
= Target HR range	126	165.2 =165

Target heart rate range = 126 – 165

oxygen uptake, and HR. In a group exercise setting, RPE can be used independent of, or in combination with, HR to monitor relative exercise intensity of most participants. It must be understood that participants on medication that alters HR can use the RPE scale to monitor relative exercise intensity. The verbal description that reflects the intensity of work is important when using either numerical RPE scale (Table 5.19). For example, a 6 – 7 is sitting and reading, an 11 is walking to the store, a 13 is beginning to breath hard, and a 15 is chasing the dog down the street. Relating real tasks in life with RPE helps participants understand how they should feel.

Dyspnea Scale — difficulty breathing by #1-4 #6-20

Dyspnea refers to difficulty in breathing or shortness of breath. The dyspnea scale is a

Table 5.19
Rate of Perceived Exertion

Perceived Exertion Scale		
6		
7 Very, very light	**Light Exercise**	*Some health benefits, but minimal fitness improvement*
8		
9 Very light		
10		
11 Fairly light		
12	**Moderate Exercise**	*Both health and fitness benefits with minimal risk*
13 Somewhat hard		
14		
15 Hard		
16	**Intense Exercise**	*For those who desire high fitness. Can precipitate heart attack in high risk*
17 Very hard		
18		
19 Very, very hard		
20 Maximal exertion		

The Borg Ratings of Perceived Exertion (RPE) Scale (Borg, 1985). The RPE scale is a reliable method to evaluate an individual's level of exertion while exercising. Individuals are asked to select a number that corresponds to their overall, general feeling of exertion. The rating should be based on total body feelings and not on leg fatigue or other localized sensations. For individuals beginning to exercise, an appropriate level of exertion is between 11 and 15 — if the RPE is greater than that, the individual should lower the exercise intensity.

subjective score that reflects the relative difficulty of breathing as perceived by the participant. Accordingly, this numerical scale can assist in monitoring exercise intensity:

+1　Mild, noticeable to participant, but not to observer

+2　Mild, some difficulty that is noticeable to observer

+3　Moderate difficulty, participant can continue to exercise

+4　Severe difficulty, participant must stop exercising

The use of this scale is for participants who have pulmonary conditions (asthma, emphysema) and those who feel limited due to breathlessness. Participants should be instructed to use the scale as a guide to their exercise intensity and in conjunction with HR and RPE. Instructors should caution participants who use this scale to reduce their intensity when breathing becomes labored (+3). If the severity of the pulmonary condition seems to worsen over time, instructors should consult with the participant's physician and recommend a more appropriate exercise setting for the participant.

Talk Test

The talk test is another subjective method of gauging exercise intensity and can be used as an adjunct to HR and RPE. When participants exercise, it is highly recommended that breathing be rhythmical and comfortable. Particularly for newer clientele, talking while exercising can indicate whether an appropriate intensity is being achieved. If the participant is "winded" and needs to gasp for breath between words when conversing, then the exercise intensity is too high and should be reduced. As higher-intensity activities are performed, it is expected that breathing rate will become faster and shallower. For higher fit-

ness levels, the use of the talk test may not be appropriate.

Application of Intensity Monitoring to the Group Exercise Setting

Whether using target HRs, RPE, dyspnea scale, or the talk test to monitor exercise intensity, there are a few practical application points to remember and share within a group exercise setting:

- If using music and measuring HR, turn off the music so the beats do not influence the counting of HRs.
- Peripheral pulses are encouraged over the use of the carotid pulse; if using the carotid pulse, press lightly.
- Check intensity toward the middle of the workout so it can be modified.
- Keep participants moving to prevent blood from pooling in the lower extremities when checking intensity.
- Utilize a 10-second pulse count if using target HRs.
- Give modifications based on results and encourage participants to work at individual levels.

Incorporate a Post-cardio Cool-down/Stretch Segment

The last few minutes of any group exercise session that contains cardiorespiratory work should be less intense, in order to allow the cardiorespiratory system to recover. Because metabolic waste products get trapped inside the muscle cells, many people experience increased cramping and stiffness if they do not cool down gradually. Cooling down enables waste products to disperse and the body to return to resting levels without injury. It is also important to cool down to prevent blood from pooling in the lower extremities and to allow the cardiovascular system to make the transition to more gradual workloads. This is especially important if some type of muscle work will follow the aerobic segment. Encourage participants to relax, slow down, keep arms below the level of the heart, and put less effort into the movements. Using less driving music, changing your tone of voice, and verbalizing the transition to the participants can create this atmosphere. Performing some static stretches at the end of this segment also works well. Participants often run off to their next commitment or go into the strength and conditioning area to perform muscle work, so they may risk missing the flexibility segment of the class if it is not put in this portion of the class format.

Muscular Strength and Endurance Segment

There are a few common principles in the muscular strength and endurance segment of most group exercise classes. They are listed below and will be reviewed in this segment.

As a group fitness instructor you should:

- Promote muscle balance and functional fitness
- Give verbal cues on posture/spinal alignment are given
- Give verbal, visual, and physical cues on posture/alignment and body mechanics
- Utilize equipment (toys) safely/effectively
- Create a motivational/instructional atmosphere

Encourage Muscle Balance and Functional Fitness

Meeting the muscular strength and endurance needs of participants in a one-on-one personal training setting is relatively easy. The program can be tailored directly to the participant, which gives personal trainers a distinct advantage. How, then, does a group fitness instructor determine what muscle groups to work and why during the muscular strength and endurance segment of the class format? Knowing how the body functions in daily movement can help focus on the appropriate exercise selection for muscle groups that are not normally used in the daily routine. Think of the group exercise class as an opportunity to balance out work from daily living. Stretching and strengthening muscles that are not regularly used can help participants attain improved muscle balance overall. This approach brings the group fitness instructor's role closer to that of individualized trainer (Kennedy, 1997). For a summary of what muscles need strengthening and stretching for improved health, see Table 5.20. This table was created by conceptualizing the muscles we use for routine living. For example, we normally pick things up using elbow flexion, which works the biceps concentrically (on the up phase). We then put things down working the biceps eccentrically (on the down phase) against gravity. Because of gravity, the triceps do not get worked a lot in daily living. In water exercise, however, the same example would produce a concentric contraction of the biceps on elbow flexion and a concentric contraction of the triceps on elbow extension due to the absence of gravity in the water. Keep in mind that the list in Table 5.20 is for functional daily living for the participants who are exercising for health and fitness. This does *not* mean the stronger muscles should not be worked in a group exercise setting; however, focus needs to be on balancing the use of weaker muscle groups and stronger muscle groups.

Verbal Cues

Since eight out of 10 Americans will have back problems during their lifetime, it is essential to teach verbal cues on posture/spinal alignment in each segment of the class and in every movement during the muscular strength and endurance segment. Here are some points to remember when teaching posture in a standing position. (The numbers below correspond to those in Figure 5.6.)

1. Head should be suspended (not pushed back or dropped forward) with ears in line with shoulders, shoulders over hips, hips over knees, and knees over ankles.

2. Arms should be suspended and hanging from the shoulder. Have participants cir-

cle the shoulder back and down. Arms should hang at the lowest point.

3. Maintain the three natural curves of the spine. A decrease or increase in the low-back curve changes the amount of compression the spine can withstand.

4. Lightly compress the abdominal muscles to help support the spinal column, especially with lifting. Compression helps to distribute weight over the entire torso, not just the low back. Extreme compression, however, restricts breathing.

5. Hips can be tucked slightly, particularly for swayback individuals, pregnant women, and participants with a large protruding abdominal area.

6. Knees should be unlocked or soft. Hyperextended knees shift the pelvis, contributing to an increased low-back curve and back strain, along with decreased blood flow to and from the legs.

Figure 5.6

Visual cues on posture/alignment

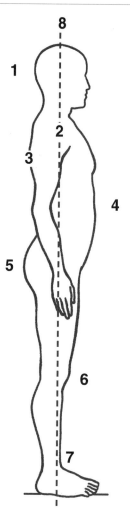

Table 5.20
Key Muscles

Muscles that need strengthening
- Anterior tibialis
- Hamstrings
- Rhomboids/middle trapezius
- Pectoralis minor/Lower trapezius
- Shoulder external rotators (teres minor and infraspinatus)
- Triceps
- Latissimus dorsi
- Gluteals
- Posterior deltoid

Stabilizers that need strengthening
- Erector spinae
- Abductors
- Adductors
- Abdominals

Muscles that need stretching
- Gastrocnemius
- Quadriceps/iliopsoas
- Upper trapezius
- Pectoralis major
- Hamstrings
- Sternocleidomastoid
- Anterior/medial deltoids

7. Feet should be a shoulder-width apart, weight evenly distributed. Participants who roll their feet to the inner or outer edges need to concentrate on keeping their weight over the entire bottom surface of each foot.

8. An imaginary plumb line dropped from the head should pass through the cervical and lumbar vertebrae, the hips, knees, and ankles.

Verbal, Visual, and Physical Cues on Posture/Alignment

Giving appropriate verbal, visual, and physical cues is one of the most important aspects of the muscular strength and endurance segment. As a general rule, in most exercises, the stabilizers will be engaged. Give several posture cues (chin up, chest out, tighten the abdominal muscles, etc.) before giving instruction on the specific muscle group to be worked. For example, when performing a latissimus dorsi strengthening exercise using exercise tubing, cue participants to soften the knees, get a good base of support with the feet apart comfortably, and contract the abdominals while keeping the spine in a neutral position. Then go on to cue the movement for the latissimus dorsi.

Looking closer at verbal, visual, and physical cues will help you understand that there is more than one way to communicate and direct movement. Verbal cues include cueing movements with appropriate terminology and instruction. For example, when performing a standing outer thigh leg lift to strengthen the gluteus medius, the following verbal cues could be included:

• Ask participants to contract the stabilizers.

• Give appropriate posture cues.

• Remind participants that the range of motion of the movement is around 45 degrees,

so lift with the side of the heel. If the toe comes up, that's hip flexion, and it works the quads/hip flexor muscles, which are already strong, so they want to take over. It is important to key into the muscle being worked for maximum effectiveness.

• Keep the movements slow and controlled and alternate sides to promote better participant comfort and balance.

Visual cues include the instructor's form. It is imperative that, when the verbal cues are given, you also perform the movement effectively. In the above example, if the instructor is saying to keep the movement at a 45-degree range of motion and the instructor is lifting higher than that, it is confusing to the participants. Whatever instructions are given need to be accentuated in the movement example by the instructor. Practice is one of the only ways to become good at being an effective visual demonstrator.

Physical cues are another way to give feedback to participants on their form. To give physical cues it is important to walk around the room and actually observe participants. A good motivator/educator rarely is at the front of the class, but moves around observing participants from different angles. Most physical cues in group exercises are given by the instructor for the participant to perform, since the instructor cannot help everyone at once. For example, when leading an abdominal curl-up exercise with the elbows behind the head, it is important to cue "elbows out to the side." If the participant can see their elbows, the pectorals are also being worked. Walk around to check on this and visually demonstrate proper alignment.

These are just a few ways to give feedback to participants on form. It is important to note what style of communication comes easier to them: verbal, visual, or physical.

Working on the area that is most difficult will help you improve. Giving and getting feedback is another important key to learning and growing. you who give a lot of feedback and ask participants for feedback on a regular basis are providing good customer service. It is important to practice student-centered learning as opposed to teacher-centered learning, especially in the area of verbal cues.

Utilize Equipment Safely/Effectively

Portable resistance-training equipment such as exercise bands, physioballs, hand-held weights, and weighted bars are to group exercise what toys are to children. They make the class more fun and provide the ability to overload the muscles in a more effective, individualized way. Some instructors actually refer to them as "toys" and the group exercise experience as "play." The most important part of having equipment is to make sure it is leveled for various abilities. Post information and tell participants to work at their own levels. Be sure to get information and education on any piece of equipment introduced. Many vendors advertise their product as the "best, most effective" device. Only instructors and participants can determine this. Analyze the need for extra equipment and be sure to test it properly before introducing it into the class. Keeping the muscular strength/endurance segment out of the aerobic portion is also important unless an interval/circuit style of class is being taught. Research has shown that the addition of light hand-held weights to the aerobic segment of a traditional hi/lo (Blessings et al., 1987; Yoke et al., 1988) and a step class (Kravitz, 1997) does not significantly increase energy expenditure. Therefore, it

is recommended that instructors do not use, nor instruct others to use, hand-held weights during the aerobic segment to enhance cardiorespiratory fitness.

Motivational/Instructional Atmosphere

It is optional to utilize music and/or the music beat during the muscular strength and endurance segment. For example, leading abdominal crunches to a musical tempo of 120 beats per minute would be fast. Always slow the tempo down to half tempo to gain control first. Then, go to the full musical tempo. Utilize music that does not have a lot of vocals so that cueing words can be heard and understood. Reduce the volume of the music and set a tone that is more focused than that of the aerobic segment. Outlined below are some general cues for muscular endurance exercises:

- Perform each exercise slowly, smoothly, and with control.
- Key into the muscle group being worked and try to relax other body parts.
- Stop when you feel tired or change to the other side or alternate sides as desired.
- Correct form is more important than the number of repetitions, keeping to the music tempo, or the amount of resistance used.
- Concentrate on breathing and work to exhale on the effort and inhale on the relaxation portion.

Flexibility Segment

There are a few common principles in the flexibility segment of most group exercise classes. They are listed below and will be reviewed in this segment.

- Stretching of major muscle groups is performed in a safe and effective manner.
- Relaxation/visualization concludes the flexibility segment.

Stretching

As mentioned earlier in this chapter, it is important to stretch the muscle groups that have been used in the group exercise activity as well as muscles that are commonly tight. For instance, after an indoor cycling class, stretching the quads, calves, and hamstrings makes sense since they are major muscles used for cycling. In a kickboxing session it is important to stretch the muscles that surround the hip since they are used in kicking movements. Keep in mind the stronger muscle groups we use all day for daily living activities (calves, hamstrings, pectorals, hip flexor, anterior deltoids). These should also be stretched.

How long should the stretches be held? Taylor (1990) suggests between 15 and 20 seconds, performing four sets. The ACSM guidelines (1998) suggest holding static stretches for 10 – 30 seconds and performing four repetitions per muscle group. It is not always possible to perform four repetitions. However, if leading a stretching-only class, this would be the ideal.

There are precautions for stretching. Ballistic (bouncing) stretching and passive overstretching can be potentially dangerous. Ballistic stretches have been shown by researchers to be significantly less effective than other stretching methods (Wallin, 1985). Passive overstretching and ballistic stretching initiate a stretch reflex. Special receptors within the muscle fiber detect sudden stretches (muscle spindles) and excessive stretching (golgi tendon organ) of the muscle. There is a complicated and continual interplay be-

tween opposing muscle groups that leads to precision of control and coordinated movement. During this interplay, if a muscle is activated by a sudden stretch *or* if continued overlengthening of the muscle fiber occurs, then the system stimulates the muscle to contract rather than lengthen and maintains the contraction to oppose the force of excessive lengthening. Simply put, if you overstretch or bounce and stretch, then the muscle shortens to protect itself. Keep pulling on a shortened muscle and it will either cramp up or rip and tear — but it will *not lengthen*. This process is often referred to as the myotatic stretch reflex. Keep in mind that this is an involuntary reflex that we do not have control over. It all happens at the spinal cord level and we cannot mentally override it no matter how hard we try.

Therefore, stretching should be comfortable. Encourage proper form by using cues like "move to the position where you can feel the muscle pull slightly, then hold; your muscles should not feel like a rubber band ready to snap; find a comfortable stretch and hold; if you are shaking, then back off the intensity of the stretch." Also, as an instructor it is important to model average flexibility so participants do not imitate form they cannot match. As with any other activity it is important to move participants ahead appropriately. Yoga is a good example of an activity that has many high-risk stretches. They are taught progressively, however, so the body adapts to them over time. Putting some of these yoga moves into a traditional group exercise setting can be dangerous.

Reminding participants of proper posture throughout stretching helps to promote overall body stability and balance and enhances the effectiveness of the stretching experience. At least two to three verbal cues are needed on every stretch to make sure body positioning is effective. For example, in a standing hamstring stretch (Figure 5.7) it is important to cue to tilt the pelvis anteriorly to lengthen the hamstring muscle. Sullivan et al. (1992) performed a study on anterior and posterior pelvic tilt positioning using two types of stretching techniques and found that the anterior pelvic position was the most important variable for enhancing hamstring flexibility.

Relaxation/Visualization

During a group exercise class, participants have been working hard, increasing the blood flow of nutrients and oxygen to the exercising muscles. Stiffness and muscular tension are now gone. As each minute of the class passes, anxieties, worries, and stressors of the day are released. Participants have now switched from logical and calculating functions to operating on spontaneity, with fluid thought. Many ideas come, but no one idea of concern stays in focus as the class moves on. The hardest part for participants is getting to an exercise class. When it is all over they usually feel good about coming. It is this feeling that keeps them coming back. They have taken time to care for themselves and thus taken another step toward healthier living. The relaxation/visualization segment is where you can help participants complete their journey. Take the last few minutes of every class to let participants experience a few moments of increased relaxation or reenergize before returning to their duties and commitments. These relaxation moments can be structured or free flowing, philosophical or quiet.

Silence or quiet, slow, soothing music might be enough. Storytelling, guided imagery, or creative visualization might help

Figure 5.7

Standing stretches

a. Low-back stretch: Round the low back by using the abdominal muscles to produce an extreme posterior tilt.

b. Hamstring stretch: Extend one leg and lean forward, using the hands for support.

c. Gastrocnemius stretch: Keep the rear foot straight and the heel on the ground. Shift the body weight forward over the front foot.

d. Soleus stretch: Shift the weight slightly to the back and bend the back knee.

e. Shoulder extensor stretch: From soleus stretch position bring clasped arms overhead and back.

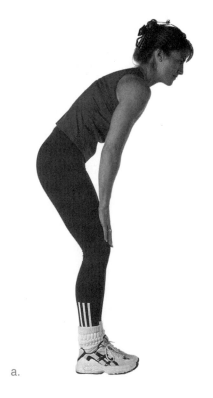

a.

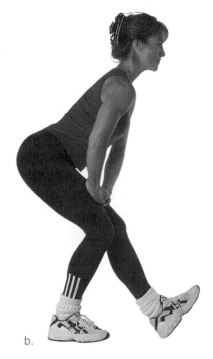

b.

deepen the sensation as you describe quiet forests, gentle breezes, a warm fire, or a cozy room. Starbursts, bright, intense sunlight, the power of a wave or waterfall might suggest the energy necessary to continue with the day's activities. Partner massage or group stories, deep breathing or progressively tightening and releasing muscle groups may help participants find any remaining tensions, areas of pain, or resistance to change. While the participants are receptive, use the time to compliment them on their hard work and reinforce their positive lifestyles or help them perform a mental exercise to increase their self-esteem and personal power. Consider reading inspirational quotes or poetry or announcements about upcoming events. Let the class in on your life outside of class to create a cohesive, family-like atmosphere. Instructors need to find a comfort area and use these last few minutes to end the exercise experience on a positive note, allowing participants to take their encounter past the allotted time.

Summary

Safe, effective, and purposeful class design requires a specific knowledge of fitness so that the appropriate overload is provided to help achieve the desired gains (see the class format summary checklist, below). Modify the different segments to meet the needs of the ever-changing fitness industry. It is important to know that group exercise carries with it a lot of power if participants feel welcome, are learning, get to know others, and feel that their time spent was worthwhile. One of the biggest challenges about being a group exercise leader is being able to balance all of these challenges. It is important that instructors move beyond emphasizing merely quantity

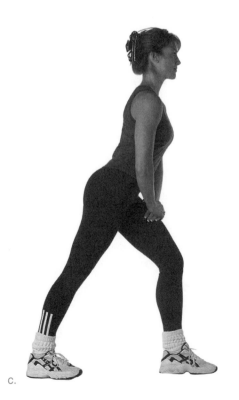

c.

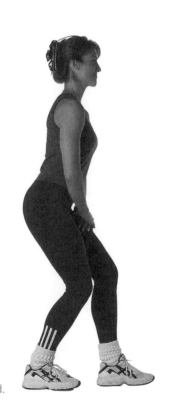

d.

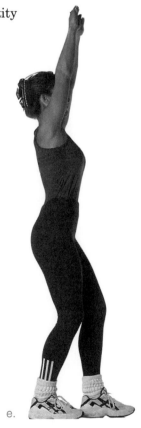

e.

fitness gains and future outcomes and understand that the real power of exercise lies in the experience itself.

Class Format Summary Checklist

Pre-class Preparation

- Knows participants' health histories and surveys new participants (see Chapter 4)
- Is available before class/orients new participants
- Discusses/models appropriate attire and footwear
- Has music cued up and equipment ready before class begins
- Acknowledges class and introduces self
- Previews class format and individual responsibilities
- Brings, and encourages, participants to bring water to classes

Warm-up Segment

- Is designed to "break a sweat"
- Focuses on rehearsal moves as a large part of the movement selection
- Includes stretches if appropriate after "breaking a sweat" and performing rehearsal movements
- Verbal directions are clear and volume and tempo of, and atmosphere created by, music are appropriate
- Instructor's form is appropriate and instructor observes participants' form and suggests adaptations for injuries/special needs

Cardiorespiratory Segment

- Promotes independence/self-responsibility
- Gradually increases intensity
- Gives impact and/or intensity options
- Builds sequences logically and progressively
- Utilizes a variety of muscle groups
- Uses music to create a motivational atmosphere

- Monitors intensity through HR and/or RPE checks
- Incorporates a post cardio cool-down/ stretch segment

Muscular Strength and Endurance Segment

- Muscle balance and functional fitness are encouraged
- Verbal cues on posture/spinal alignment are given
- Verbal, visual, and physical cues on posture and alignment and body mechanics are appropriate
- Utilizes equipment (toys) safely/effectively
- Creates a motivational/instructional atmosphere

Flexibility Segment

- Stretching of major muscle groups is performed in a safe and effective manner
- Relaxation/visualization concludes the flexibility segment

References

Alter, M. (1996). *Science of Flexibility.* Champaign, Ill.: Human Kinetics.

American College of Sports Medicine. (1998). *ACSM's Resource Manual for Guidelines for Exercise Testing and Prescription*, 3rd ed. Chapter 56: Specificity of exercise training and testing by Durstine and Davis, p. 476. Philadelphia: Williams and Wilkins.

American College of Sports Medicine. (1998). The Recommended quantity and quality of exercise for developing and maintaining cardiorespiratory and muscular fitness, and flexibility in healthy adults. *Medicine & Science in Sports & Exercise,* 30, 6, 975 – 991.

Astrand, P. & Rodahl, K. (1977). *Textbook of Work Physiology.* New York: McGraw-Hill.

Bain, L., Wilson, T., & Chaikind, E. (1989). Participant perceptions of exercise programs for overweight women. *Research Quarterly,* 60, 2, 134 – 143.

Blahnik, J. & Anderson, P. (1996). Wake up your warm up. *IDEA Today,* June 1996, 46 – 52.

Blessing, D., Wilson, D., Puckett, J., & Ford, H. (1987). The physiologic effects of eight weeks of aerobic dance with and without hand-held weights. *American Journal of Sports Medicine*, 15, 5, 508-510.

Borg, G. (1982). Psychophysical bases of perceived exertion. *Medicine & Science in Sports & Exercise*, 14, 377 – 381.

Boutche, S. & Trenske, M. (1990).The effects of sensory deprivation and music on perceived exertion and affect during exercise. *Journal of Sport & Exercise Psychology*, 12, 167 – 76.

Crawford, S. & Eklund, R. (1994). Social physique anxiety, reasons for exercise, and attitudes toward exercise settings. *Journal of Sport & Exercise Psychology*, 16, 70 – 82.

Dunbar, C., Robertson, R., Baun, R., Blandin, M., Metz, K., Burdett, R., & Goss, F. (1992). The validity of regulating exercise intensity by ratings of perceived exertion. *Medicine & Science in Sports & Exercise* 24, 1, 94 – 99.

Evans, E. & Kennedy, C. (1993). The body image problem in the fitness industry. *IDEA Today*, May, 50 – 56.

Frangolias, D. & Rhodes, E. (1995). Maximal and ventilatory threshold responses to treadmill and water immersion running. *Medicine & Science in Sports & Exercise*, 27, 7, 1007 – 1013.

Gfeller, K. (1988). Musical components and styles preferred by young adults for aerobic fitness activities. *Journal of Music Therapy*, 25, 28 – 43.

Girouard, C. & Hurley, B. (1995). Does strength training inhibit gains in range of motion from flexibility training in older adults? *Medicine & Science in Sports & Exercise*, 27, 10, 1444 – 1449.

Golding, L., Meyers, C., & Sinning W. (1986). *The Y's Way to Physical Fitness,* 3rd ed. Champaign, Ill: Human Kinetics.

Goleman, D. (1998). *Working with Emotional Intelligence.* New York: Bantam Books.

IDEA. (1997). Recommendations for music volume in fitness classes. *IDEA Today*, June 1997, p. 50.

Kennedy, C. (1997). Exercise analysis, *IDEA Today*, January 1997, 70 – 73.

Kravitz, L., Heyward, V., Stolarczyk, L., & Wilmerding, V. (1997). Does step exercise with handweights enhance training effects? *Journal of Strength & Conditioning Research*, 11, 3, 194 – 199.

Kravitz, L. (1994). The effects of music on exercise. *IDEA Today,* October 1994, 56 – 61.

McLean, K. & Skinner, J. (1992). Validity of FUTREX-5000 for body composition determination. *Medicine & Science in Sports & Exercise*, 24, 253 – 258.

Nardini, M., Raglin, J., & Kennedy, C. (1999). Body image disordered eating. Obligatory exercise and body composition among women fitness instructors. *Medicine & Science in Sports & Exercise*, May 1999 (abstract).

Parker, S., Hurley, B., Hanlon, D., & Vaccaro, P. (1989). Failure of target heart rate to accurately monitor intensity during aerobic dance. *Medicine & Science in Sports & Exercise*, 21, 2, 230 – 234.

Pate et al. (1995). Physical activity and public health: A recommendation from the Centers for Disease Control and Prevention and the American College of Sports Medicine. *Journal of the American Medical Association*, 273, 5, 402 – 407.

Roach, B., Croisant, P., & Emmett J. (1994). The appropriateness of heart rate and RPE measures of intensity during three variations of aerobic dance. *Medicine & Science in Sports & Exercise*, 26, 5, (Supplement) (Abstract #24).

Robertson, R., Goss, F., Auble, T., Cassinelli, D., Spina, R., Glickman, E., Galbreath, R., Silberman, R., & Metz, K. (1990). Cross-modal exercise prescription at absolute and relative oxygen uptake using perceived exertion. *Medicine & Science in Sports & Exercise*, 22, 5, 653 – 659.

Rozenek, R. & Storer, T. (1997). Client assessment tools for the personal fitness trainer. *Journal Strength & Conditioning*, 52 – 63.

Shellock, F. (1983). Physiological benefits of warm-up. *Physician & Sportsmedicine*, 11, 134-39.

Staum, M. (1983). Music and rhythmic stimuli in the rehabilitation of gait disorders. *Journal of Music Therapy*, 20, 69 – 87.

Sullivan, M., Dejulia, J., & Worrell, T. (1992). Effect of pelvic position and stretching method on hamstring muscle flexibility. *Medicine & Science in Sports & Exercise* 24, 12, 1383 – 1389.

Taylor, D., Dalton, J., Seaber, A., & Garrett, W. (1990). Viscoelastic properties of muscle-tendon units: the biomechanical effects of stretching. *American Journal of Sports Medicine*, 18, 300 – 309.

Wallin, D., Ekblom, B., Grahn, R., & Nordenborg, T. (1985). Improvement of muscle flexibility. A comparison between two techniques. *American Journal of Sports Medicine*, 13, 4, 263 – 268.

Walter, J., Figoni, F., & Andres, F. (1995). Effect of stretching intensity and duration on hamstring flexibility. *Medicine & Science in Sports & Exercise*, 27, 5, Supplement S240.

Westcott, W. (1991). Role-model instructors, *Fitness Management*, March, 48 – 50.

YMCA. (2000). *YMCA Fitness Testing and Assessment Manual*. Champagne, Ill.: Human Kinetics.

Yoke, M., Otto, R., Wygand, J., & Kamimukai, C. (1988). The metabolic cost of two differing low impact aerobic dance exercise modes. *Medicine & Science in Sports & Exercise*, 20, 2, (Supplement) (Abstract #527).

Suggested Reading

American College of Sports Medicine. (1998). A*CSM's Resource Manual for Guidelines for Exercise Testing & Prescription*, 3rd ed. Philadelphia: Williams & Wilkins.

American Council on Exercise. (1996). *Personal Trainer Manual*. San Diego: ACE.

Getchell, B., Mikesky, A., & Mikesky, K. (1998). *Physical Fitness: A Way of Life*. Boston: Allyn and Bacon.

Howle, E. & Franks, B. (1997). *Health Fitness Instructor's Handbook*. Champaign, Ill: Human Kinetics.

Jordan, P. (1997). *Fitness Theory and Practice*. Sherman Oaks, Calif: Aerobics and Fitness Association of America, p. 5 – 30.

Kennedy, C. & Yoke, M. (2000). *Exercise Leadership*. Champaign, Ill: Sagamore Publishing.

Neiman, D. (1999). *Exercise Testing and Prescription*, 4th ed. Mountain View, Calif.: Mayfield Publishing.

McArdle, W., Katch, F., & Katch, V. (1996). *Exercise Physiology*, 4th ed. Philadelphia: Williams and Wilkins.

Chapter 6

In This Chapter:

Lorna Francis, Ph.D., previously a physical education professor at San Diego State University, is an internationally recognized speaker and the author of several fitness books. An ACE-certified instructor, Dr. Francis is an emeritus member of ACE's board of directors and was co-recipient of the 1989 IDEA Lifetime Achievement award.

Richard J. Seibert, M.A., M.Ed., is a fitness industry consultant and ACE-certified group fitness instructor, is an internationally recognized speaker and author specializing in instructor training, contributed toward the development and delivery of ACE's Practical Training Program, and has served on ACE's professional development committee.

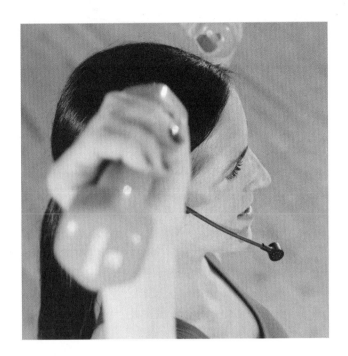

Teaching a
Group Exercise Class

By Lorna L. Francis and Richard J. Seibert

Each year more than 8 million people participate in some form of group exercise class. They go to indoor cycling, water aerobics, cardio kickboxing, yoga, and many other forms of group exercise. In every one of these situations, they rely on a group fitness instructor to help them learn and perform the necessary movements to be successful. The success of the class depends on the instructor's ability to apply sound instructional principles and practices. In fact, effective teaching may well be the most important aspect of the group fitness instructor's role. Inadequate leadership is often cited by participants as a reason for dropping out of formal exercise programs.

Unfortunately, many people believe that teaching is intuitive and spontaneous. However, an intuitive and spontaneous approach to teaching often results in ineffective leadership. Over the years, researchers have provided valuable information to help instructors effectively plan and implement their programs. Scientific investigation of teaching techniques has led to an under-standing of the phenomenon of teaching and its impact on learning behavior. More importantly, when followed, teaching tech-niques provide the instructor with the necessary means to transfer their fitness knowledge, skill, and enthusiasm to their exercise participants. The purpose of this chapter is to provide you with a sound teaching foundation by exploring the ele-ments of effective teaching and how they apply to a group fitness setting.

Systematic Class Design

Instructors need to follow a simple sys-tem in order to target the correct audi-ence, design an effective class, and teach the correct exercises. The system works well in the correct order of applica-tion, and, conversely, can be disastrous when the instructor reverses the order of application. In order to teach the right class to the right set of participants, you must first understand the exercise partici-pants. Next, the overall goals and objec-tives of the class should be determined to aid in exercise selection. After the class is over, you must determine the quality of the class. More specifically, you must eval-uate how well the students met the goals and objectives of the class.

By reversing the order of application, you may design the class around a set or style of movements. This method of class design can discourage class participation except for those few participants who hap-pen to be successful with the movements. In this way, you are determining the class through the selection of movements rather than determining the movements based on the class.

Understanding the Exercise Participant

Many instructors do not appreciate the complexity of the process required to learn a new exercise or movement pattern. In a matter of seconds, the student must perceive and react to the proper cues, remember similar situations and instruction on what to do, determine the proper strategy and make the correct response, and, finally, through feedback, determine whether he or she performed the exercise correctly. This section exam-ines the learning process and describes learning strategies that will facilitate the teaching of motor skills.

Magill (1980) defines learning as an "in-ternal change in the individual that is in-ferred from a relatively permanent improve-ment in performance of the individual as a result of practice." Instructors can therefore infer that learning has occurred when a person's performance shows less variability over time.

Learning takes place in three domains of human behavior: cognitive, affective, and mo-tor. All three domains are important in the fitness field.

The **cognitive domain** describes intellec-tual activities and involves gaining knowl-edge. Studies have shown that education within an exercise program positively affects motivation and exercise compliance. There-fore, competent instructors should remain up-to-date on the latest research in exercise and related fields in an effort to inform their students and to respond intelligently to their questions or concerns.

The **affective domain** describes emotional behaviors. Motivation to exercise depends on a person's feelings about exercise. Instructors are therefore instrumental in helping participants develop positive attitudes toward exercise.

Finally, the **motor domain** refers to those activities requiring movement. Learning motor skills is the foundation of exercise classes.

Within the fitness profession, the motor domain has been heavily emphasized and limited attention has been given to the affective and cognitive domains. However, research has shown that teaching within all three domains is critical to exercise compliance.

Stages of Learning

To teach effectively, you must be aware of the various stages of learning. One of the most commonly cited learning models was developed by Fitts and Posner (1967), who theorized that there are three stages of learning for a motor skill: cognitive, associative, and autonomous. Within the **cognitive stage of learning**, learners make many errors and have highly variable performances. They know they are doing something wrong, but they do not know how to improve their performance. At this stage, participants seem terribly uncoordinated and consistently perform exercises incorrectly. Those in the **associative stage of learning** have learned the basic fundamentals or mechanics of the skill. Their errors, tend to be less gross in nature and they can now concentrate on refining their skills. During this stage, exercise participants are able to detect some errors, and the instructor needs to make only occasional corrections. During the **autonomous stage of learning** the skill becomes automatic or habitual. Learners can now perform without thinking and can detect their own errors. Driving a car, for example, is a very com-

plex motor skill that over time is performed in the autonomous stage. The driver often is concentrating elsewhere and is able to recognize when mistakes are made.

The type and amount of information that exercise participants can understand depend on their current stage within the learning process. Beginning aerobic exercisers may be concentrating fully on performing the skill correctly. They may forget to perform even the most basic tasks, like breathing regularly or watching out for obstacles. Because beginners are less skilled at determining what information they must attend to, you must provide them with specific information about what is important. For example, since maintaining appropriate posture is necessary to properly execute many exercises and movement patterns, you must constantly remind beginners to maintain correct exercise posture. Advanced aerobic exercisers are more likely to understand and respond to fine motor skill adjustments. For example, relaxing a grip or contracting an antagonist muscle group has more meaning to an advanced exerciser. However, advanced participants may require more information when a routine or sequence has changed from a habitual pattern. To employ appropriate teaching strategies, you must be aware of each participant's stage of learning.

The following instructor guidelines will facilitate the movement of the exercise participants from the beginner level to the advanced level.

1. *Enhance motivation to learn.* Wlodkowski (1984) describes how a motivated learner will surpass a nonmotivated learner in performance and outcome. Without motivation there is little effort and participation. Simply stated, instructors need to

develop classes that strongly appeal to their participants. Avoid the pitfall of developing classes that have greater appeal to themselves than to their participants.

2. *Progress gradually from simple to complex.* It is important to ensure that exercise participants master movements and movement patterns in their simplest forms before moving on to complex movements. For example, if a participant is displaying poor posture and form during standing lunges, it would be ill advised to move on to standing lunges utilizing additional resistance.

3. *Offer feedback:* Participants tend to view corrective feedback as informative rather than critical, especially when they can use the feedback to improve performance. Feedback that focuses on successes and errors evenly can help move the participants into an advanced stage in which they can monitor their own performance. A more thorough discussion of feedback is provided at the end of this chapter.

Participant Needs

Many group fitness classes are composed of participants with varying levels of fitness and skill. In smaller communities, special populations, such as pregnant, obese, or people with disabilities, are mainstreamed into regular group fitness classes. This state of affairs presents a challenging teaching environment for instructors. To effectively plan a group exercise class, it is important that you first be familiar with the health history and fitness level of each class participant. Having this information will help

you develop modifications to the exercise plan that can reduce a participant's risk of developing health complications during exercise. For example, participants with a history of high blood pressure should be reminded not to perform static strength exercises and to avoid holding the arms at or above shoulder level for an extended period of time. A pregnant woman should be advised not to perform exercises on her back after the fourth month of pregnancy. Mainstreaming special populations can be done as long as these individuals are apprised of specific exercise modifications and are periodically reminded of those modifications during the class session. For more information on modifying exercise for special populations see Chapter 8.

Designing Instruction

Establishing Class Goals

The effective use of goal-setting facilitates both learning and performance of motor skills. The competent group fitness instructor establishes **program goals** and aids participants in developing their personal goals. Program goals should reflect what you expect students to gain from the program. Examples of program goals might include the following:

1. The participant will maintain adequate aerobic fitness, or increase it, in order to acquire cardiorespiratory health benefits.

2. The participant will maintain adequate and specific joint range of motion, or increase it, in order to prevent muscle imbalances and to provide appropriate range of motion for exercise movements.

3. The participant will maintain adequate and specific muscular strength, or in-

crease it, in order to prevent muscle imbalances and to provide adequate strength to effectively perform exercise movements.

Lesson Planning

Planning and class preparation result in the efficient use of time, smooth progression of activities, and greater program variety. Often instructors who do not plan their lessons present the same music, exercises, and movement patterns day in and day out. Participants and instructors alike become bored with this daily routine.

It is particularly important that inexperienced instructors write out their daily class activities. While experienced instructors may no longer need to write a daily lesson plan, they should at least spend time before each class mentally preparing class activities. A daily lesson plan should consist of class objectives, planned activities and the time allotted for each activity, necessary equipment, and patterns of class organization. Figure 6.1 contains a sample lesson plan that can be modified to meet the needs of individual instructors and the objectives of specific classes.

Class Objectives

Just as group fitness instructors need to establish program goals, they also need to develop more specific objectives for each class meeting. **Class objectives** state what you expect your participants to accomplish during each exercise session. The following are examples of class objectives:

1. The participant will maintain or increase **cardiorespiratory fitness** by exercising aerobically for 15 to 30 minutes at an intensity of 50% to 75% maximal heartrate reserve.

2. The participant will increase or maintain adequate and specific flexibility by performing the following stretching exercises to their fullest range of motion: hamstrings, quadriceps, and so on.

3. The participant will increase or maintain adequate and specific strength and endurance by performing eight to 12 repetitions of the following exercises: curl-ups, prone shoulder and hip extensions, and so on.

Objectives help you focus on the purpose of each selected exercise and activity. In fact, novice instructors should list the purpose of each strength and flexibility exercise used in their classes. Knowing the purpose and benefits of each exercise will help you select appropriate class activities.

Class Activities and Time Allocations

Class activities are planned to meet the objectives of each component part of an aerobics class. Component parts of a class include:

1. Warm-up and prestretch
2. Aerobic conditioning
3. Aerobic cool-down
4. Resistance training
5. Post stretch

Strength and flexibility exercises should be carefully planned. Specific stretching and resistance training exercises are discussed in Chapter 2. The selection of music and movement patterns for the warm-up, aerobic conditioning, and cool-down segments of the class is one of your most challenging tasks. This very important activity is addressed in greater detail later in this chapter.

The time allotted for each activity varies according to the total class time available and according to the specific nature of the

Figure 6.1
Sample Lesson Plan

Class: Aerobic Exercise   **Date:**   **Time:** 9 – 10:15 a.m.

Class Objectives:

1. Participants will improve or maintain cardiorespiratory fitness by performing aerobics movements for 15 to 25 minutes at 50 to 75 percent HR reserve.

2. Participants will improve or maintain flexibility by performing specific stretching exercises, holding for 10 seconds at maximum range of motion.

3. Participants will improve or maintain strength by performing specific strength exercises for three sets of 12 repetitions.

Activities	Time (minutes)	Patterns of Class Org.	Equipment	Music	Comments
Warm-up	5	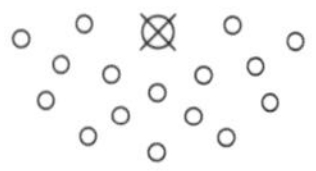		Will vary according to season, age group and participant interest. 120 – 140 bpm	Slow and controlled rehearsal
Preaerobic stretch (*Pectoralis major, hamstrings, hip flexors, erector spinae, quads, gastrocnemius*)	5	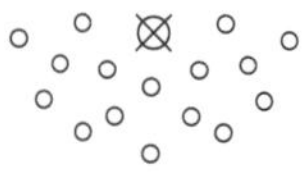		120 – 140 bpm	Utilize active stretching rather than deep static stretching
Aerobic exercise (*Freestyle technique using a linear progression*)	25	(same as above)		120 – 140 bpm	Take ExHR. Check ExHRs with a show of hands
Cool-down	4	(same as above)		120 – 140 bpm	Take recovery HR
Muscle strengthening (*Curl-ups, toe-raises, prone hip extension, tricep extension, scapulae adduction*)	20	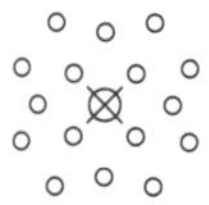	Mats, rubber bands	110 – 130 bpm	Slow and controlled; breathe on exertion
Postaerobic stretch (*Same muscle groups as preaerobic stretch*)	10	(same as above)	Towels	100 bpm	Stretch to the point of tightness, not pain
Final note	1				Give praise/ encouragement

bpm = beats per minute; HR = heart rate

activity. Some activities will naturally require more time than others. Minimum and maximum time requirements for the warm-up, aerobics, and cool-down segments are discussed in Chapter 5. The time allotted for stretching and strengthening depends on the number of exercises to be performed.

Beginning and ending class on time is also important. Instructors who methodically plan their lessons will know the precise length of time for each activity. However, since unforeseen events, such as a tape deck malfunction, do occur, the competent instructor needs to be flexible and able to improvise at the last minute if necessary.

Patterns of Class Organization

Group fitness classes should be arranged to ensure the safety of participants and to enable everyone to hear the instructions and see the demonstrations. Patterns of class organization refer to the formations used by instructors to provide their students with maximum opportunities for learning and performing. In a typical group fitness class formation, the instructor stands at the front of the room and participants face him or her. While this formation can be effective, it has one major disadvantage. Usually the enthusiastic, experienced participants stand in the front of the room while the less experienced stay in the back. The result is a potentially unsafe situation, because it is difficult for an instructor to observe those in the back of the room. To resolve this problem, you can periodically move from the front to the sides and to the back of the class, asking participants to turn and face you in each new position. It is further recommended that you keep the level of complexity low when turning the class toward the back. The back row is likely to feel uncomfortable with the rest of the class behind them.

It is common for group indoor cycling classes to be laid out in a circular or horseshoe pattern. The instructor is at one end of the room and participants form a single or double circle around them. Group fitness instructors using this formation should change their point of focus to observe each person in class.

Facility and Equipment Considerations

Not all instructors can choose the facility in which they teach. Ideally the exercise facility should have the following:

1. Good ventilation, with a temperature range of 60 to 70° F.

2. A floor that will effectively absorb shock and will control undesirable medial-lateral motions of the foot. A hardwood sprung floor is ideal.

3. Sufficient space for each student to move comfortably (with arms outspread, each participant should be able to take two large steps in any direction without touching another student).

4. Mirrors for participants to observe their own exercise positions and postures.

5. In large classes, a raised platform for the instructor.

6. Access to drinking water.

Equipment needs include music tapes, tape deck and speakers, microphone, mats, and some form of resistance-training equipment, such as weights, pads and gloves, tubes, or rubber bands. Equipment for additional activities, such as circuit training, might include balls, hoops, jump ropes, and steps.

Always arrive early to check that all equipment is in working order before class begins. Class time should never be spent cueing tapes or searching for equipment.

One of the most important pieces of aerobics equipment is the sound system. Although instructors rarely have the opportunity to select the sound system, they should be familiar with the basic features of the equipment they are using. Before you begin your classes, always check the proper setting of the volume, bass, treble, and pitch controls. According to Price (1990), audiologists recommend that group fitness instructors keep their music volume under 85 decibels (normal conversation ranges from 60 to 70 decibels, an alarm clock ringing 2 feet away is about 80, a chainsaw is 100, while a jet plane takeoff is around 120). The Occupational Safety and Health Administration (OSHA), which regulates noise standards for workers, states that ear protection must be provided for workers if noise level on the job averages 90 decibels over an eight-hour period. Extended exposure to sound levels at 85 to 90 decibels and above can eventually damage a person's hearing. Instructors who use loud music are not only at risk of damaging their own hearing and that of their participants, but they are also much more likely to suffer from voice injury, as they find themselves having to shout over loud music.

In addition to keeping the music volume at an appropriate level to protect the hearing of class participants, audiologists recommend that instructors turn up the bass and lower the treble, since high frequencies can be more damaging than low frequencies (Price, 1990). A higher bass setting can also be beneficial for class participants who have difficulty hearing the underlying beat. If a tape deck has pitch control (a feature that allows you to speed up or slow down the music tempo), it should be checked for proper positioning before class begins (the center position usually indicates normal speed). Nothing is more frustrating for an instructor than to begin a class and find that the music is much slower or faster than anticipated. Instructors should attempt to minimize the use of the pitch control, because extreme changes in the speed of the music distort the sound. If you find yourself constantly pitching the music speed up, you might want to consider selecting music that is performed at a faster tempo.

Selecting Appropriate Exercises

An effective group fitness instructor must develop skills to determine which exercises and movement patterns are effective and safe to use in the exercise class. A thorough knowledge of exercise science is essential in this decision-making process. An **exercise evaluation** must be done for each movement pattern to determine its effectiveness and safety. To determine exercise effectiveness, ask yourself, "Does this particular exercise do what it is supposed to do?" In other words, what is the purpose of the exercise and does it meet the intended objective? When considering stretching exercises, you must ask, "Does this particular exercise effectively stretch the muscle(s) it is supposed to stretch?"

For example, while it is possible to stretch the erector spinae and hamstrings using a straight-legged sitting toe-touch exercise, class participants with tight erector spinae or tight hamstrings may be unable to put sufficient stretch on the targeted muscles. Compound stretches, where several major muscle groups are being stretched at the same time, do not isolate a specific muscle or muscle group. Therefore, two different stretches might be used: one that targets the hamstrings and one that targets the erector spinae.

When considering the effectiveness of strength exercises, you must ask, "Does this exercise strengthen the intended muscle(s)?" Some group fitness instructors are confused about the direction in which the resistance is being applied when evaluating certain strength exercises, and consequently they tend to teach exercises that do not target the intended muscle group. For example, holding a rubber band in the right hand above the head while pulling the band down toward the hips with the left hand (lat pull-down), will help to strengthen the latissimus dorsi. However, performing this same movement with a hand-held weight will strengthen the deltoids. Knowledge of muscles and their actions and an understanding of the direction in which the resistance is being exerted is valuable in helping you select effective strength exercises.

If an exercise does not fulfill your objective, it should not be selected for inclusion in the group fitness class. If an exercise is determined to be effective, you must then decide if it is safe. "Does the selected exercise cause pain in the joints or does it put unnecessary stress on other vulnerable parts of the body?" For example, while unsupported, sustained forward flexion in a standing position is often used to stretch the hamstrings, this particular position can be hazardous to the lumbar spine. Therefore, a safer alternative for stretching the hamstrings should be considered. While in many instances you will probably choose to reject an exercise that is determined to be unsafe or contraindicated, there are times when the benefits of an exercise outweigh the risks. For example, to effectively stretch the quadriceps it is necessary to apply an external force to move the heel of the foot toward the buttocks. This position can be mechanically stressful to vulnerable structures of the knee. However, if the exercise is performed with care, the benefits often outweigh the risk for participants with healthy knees.

Your ability to evaluate the effectiveness and safety of exercises will improve as you learn more about the functional anatomy of the human body and the many factors that can affect efficient human movement.

You must also be familiar with the specific mechanics of each exercise. For example, when using rubber bands, there is a natural tendency to hyperextend the wrist joints when flexing and extending the elbow joint (this gives the exerciser a mechanical advantage). Since wrist hyper-

extension puts considerable stress on the tendons that cross the wrist joint, class participants must be frequently reminded to maintain a neutral wrist position. Careful attention must be given to avoid shoulder impingement. This condition can occur when class participants repeatedly use lateral movements of the arms above shoulder level with the palms facing downward (with or without weights). Students must be encouraged to turn the palms upward as the arms are raised above shoulder level. When performing lunging or squatting exercises, it is advisable that the load-bearing knees are not flexed deeper than 90 degrees. Squatting beyond 90 degrees places high levels of compression stress on the back of the kneecaps.

These are but a few examples of common technique errors performed by exercise participants. To effectively teach and correct exercises, you must have a good understanding of sound mechanics for every exercise you select.

Selecting Appropriate Teaching Techniques

To become proficient at teaching group exercise, you must be familiar with methods for selecting appropriate exercises and movement patterns, analyzing exercise skills, and modifying exercise for various fitness levels and special populations. You must also be knowledgeable concerning techniques for increasing participant motivation and exercise adherence (see Chapter 7). The following section addresses these important teaching strategies.

Teaching Styles

The teaching style chosen is an important factor in determining the your success in effectively presenting class activities. You should be familiar with a variety of teaching styles. Mosston (1981) has identified eight specific teaching styles. Each accomplishes a different set of objectives, and it is both possible and desirable to use several styles in an aerobics class. The five styles directly applicable to an exercise class are command, practice, reciprocal, self-check, and inclusion. Each style is described and discussed in terms of its practical application to aerobic exercise.

An instructor using the **command style of teaching** makes all decisions about posture, **rhythm**, and duration, while participants follow his or her directions and movements. This style is most appropriate when instructors want to achieve the following objectives:

- Immediate participant response
- Participant emulation of instructor as role model
- Participant control
- Safety
- Avoidance of alternatives and choices
- Efficient use of time
- Perpetuation of aesthetic standards

The command style has been perhaps the most commonly used style in group fitness classes. While this style is particularly suited to warming up, cooling down, and learning new routines and exercises, it leaves no room for individualization. The participant has little say in decisions about personal physical development and few opportunities exist for social interaction. To achieve these objectives, an instructor must rely on other teaching styles.

The **practice style of teaching** provides opportunities for individualization and includes practice time and private instructor feedback for each participant. While all exercisers are working on the same task, individual

participants can choose their own pace and rhythm. The practice style is particularly suited for classes where the fitness level of participants varies greatly. Using this style, instructors can encourage students to perform the maximum repetitions suitable to their skill or fitness level. The real key is that once instructors determine the task, such as curl-ups, they are free to move around and give individual feedback where necessary. A disadvantage to this style is that not all participants are sufficiently motivated to achieve their maximum potential.

The **reciprocal style of teaching** involves the use of an observer or a partner to provide feedback to each participant. This style enables everyone to receive individual feedback, an often impossible task for the instructor. The reciprocal style can best be used for fitness assessment. For example, tests evaluating posture, girth measurements, strength, and flexibility can be quickly administered by partners. Using a criteria card that describes the test, the criteria for passing, and the performance level achieved allows students to monitor their own progress. A sample criteria card is presented in Figure 6.2. Aside from providing the participant with important feedback, the reciprocal style encourages social interaction, which is one reason people choose to participate in organized exercise programs. One major disadvantage of this style is that the observer or partner may not provide appropriate feedback.

The **self-check style of teaching** relies on participants to provide their own feedback. Participants perform a given task and then record the results, comparing their performance against given criteria or past performances. This style lends itself nicely to the recording of **target heart rate**, **recovery heart rate**, and number of floor-exercise rep-

Figure 6.2
Sample criteria card

Name_____

Test	Passing Criteria	Performance Level		
		1	2	3
		Date: _____	_____	_____
Flexibility *Hamstrings**	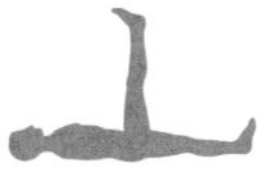 Leg raised to vertical	_____	_____	_____
*Quads**	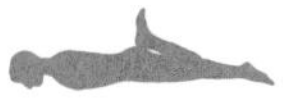 Heel touching buttocks	_____	_____	_____
Strength *Sit-ups (1 min)*	Males Age <35 35-44 >45 45+ 40+ 25+	_____	_____	_____
	Females Age <35 35-44 >45 40+ 30+ 15+	_____	_____	_____
Cardiovascular *3-min step test HR*	Males Females <105 <116	_____	_____	_____
Body Composition *Percentage body fat*	Males Females <19% <26%	_____	_____	_____

*Draw the leg position of the exerciser being tested.

etitions. Instructors must provide a record card for each participant. A sample record card is presented in Figure 6.3. Because a key component of motivation and exercise compliance is self-monitoring of progress, it is desirable to incorporate the self-check style into every exercise program.

The **inclusion style of teaching** enables multiple levels of performance to be taught within the same activity. Perhaps one of the most significant problems facing the group fitness industry is teaching multiple skill and fitness levels in the same class. Skill and fitness level can vary in each segment of the exercise class, including stretching, strengthening, and aerobic work. Class should be designed to incorporate all levels so that each person can achieve maximum success. During the stretching and strengthening segments of the program, the instructor can offer alternate positions for the different levels. For example, during abdominal work the participant with weak abdominal muscles can choose to do pelvic tilts, while the person with stronger abdominals can perform curl-ups. The instructor can also offer different levels of difficulty during the aerobic segment. For example, beginners to kickboxing

Figure 6.3

Sample
record card

Name_____   Date_____

Resting Heart Rate_____   Target HR Zone _____ to _____

Activity	
Aerobic exercise HR	158
Aerobic exercise recovery HR	118
Curl-ups (Body weight)	20-20-20 (3 sets of 20 reps)
Leg lifts (5 lbs)	12-12-10
Shins (rubber bands)	12-10-10

can perform front kicks while the more advanced participants can perform front kicks followed by blocks and punches. Instructors periodically need to demonstrate each level of movement, spending more time on the patterns for beginners.

Teaching Strategies

When teaching an exercise or movement pattern, you should determine which teaching approach will be most effective. You can use the following strategies separately or in **combinations**. You should also use redundancy to help the participants learn the movements more deeply.

Slow-to-fast

The **slow-to-fast teaching strategy** allows participants to learn complex movement at a slower pace. Also known as rhythmic variation, this technique emphasizes the proper configuration of a movement pattern. For example, if you were teaching a box step (left foot forward, right foot across left foot, left foot backward, right foot to the right), instead of performing individual steps on each beat of the music, 2 counts would be taken for each foot placement, thus taking 8 counts to complete the move-

ment pattern. The amount of time taken to perform the movement is increased so that the entire skill can be taught in sequence. Once participants have learned to perform the movement correctly, they can perform the movement on the beat. Because this strategy may reduce **exercise intensity**, you should refrain from using this strategy for extended periods of time during the peak of the aerobic segment of class.

Repetition Reduction

The **repetition reduction teaching strategy** involves reducing the number of repetitions that make up a movement sequence. It is used for a movement pattern that has two or more distinguishable parts. For example, if you wanted to use a combination of one jumping jack and two alternating punches, he or she might begin the sequence with four jumping jacks and eight alternating punches, reducing the movement pattern to two jumping jacks and four alternating punches, finishing with one jumping jack and two alternating punches. This technique allows participants to master each movement within a sequence. It should be noted that in the example above, the number of music beats for the jumping jacks equals the number of beats needed to perform the punches. In this way, the movement fits smoothly into music written in 8 count phrases.

Spatial

The **spatial teaching strategy** is commonly used when introducing participants to a new body position. During the strength-training segment of the class, begin each new exercise by reviewing the proper alignment. You might say, "Begin with your feet about shoulder width apart, knees slightly bent, spine straight with supportive abdominals, hands hold the dumbbells with the palms facing the body, elbows slightly bent, shoulders down, and head looking straight ahead." Note that the direction of alignment cues was given in a toe-to-head direction in order to prepare the class for a lateral dumbbell raise. The same cues can be offered in a head-to-toe sequence.

Part-to-whole

The **part-to-whole teaching strategy** breaks a skill down into its component parts and each part is practiced. You should teach each part in its simplest form. Once participants have mastered each component, they can be placed in proper sequence. When breaking movements down into parts, it is important to note any critical or advanced components. For example, a movement pattern may require pivoting on one or both feet. In this case, you should make sure that the class can perform the pivot safely before adding the pivot into the movement pattern. The simplest way of using the part-to-whole teaching strategy is the "add on method." After introducing a movement pattern, "A," a new part is practiced and then added to make "A + B." After movement pattern "A + B" is

mastered, a new movement, "C," is practiced and then added to the existing pattern to make "A + B + C." Additional parts are added to make a sequence of movements patterns.

Simple-to-complex

The **simple-to-complex teaching strategy** treats a sequence of movement patterns as a whole, with small changes occurring at the pace of the class. Using this advanced strategy, small amounts of complexity are added to a simple movement combination in order to slowly challenge the exercise participants. As an example, a movement pattern, "A + B," is introduced in its simplest form. Movement "A" is 16 counts of abdominal curls, and movement "B" is 16 counts of alternating oblique curls. Movements "A + B" are repeated until the entire class can perform them correctly. Movement "A" is then made more complex by adding a rhythmic variation to it of 1 count up and 3 counts down. This 16 count variation of "A" is followed the original 16 "B" count movement. The added level of complexity is repeated until the entire class can perform it correctly. At this time, the instructor maintains the 16 count variation of "A" followed by an optional advanced movement variation for "B" in which the opposite knee lifts during the alternating oblique curl. This strategy is well suited for mixed level classes as it allows each participant to progress to a level that is comfortable for them.

Preparing and Teaching Class Activities

The majority of a group fitness instructor's preparation time is spent selecting music and developing movement patterns. The purpose of this section is to explain music selection, to explore different choreographic techniques, and to become familiar with successful cueing skills.

Selecting Music

Music not only provides the timing for exercise movements, it also makes a class enjoyable and it helps to motivate participants. Because music plays an important role in most group exercise programs, you should be familiar with its fundamental elements.

The music **beat** is the regular pulsations that have an even rhythm and occur in a continuous pattern of strong and weak pulsations. Strong pulsations are called the **downbeat** while weaker pulsations are called the **upbeat**. A series of beats forms the underlying rhythm of a song. The rhythm is the regular pattern of sound that is heard when listening to music. A **meter** organizes beats into musical patterns or measures, such as four beats per measure. A **measure** is a group of beats formed by the regular occurrence of a heavy **accent** on the first beat or downbeat of each group. Most aerobics routines use music with a meter of 4/4 time (the first "4" indicates 4 beats per measure while the second "4" shows that the quarter note gets the beat).

To successfully choreograph movement patterns, you must be familiar with your music. Determining music **tempo** is the first requirement. The tempo, or speed, of the music determines the progression as well as the intensity of exercise. The beats per minute (bpm), or music tempo, for a song can be determined by counting each beat for one minute. Using experience and common sense, instructors have adopted general guidelines for selecting the appropriate music tempo for the various component parts of an aerobics program. Slow tempos under 100 bpm without a strong

underlying beat are generally used for post-stretching, while tempos from 120 to 140 bpm are frequently used for warm-ups, pre-stretch, and cool-downs. Muscle-strengthening exercises are often performed to tempos of 110 to 130 bpm. The tempo for strengthening exercises should be slow enough for participants to control their movements. Aerobic activities are generally performed at a tempo of 120 to 160 bpm. Instructors must be cautious when choosing music speeds over 150 bpm because participants need to move quickly at higher tempos.

Encouraging students to perform smaller movements will help them preserve the control necessary for safety when using high music speeds. Beginners should never be expected to move at fast speeds because they are not yet proficient enough to perform quick movements under control. Another consideration with fast-paced music is that participants with long arms and legs need more time to cover the same spatial area as participants with shorter limbs. For example, people with short arms can bring their arms above their heads more quickly than can people with long arms. Consequently, participants with long arms often appear to be uncoordinated unless they bend their elbows to keep in time with the instructor and the music.

After determining the tempo, it is useful to break down the music into musical phrases. According to Bricker (1991), "as letters of the alphabet combine to form sentences, so beats of music combine to form measures, and measures combine to form phrases. A **phrase** is composed of at least two measures of music. To learn to recognize musical phrases, imagine where you would pause for breath if you were singing a song." Shyba (1990) likes to think of a musical "sentence" as a group of four phrases (usually 32 counts). Shyba recommends that instructors indicate on a piece of paper each musical phrase with a pen stroke crossing the set out with the last phrase in the sentence (卌). Therefore, if you were listening to 32 measures (four beats per measure) making up 16 musical phrases (eight beats per phrase) or four musical sentences (32 beats per sentence), there would be four sets of three vertical pen strokes crossed by 1 diagonal pen stroke (each pen stroke representing an 8-count phrase: 卌 卌 卌 卌). Musical phrasing is ideal when it groups into musical sentences of 32 counts. However, there are times when a phrase may be subdivided, and it becomes awkward if you are is in the middle of a 32-count combination when the musical phrasing becomes inconsistent. Shyba (1990) recommends that instructors use phrasing inconsistencies to introduce a new step or to perform simple free-form footwork until the musical sentences establish themselves.

When choreographing movements to music, take care to begin the movement pattern on the downbeat of the measure (the first count of the measure). Combining 8-count movements, such as eight marches or four jumping jacks to make up a 32-count combination (Figure 6.4), will help participants anticipate movement changes on the downbeat, thus giving them a feeling of success.

While many movement patterns are performed on each beat of the music, it is possible to change the rhythm of the movement so that it is being performed double time to the basic beat (one and two and three and four and), half-time (2 counts per movement), or in **syncopation**, where the accent is temporarily displaced from the naturally

Figure 6.4
A sample 32 count movement pattern

Phrase Number (8 counts)	Music	Movement
#1	Mary had a little lamb,	8 march forward
#2	Little lamb, little lamb,	4 jumping jacks
#3	Mary had a little lamb,	8 march back
#4	Whose fleece was white as snow.	4 jumping jacks

occurring accent in the music (one AND two AND, with the accent occurring on the AND rather than on one or two).

The rhythm of the music can often dictate the style of movement. You will find it easiest to work with music that has a steady rhythm and a strong beat. The type of music selected will depend on the demographics of the exercise group and your creativity. Staying open-minded is important. You must not rely exclusively on your personal music preferences. The music selected should reflect, in part, the interests of the age group. For example, young people may enjoy Top 40 pop, while an older group may prefer swing or big band music. Age should not be the only criterion for selecting music, however. In some parts of the country, gospel, folk, and country music are more appealing than rock 'n' roll. Instructors may also want to consider the time of the year. At Christmas, for example, participants may be delighted to exercise to "Rudolph the Red-Nosed Reindeer." For further variety, you can select music for special "theme days" — square dance, clogging, and polka music for a country music day or cha-cha, rumba, and samba music for a Latin music day. The greater the variety of music, the more enjoyment most participants will derive from a group fitness program.

With some types of group fitness instruction, the music is used to set a mood rather than to mark movement patterns. In these cases, selecting music written in 8 count phrases with regular rhythms and beats is unnecessary. Indoor cycling, stretching, and yoga classes are just some of the classes that traditionally use music to enhance the mood of the exercise rather than to synchronize movements.

To keep participants interested, change music frequently. If you have trouble staying current with music selections, there are national music organizations that manufacture music tapes for aerobics classes. In addition, you can ask regular participants for music suggestions.

Choreography

The types of movements selected should reflect the goals and objectives of the class. The first consideration is whether the selected movement or the sequencing of movements is safe. Other chapters in this manual address contraindicated exercises, but for review purposes, keep in mind the following general guidelines when selecting choreography:

1. Avoid movements that result in hyperextension of any joint.
2. Avoid excessive repetitions on one weight-bearing leg. Alternate legs frequently.
3. Avoid flinging the limbs at any time.
4. Make sure lateral foot movements are well-controlled to avoid tripping or falling (especially on carpet).
5. Avoid contraindicated positions such as sustained and unsupported forward flexion.
6. Avoid stretching muscles ballistically while performing movement patterns.
7. Avoid changing direction rapidly. Transitions between complex step patterns may require a movement sequence in place before changing direction.
8. Avoid continuous movement that requires participants to remain on the balls of their feet for extended periods.
9. Avoid holding the arms at or above shoulder level for an extended period of time. Vary frequently low-, mid- and high-range arm movements.
10. Balance routines so that the same movements are performed equally on both sides of the body.

Choreographic Methods

Two basic choreographic methods, known as **freestyle choreography** and **structured choreography**, are used to combine movement patterns and music. The structured method uses choreographed movements that are formally arranged and repeated in a predetermined order, usually to the same piece of music each time the routine is used. Examples of structured programs are those of the STEP Company's "Body Pump" and Judi Sheppard Missett's "Jazzercise."

The freestyle method uses movements that are built and sequenced by the instructor during the exercise class. The pacing is often dependent on the success participants demonstrate with the sequences as well as the complexity of the movement patterns or combinations. Freestyle movements can be sequenced either by using a **linear progression** or by placing movements into patterns or combinations. A linear progression consists of one movement that transitions into another without cycling sequences. By changing only one variable at a time, such as arm or leg movement, direction of movement, or rhythm, students can practice movement patterns without the pressure of remembering sequences. Linear progressions are particularly useful for introducing new moves and for adding variations. The following is an example of a linear progression in which only one element of variation is changed at any one time:

Base movement: Knee-lift in place for 8 counts (four knee-lifts)

Add arms: Arm curls for 8 counts

Add direction: Travel forward for 8 counts; travel backward for 8 counts

Change the arms: Overhead press for 16 counts (still traveling)

Change the legs: Hamstring curls (same arms) for 16 counts (still traveling)

Change the arms: Push down for 16 counts (still traveling)

When using a freestyle approach, it is important to use effective teaching strategies so that class participants can successfully follow the choreography to maintain appropriate levels of exercise intensity. Copeland (1991) recommends that instructors start with a base move, such as marches or step-touches, and change only one element of variation at a time. Examples of elements of variation recommended by Copeland include planes, levers, direction, and rhythm. Variations in planes include the horizontal or transverse plane, which divides the body into lower and upper parts and includes rotation around the long axis of the body; the frontal plane, which divides the body into anterior and posterior parts and includes abduction and adduction; and the sagittal plane, which divides the body into right and left sides and includes flexion and extension. You can change the arms from lateral raises (frontal or lateral plane) to arm curls (sagittal plane).

Lever variations refer to the length of a lever or limb (short, long). Changing from an arm curl (short arm lever) to frontal raises (long arm lever) is an example of a lever variation. Directional variations add the element of travel, allowing participants to move forward, backward, left, right, diagonally or in a circle. Variations in rhythm involve changing the rhythm of a movement. For example, varying a jumping jack to a slow jumping jack changes the rhythm of a similar movement.

Combinations are defined as two or more movement patterns combined and repeated in sequence several times in a row. The following is an example of a combination:

Four lunges in place with upright rows — 8 counts

Four knee lifts traveling forward with overhead presses — 8 counts

Four jumping jacks with arms lifting laterally — 8 counts

Eight runs traveling backward with chest presses — 8 counts

According to Copeland (1991), "There are many advantages to using patterns in your choreography. The human mind instinctively arranges events into patterns, so they allow the mind to relax and easily anticipate what will happen next. This repetition allows…students to commit to the movement more fully and to maintain a steady-state workout." However, you must select movement patterns carefully. Complex routines can slow down the class and confuse participants, particularly in a beginning or multilevel class.

Finally, when putting the class together, movement patterns can be taught using a combination of teaching strategies. For example, you may teach an oblique curl using the fast to slow teaching strategy, then add an abdominal curl movement using a part to whole teaching strategy to create a sequence of 32 counts of oblique curls followed by 32 counts of abdominal curls. You can then reduce the repetitions to 16 counts of oblique curls and 16 counts of abdominal curls to create the final movement pattern.

To keep track of the movement patterns or choreographed routines, it is helpful to maintain a card file or notebook to record specific movement patterns and teaching strategies. Before teaching a new routine or series of movement patterns to a class, practice (preferably in front of a mirror) until the movement patterns are memorized and transitions and cues have been worked out. Practicing routines or combinations in advance helps instructors determine whether the sequence of movement patterns flows smoothly.

A slow progression is important to help participants learn a skill effectively and to avoid musculoskeletal injuries. Encourage beginners to start slowly and progress gradually. In addition, movements must be selected so that most participants are successful. Some participants will learn new steps more quickly than others. Be patient and supportive of slower learners, reminding them that they will improve with practice. And always try to be available before and after class for individual help.

It is important that all movement patterns are effectively and safely sequenced to ensure smooth and comfortable transitions. A simple transition is one between two movements that are closely related. Simple transitions involve changes using either the legs or the arms. For example, punching up easily transitions into punching front. As the number of variations between movement patterns increases, so does the difficulty of the transition. Also, changing both legs and arms at the same time increases the difficulty of the transition.

The way you sequence movements should be based on **physiological**, **biomechanical**, and **psychological balance** (Copeland, 1991). Intensity and duration are two physiological considerations when sequencing movements. To help class participants maintain heart rates within their training zones, the relative intensity level of each movement must be balanced. For example, if you choose a high-intensity movement, such as jumping jacks or high-impact lunges, the next movement should be less intense, for example, marches. If an exercise class is of long duration, too many high-intensity movements may fatigue participants before the end of the session.

Biomechanical balance is achieved by balancing the musculoskeletal stress of various movements. For example, if you select a movement that is performed on one leg at a time, care must be taken to change the support leg before it is overly stressed. Similarly, if a movement is highly stressful to a joint, such as jumping jacks, the next movement should not stress that same joint. Finally, be careful not to use too many complex movements if you are striving to achieve psychological balance. According to Copeland (1991), "Movement that is too complex is not only frustrating for the student but has a direct effect on the physiological and biomechanical balance. Form, technique and safety can be compromised."

Cueing

Cueing is a crucial part of teaching group exercise classes. It serves as a warning system that allows class participants to follow movement patterns with ease and confidence. The success with which students perform movement sequences in a smooth and continuous manner depends on your ability to effectively cue changes in movement patterns.

When leading group exercise, face the class as often as possible, using mirroring techniques, such as moving to the participants' left when directing them to the right. You can only monitor class safety by watching all participants at all times. All cues should be precise and timely.

Transitions play an integral part in cueing. If the transition is closely related, then the amount of information should be small. A long cue is only necessary when the transition is difficult and involves a movement that is unrelated. The content of the cue may include the body part, the action, the direction, and/or any elaboration necessary to understand the movement. See Table 6.1 for samples of movement cues.

Once the movement cue has been described, place the cue into the music using the following formula: "4 (gap) 3 (gap) tell me what to do (gap)." The cue begins on the heavy down beat of the beginning of the phrase. The final gap represents the time between when the movement cue ends and the new movement begins. The final gap can be filled with a clap or vocal sound, like "hup" or "go."

Table 6.1
Samples of movement cues

Body part	Action	Direction	Elaboration
Arms	Reach	Up	2 times
Hands	Push	Side	In place
Shoulders	Press	Front	Right
Knee	Lifts	Back	Forward
Foot	Taps	Diagonal	Double time
Head	Roll	Down	Slowly

Figure 6.5
Verbal cues and timing

Music Counts	1	2	3	4	5	6	7	8
Example #1	4		3		arms	press	up	
Example #1 - *modified*					arms	press	up	Clap
Example #2	4		3		alter-	nate the	arms	
Example #2 - *modified*					alter-	nate the	arms	HUP!

For example, to introduce an arm pattern, use a cue similar to the following: "4 (gap) 3 (gap) arms press up (gap)." To modify or make a small change to the arm pattern, use "4 (gap) 3 (gap) alternate the arms (gap)." To view the timing of the cue, refer to Figure 6.5

Using this formula, you can plug in the important descriptive words to guide the exercise participant into the next movement. Once the movement is established, only small cues are necessary if the changes are closely related.

Here are some additional guidelines for effective cueing:

1. Count down, 4, 3, 2…rather than up, 1, 2, 3,…
2. Avoid words with more than one meaning, like "out."
3. Refer to objects around the room to help with directional cues. The cue "face the window" may have more meaning than "turn right."
4. Count out difficult rhythms (e.g., 1 - and - 2 - 3- and 4).
5. Be consistent with names of movements and timing of cues.
6. Avoid tagging on extra words with little meaning, such as, "now take it to a…" or "I wanna see a…"

As students become proficient at executing movement patterns, they will need fewer verbal cues from exercise instructors. Instead of cueing every movement, you can limit verbal cues to transitions between movements. Visual cues are also helpful to communicate movement expectations. The use of visual cues has several advantages, including lowering the risk of voice injury, allowing you to communicate in facilities with poor acoustics or with a large number of class participants, and providing opportunities for the hearing-impaired to join an aerobics program. There are currently two formalized sets of visual cues in use among exercise instructors (Figures 6.6 and 6.7).

According to Webb (1989), who promotes a series of hand/arm visual cues called the Aerobic Q-Signs (Figure 6.6), verbal cues can be used to call out the name of the step while visual cues are used to indicate the direction or number of repetitions. Webb recommends that instructors practice visual cue signs in front of a mirror, making sure that visual cues are given 4 counts before the movement change is to occur. She also suggests that instructors introduce a few signs at a time into their classes so that participants can gradually adapt to their use.

Oliva (1988) promotes visual cues based on the principles of Visual-Gestural Communication and American Sign Language to include persons who are deaf or hard of hearing (Figure 6.7). Oliva maintains that visual cues must be "visually logical" and clearly visible to viewers. For example, instructors should indicate lower-body moves by patting the lead leg. A strong distinction needs to be made between moves that travel and moves that simply change direction (within one step of original position). Specific visual cues that match specific low-impact foot-moves are available (Oliva, 1988). Oliva recommends that visual cues for turns should be indicated directly above the floor space that the turn will cover. Finally, the timing and command sequence for visual cues should be the same as for verbal cues.

The use of verbal and visual previews are particularly useful when introducing a complex movement pattern. Each of these previews is given by the instructor while the class continues to perform the movement that they are currently performing. When using a verbal preview, the instructor explains in detail the next step or arm pattern. When using a visual preview, the instructor demonstrates the next movement sequence,

Figure 6.6

Aerobic Q-signs
(Source: Webb,
1989.)

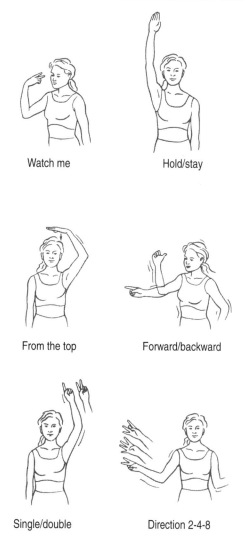

Watch me   Hold/stay

From the top   Forward/backward

Single/double   Direction 2-4-8

while the class continues to perform the current movement.

When using verbal cues, it is imperative that you learn to use your voice properly to avoid vocal injuries. According to MacLellan, Grapes, and Elster (1980), voice injuries among aerobics instructors occur from "the improper use of the voice, interference of muscular tension with vocalization, attempts at projection over loud music, and a poor work environment." They recommend the following techniques to prevent voice injury:

1. Keep cues short and avoid unnecessary vocalization.
2. Keep music at a decibel level that does not require you to shout over the music.
3. Frequently take small sips of water to keep the vocal mechanism lubricated.
4. Avoid cueing in positions that inhibit abdominal breathing (such as during curl-ups) or constrict the vocal tract (such as when performing push-ups). It is preferable to give the cues before the exercise is executed.
5. When using a microphone speak in a normal voice.
6. Do not lower the pitch of the voice to sound louder as this leads to vocal fatigue (producing a hoarse, weak, and strained voice).
7. Avoid frequent clearing of the throat.

Analyzing Performance and Providing Alignment Cues

An important role of the exercise instructor is to effectively analyze the movement skills of class participants. An exercise that is performed incorrectly will not achieve the desired goal, but more importantly, improper exercise execution could result in injury. Body alignment is crucial to proper exercise exe-

cution. You must therefore have a thorough knowledge of appropriate body alignment.

Most exercises require exercise participants to maintain a neutral pelvis. Class participants should be frequently reminded of mechanically sound posture — neutral head, shoulders back, chest up, neutral pelvis, and relaxed knees (standing posture). For more information on proper body alignment see Chapter 2.

When teaching exercises, communicate important alignment and execution cues. It is also recommended that you walk around

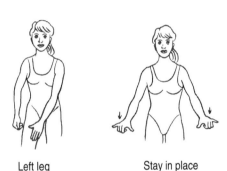
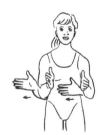
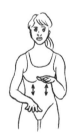
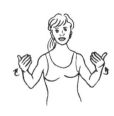
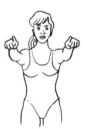

Left leg   Stay in place

Shift to face this direction   March in place

Move it forward   Move it back

Figure 6.7
Visual cues for exercise classes (Source: Oliva, 1988)

the room as much as possible to make appropriate corrections. This is particularly important during the muscular strength and poststretch phase of the exercise class. Unless you provide appropriate feedback, few participants, especially beginners, will have any idea that they are not performing an exercise properly.

Be very cautious with hands-on corrections. Pushing a participant's limb into proper position during a stretch could result in a serious injury for the exerciser, especially if he or she is inflexible. As a rule of thumb, you should not perform hands-on corrections for exercises that require the manipulation of a muscle being stretched. Instead, demonstrate proper execution of the exercise and offer verbal corrections. However, if a participant is hyperextending a joint, for example, it might be beneficial for you to lightly touch the exerciser's knees or elbows as a reminder to soften them. Common sense must always be applied when making decisions about whether to physically correct an inappropriate exercise position.

The most common modification that has to be addressed by group fitness instructors is that of modifying exercise intensity to provide safe and effective activity for all fitness levels. Factors that affect exercise intensity include music tempo and the size of arm and leg movements. In a multilevel program, the speed of music must be selected to accommodate the less-fit individuals in the class. It is hazardous for individuals with a poor level of fitness to exercise to fast music. However, the person with a higher level of fitness can manipulate the exercise by performing larger leg and arm movements to increase exercise intensity. You can assist this process by demonstrating

movement modifications for each level of fitness found in the class.

One way to meet the intensity needs of each level of fitness is to be familiar with the energy expenditure for different types of movements. For example, the following is a four-level system based on the fact that locomotion and large leg movements increase energy expenditure.

- *Level one:* small leg motions, in place
- *Level two:* small leg motions, traveling
- *Level three:* large leg motions, in place
- *Level four:* large leg motions, traveling

Using this system, advanced participants can be shown how to increase intensity by increasing the leg motions and the amount of traveling. Likewise, beginner participants can be shown how to decrease intensity by decreasing the leg motions and the amount of traveling.

Arm movements can also be adjusted, though to a lesser degree than leg movements, in order to increase or decrease intensity. While it is true that an overhead press is more intense than an arm curl, this is because the arm curl is performed with a shorter lever and therefore requires less energy expenditure to perform than an overhead press, which moves from a shorter lever to a longer lever. However, side laterals (a long-lever exercise that involves shoulder abducting to shoulder height with the elbows extended) require about the same energy expenditure as an overhead press, even though side lateral raises are performed at a lower level than an overhead press.

Teaching to two or three levels requires some skill on the part of the instructor, who needs to demonstrate each of the levels every time a new movement is introduced. While it is tempting to spend most of your time demonstrating the more intense version of a movement, it is probably the least-fit or beginner student who requires constant visual cues. It is not surprising that deconditioned individuals (who, more often than not, are also less skilled at movement performance) emulate the more intense choreography being demonstrated by the instructor, even when the instructor tells participants to move at their own pace. Unfortunately, beginning level participants are not skilled enough to perform movements without visual cues. After intensity options are given and each of the levels has been demonstrated, you should come back to performing to the level of the beginner participants. Do not forget that your primary objective as an exercise leader is to teach rather than to perform.

It is the responsibility of both the instructor and the participant to monitor exercise intensity. You control intensity according to the music tempo selected and the types of movements demonstrated. The participant manipulates the exercise intensity by controlling the size of the movements performed. Encourage beginners to take their heart rates (HR) frequently, and they should also be aware of the progress participants are making. One approach is to ask for a show of hands for those above, below, and within their target HR range. Advise those participants who are above their target zone to keep their feet closer to the ground and reduce the size of their arm movements. Those students exercising below their target zone should be encouraged to take larger steps and increase the size of their arm movements if they are ready to do so.

You must make sure that exercise HRs can be reported in a nonthreatening and noncompetitive environment to ensure honesty. Accurate reporting is particularly important for participants who must maintain strict exercise HRs due to specific medical conditions.

To avoid injury, it is extremely important that participants adjust the intensity of their movements to their cardiorespiratory fitness level. Within a multilevel class, beginners should be encouraged to progress slowly in both the intensity and duration of exercise. After deconditioned exercisers have reached their aerobic goal for the day, request that these individuals lower the intensity by "walking" through the rest of the movements while more experienced participants continue to exercise at a higher intensity. Be very careful not to give conflicting messages to participants. If everyone is expected to work at his or her own intensity level, you must avoid general phrases such as, "Get your feet up higher," "Push through it," or "Just do one more." Participants will feel compelled to work at higher intensities regardless of whether they are ready to do so.

Evaluating Performance

Providing Feedback

During class, the group fitness instructor has many opportunities to provide immediate **feedback** to the participants. Wlodkowski (1984) defines feedback as information learners receive about the quality of their performance on a given task. Generally speaking, feedback should be informational, based on performance standards, specific, and immediate. In this way the feedback can be used to either reinforce their performance or to make the necessary corrections to improve their performance.

Informational Rather than Controlling

Feedback is for the participant's benefit not the instructor's. Therefore, it should be filled with information about the participant's performance and not the exercise instructor's need to be pleased. You should act like a mirror, reflecting the information about the performance back to the participant. Feedback that is perceived as pressure to perform or to please the instructor can ultimately decrease motivation to perform (Ryan, 1982). For example, "Your knee is at belt level, that is just the right place" or, "Your knee is at chest level, move it down to belt level" are better than, "I am so pleased you got it right" or, "I'd like it better if you lowered your knee to belt level."

Once a participant has made an improvement in performance, a positive statement like "that's it" or "now you have it" can help reinforce the new performance. Kaess and Zeaman (1960) have demonstrated that positive feedback (i.e., knowledge that one is right) is more effective than negative feedback (knowledge that one is wrong). Instructors should seek to find positive performances from each participant throughout the class.

Based on Performance Standards

An instructor relies on kinesiological principles, past experience, and aesthetic standards to determine the correctness of a performance (Mosston, 1981). Kinesiological principles are used to determine which postures and movements are mechanically correct. For example, curl-ups are performed with the knees bent to reduce stress on the lower back and to isolate the abdominal musculature. Past experience is often used to correct a movement based on subtleties accumulated from observing many exercisers perform the same movement. Experienced

instructors can often find just the right word or phrase to correct consistently inappropriate performances. Aesthetic standards are used to correct movements and postures determined to be culturally attractive. Aerobics movements are often corrected on the basis of aesthetic standards.

Specific

Feedback should be specific for the same reason movement cues should be. Exercise participants cannot correct mistakes unless they are clear about their errors and the correct performance standards. A nonspecific statement like, "you did that great," may not clearly communicate what was great about the exercise. Instead, use the specific details of the performance standard to explain what you observed. For example, "You kept breathing throughout the exercises. Great job!"

Immediate

Delivering feedback as soon as possible allows the exercise participant to make a connection between the performance and the feedback. It also can be applied right away. If the feedback is delivered later, the exercise participant may not be as motivated to apply the information.

In addition to feedback regarding what was observed compared to the performance standard, you may add rationales and corrective teaching statements. A rationale explains why the performance is important. As discussed earlier, it addresses the cognitive domain and can positively affect motivation and exercise compliance. For example, "You are stopping your arms at shoulder level (*what you observed*), that's perfect (*performance standard*), because it reduces the stress on the shoulder joint (*rationale*)."

Together, this feedback increases motivation and moves the exercise participant more deeply into the autonomous stage of learning.

When participants are learning a new skill, you may also need to offer corrective teaching statements. Corrective teaching statements provide the participant with the necessary information to improve performance. For example, "Joe, your knee is moving beyond your ankle during the lunge segment of class (*what you observed*); next time stop the knee as it approaches the point directly over your ankle (*performance standard*). This will reduce the amount of stress you place on your knees (*rationale*). A good visual cue is to look down at your knee during the exercise, and if you can see your shoelaces, you know you have not gone too far (*corrective teaching*)."

A person can attend to only a few cues at any given moment. Therefore, when giving feedback, limit the number of corrections offered at any one time. Positive reinforcement is very important in the early stages of learning. Use positive **value statements** when participants make a good attempt even if the performance is not yet correct. Appropriate feedback should always be given in a friendly manner. If several participants are performing a move incorrectly, you can give feedback to the entire class. However, if one person consistently performs an exercise or movement incorrectly, you should talk to that person privately, either when other class participants are working individually or after class.

The effective group fitness instructor monitors participants' progress toward personal goals through periodic testing. Each aerobic exercise participant should be evaluated initially to establish a baseline by which to measure progress. Physiological measures such as cardiorespiratory fitness, body composition, strength, and flexibility are described in Chapter 5.

Instructors can work with exercise participants and other fitness professionals, such as personal trainers, to periodically measure progress. If there is no access to these services, you should attempt to use valid tests that can be easily administered either by partners or by the participants themselves. Providing criteria cards that indicate test directions, criteria for passing, and performance level achieved by exercisers saves valuable class time and can serve as a motivational tool for participants (Figure 6.2).

In addition to periodic testing, you should encourage participants to monitor their daily accomplishments. Most fitness facilities provide program cards or access to computer programs designed to record daily exercise participation. If these services are not provided, a simple record card can be used to keep track of daily progress (see Figure 6.6). Items such as heart rate (resting, exercise, and recovery) and the number of floor-exercise repetitions can be regularly monitored and recorded by participants themselves. Criteria and record cards should be stored in an alphabetized file that is available to participants at each class meeting. Remind participants to pick up their cards, record the appropriate information, and refile them before leaving class.

It is important that you stay aware of your students' progress toward their goals by periodically examining participants' record cards and through one-on-one interaction with participants either before, during, or after class. If a participant is not showing progress, it is your responsibility to help determine the problem. It may be that unrealistic goals have been set or there has been an attendance problem. Showing genuine concern for students encourages long-term participation in a formal exercise program.

Summary

Effectively teaching an group fitness class is a challenge to every group fitness instructor. Competent teachers carefully design their programs and employ sound teaching principles; they develop sound strategies to motivate their participants to continue exercising: and they remain abreast of current health, nutrition, and fitness information and trends. The extra work that is required to become an effective teacher will be repaid many times over when you earn your students' respect by providing safe, fun, and well-structured aerobics classes. Demonstrating expertise in the fitness industry will provide you with many professional opportunities and with the personal satisfaction of contributing to the well-being of so many participants.

References

Bricker K. (1991). Music 101. *IDEA Today,* 3, 55 – 57.

Copeland C. (1991). Smooth Moves. *IDEA Today,* 6, 34 – 38.

Dishman, R.K. (1986). Exercise compliance: A new view for public health. *The Physician and Sportsmedicine*, 14, 127 – 43.

Fallon, D.J. & Kuchenmeister, S.A. (1977). *The Art of Ballroom Dance*. Minneapolis, Minn.: Burgess Publishing Company.

Fitts, P.M. & Posner, M.I. (1967). *Human Performance*. Belmont, Calif.: Brooks/Cole.

Franklin, B.A. (1986). Clinical components of a successful adult fitness program. *American Journal of Health Promotion*, 1, 6 – 13.

Griffith, B.R. (1992). *Dance for Fitness*. Minneapolis, Minn.: Burgess Publishing Company.

Harris, J.A., Pittman, A.M., & Waller, M.S. (1978). *Dance A While*. Minneapolis, Minn.: Burgess Publishing Company.

Institute for Aerobic Research. (1988). Creative Choreography with Candice Copeland. *Reebok Instructor News,* 6, 7.

Kaess, W. & Zeaman, D. (1960). Positive and negative knowledge of results on a Pressey-type punchboard. *Journal of Experimental Psychology*, 60, 12 – 17.

MacLellan, M.A., Grapes, D., & Elste, D. (1980). Voice injury. *Aerobic Dance-Exercise Instructor Manual*, San Diego, Calif. American Council on Exercise.

Magill, R.A. (1980). *Motor Learning*. Dubuque, Iowa: Wm. C. Brown Company.

Milgram, S.(1956). *Obedience to Authority: An Experimental View*. New York: Harper & Row.

Mosston, M. (1981). *Teaching Physical Education*. Columbus, Ohio: Charles E. Merrill Publishing Company.

Nieman, D.C. (1986). *The Sports Medicine Fitness Course*. Palo Alto, Calif.: Bull Publishing Company.

Oliva, G.A. (1988). *Visual Cues for Exercise Classes*. Washington, D.C.: Gallaudet University.

Price, J. (1990). Hear today, gone tomorrow? *IDEA Today,* 5, 54 – 57.

Rasch, P.J. (1989). *Kinesiology and Applied Anatomy*. Philadelphia, Pa.: Lea & Febiger.

Rogers, C. (1961). *On Becoming A Person*. Boston, Mass.: Houghton Mifflin Company.

Ryan, R.M. (1982). Control and information in the intrapersonal sphere: An extension of cognitive evaluation theory. *Journal of Personality and Social Psychology*, 43, 3, 450 – 461.

Shyba, L. (1990). Finding the elusive downbeat. *IDEA Today,* 6, 27 – 29.

Siedentop, D. (1983). *Developing Teaching Skills in Physical Education*. Palo Alto, Calif.: Mayfield Publishing Company.

Webb, T. (1989). Aerobic Q-Signs. *IDEA Today,* 10, 30 – 31.

Wlodkowski, R.J. (1984). *Enhancing Adult Motivation to Learn*, San Francisco, Calif.: Jossey-Bass.

Chapter 7

In This Chapter:

Deborah Rohm Young, Ph.D., assistant professor of medicine at The Johns Hopkins School of Medicine and faculty member of the Welch Center for Prevention, Epidemiology, and Clinical Research, researches the health benefits of physical activity.

Abby C. King, Ph.D., associate professor of health research and policy and medicine at Stanford Medical School and senior scientist at the Center for Research in Disease Prevention, has written extensively on the behavioral determinants of exercise.

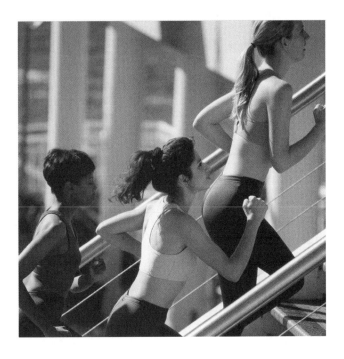

Adherence and
Motivation

By Deborah Rohm Young and Abby C. King

Given that it is difficult to pick up a newspaper or magazine without finding an article discussing the benefits of regular physical activity, it is little wonder that most Americans know that regular physical activity is desirable. Adults are indeed aware of the health and psychological benefits associated with exercise, yet this knowledge is rarely transferred into action. About 60% of American adults do not get the minimum amount of recommended physical activity. About one-quarter are completely sedentary. Nearly 50% of those who start an exercise program drop out within the first 6 months.

Often adults do not know how to start their own exercise program, where to get sound advice on beginning a program, or are fearful of failing because of previous experiences with exercise. Fitness instructors are in a fortunate situation, as they do not have to convince people to attend their workout; participants have taken the first step by finding an exercise class and committing themselves to attending at least once. The instructor's challenge is to encourage continued participation.

The most common reasons given for not continuing an exercise program are lack of time and boredom. The time-constraint reason is intriguing; those who exercise regularly also cite lack of time as an ongoing problem for them. But these individuals fit regular exercise into their daily schedules. How do they avoid letting their time pressures short-circuit their exercise program? What "tricks" do they use to motivate themselves? Regular exercisers also report facing boredom yet they continue with their program. How are they different from those who let boredom drive them out of aerobics classes?

Researchers who have studied exercise **adherence** issues have begun to formulate answers to these and other questions regarding the motivational aspects of regular exercise. The group fitness instructor who incorporates motivational techniques into each exercise class has a unique opportunity to help participants develop positive attitudes toward, and to stay involved in, regular physical activity and exercise throughout their lives.

This chapter discusses characteristics often found in exercise program participants and dropouts. Knowing about the factors that influence exercise adherence and determining who are the least likely to attend regularly and who may drop out can be crucial in the development and implementation of strategies to maximize adherence.

Numerous studies have confirmed the effectiveness of using such motivational strategies, but often these strategies are not implemented in the "real world." This chapter identifies characteristics of instructors that help maintain adherence and details the strategies necessary to enhance adherence to regular class participation. Ad-

ditionally, skills needed to help participants maintain exercise programs during "high-risk" times, such as vacations, holidays, and when under pressure at work or home, are presented.

Major Factors Influencing Exercise Adherence

What is exercise adherence? Although exercise adherence has been defined in a number of ways, for the purpose of this chapter it will be defined as the amount of exercise performed during a specified period of time compared to the amount of exercise recommended. The amount of exercise can refer to the frequency, intensity, or duration or some combination of these three dimensions.

There are a number of factors associated with exercise adherence. They often are categorized as personal, program, and environmental factors. This categorization scheme highlights the many different influences on physical activity behavior.

Personal Factors

To effectively motivate participants, it is helpful to be aware of characteristics that appear to be associated with exercise adherence as well as dropout. Although not every person exhibiting a particular characteristic may adhere to or drop out from the class, understanding these characteristics may help the exercise instructor to "flag" those potentially at risk and provide them with extra assistance early in the program.

Some unique characteristics exist in those who tend to adhere to physical activity programs. One is that such individuals are more likely to have previously participated in exercise programs. Additionally, physical and psychological/behavioral skills necessary to exercise appropriately and regularly (e.g., physical coordination, good time-management skills); a participant's self-efficacy (confidence in being able to exercise); an ability to perceive exercise as enjoyable; and the participant's ability to overcome typical barriers to exercise such as travel, injury, illness, competing demands on time, and high-stress periods have all been associated with increased adherence to exercise programs.

Although some of these factors may be lacking in some participants and may be difficult to develop, others, such as perceptions of the enjoyability of exercise, are more amenable to change. By asking participants what they did and did not like about previous programs in which they may have participated and why they discontinued these previous programs, the group fitness instructor can adjust the current program to optimize its enjoyability for all participants. Later in this chapter, additional ways to develop skills that participants need to maintain good exercise habits are presented in detail.

Individuals identified in the scientific literature to be at increased risk for dropout include smokers, people with lower socioeconomic status, and the overweight. A brief interview of new participants can identify those with health habits and prior exercise experiences that place them at risk for dropout.

When a participant at increased risk for dropout is identified, extra monitoring is desirable, particularly for signs of overexertion. A high-risk participant trying to exercise at an overly vigorous pace is twice as likely to drop out. Given the strong desire to conform to the larger group, simply telling participants not to overexert themselves may not be enough if the majority of the class is exer-

cising at a high-intensity level. This is particularly applicable to aerobics or other classes in which the group tendency is to exercise at the same intensity as the instructor. If the class consists of participants with varying abilities, it is useful to present both a more difficult and an easier version of each routine. If possible, having a co-leader or experienced class member actually demonstrate a lower-intensity version of the routine at the same time that the higher-intensity version is being demonstrated may decrease the chance that participants will overexert in trying to keep up with the more vigorous routine. Introducing the **rating of perceived exertion (RPE)** scale (Borg, 1982) (Figure 7.1) to new participants and instructing them how to monitor the intensity of their workout will help prevent them from overexertion. In general, a new participant,

Figure 7.1

The Borg Ratings of Perceived Exertion (RPE) Scale (Borg, 1985). The RPE scale is a reliable method to evaluate an individual's level of exertion while exercising. Individuals are asked to select a number that corresponds to their overall, general feeling of exertion. The rating should be based on total body feelings and not on leg fatigue or other localized sensations. For individuals beginning to exercise, an appropriate level of exertion is between 11 and 15 — if the RPE is greater than that, the individual should lower the exercise intensity.

Perceived Exertion Scale	
6	**Light Exercise**
7 Very, very light	*Some health benefits, but minimal fitness improvement*
8	
9 Very light	
10	
11 Fairly light	
12	**Moderate Exercise**
13 Somewhat hard	*Both health and fitness benefits with minimal risk*
14	
15 Hard	
16	**Intense Exercise**
17 Very hard	*For those who desire high fitness. Can precipitate heart attack in high risk*
18	
19 Very, very hard	
20 Maximal exertion	

regardless of risk for dropout, should keep his/her RPE below 14 – 15 until accustomed to the workout. Including short breaks during class also may help to maintain exercise involvement for the participant at increased risk for dropout.

It is imperative that the instructor maintain a noncondescending attitude toward all participants, including those with suboptimal health behaviors. Although it may be difficult for some fitness instructors to understand why individuals hold on to those extra pounds or continue smoking in light of overwhelming health risks associated with these behaviors, it must be remembered that every individual has unique priorities and behavior patterns in life. Rather than chastise for a perceived bad habit, the instructor should praise positive behaviors and provide a good example.

Program Factors

Factors specific to the exercise program can also affect participant adherence. Convenience of the exercise class is often cited as a determinant of adherence. Classes should be scheduled, if possible, during times of the day when most participants potentially have free time. It is also beneficial if classes are scheduled at a variety of times so that there is an alternate class the participant can attend if unforeseen circumstances require that a participant miss a class.

To maximize adherence, classes should be no longer than 60 minutes. Programs any longer than that are perceived to be too time-consuming by many participants, while programs much shorter are often considered not worth the effort. The exercise routine itself also impacts adherence. If the routine is either too easy or too hard for the participant, or not varied enough to

prevent boredom, chances for dropout are increased. Some popular forms of group exercise, such as aerobics and kick boxing, require physical coordination that may be intimidating to new participants. Spending time with new participants to demonstrate the movements helps them learn the sequencing and provides the added benefit of making them feel special. The perceived friendliness of class members can be an additional boost to adherence. When new participants feel welcome, it is easier for them to return to subsequent classes.

Environmental Factors

Environmental factors — the ambience of the exercise site, cues and reminders for exercise, weather conditions, time limitations, and the amount of support and **feedback** that is provided — can all influence whether a participant maintains the exercise program.

A well-lit exercise room decorated in a pleasant motif and of sufficient size to accommodate class members, along with an adequate cooling/heating system, is preferable to a hot, dark, smelly, gym-like environment. Exercise equipment that may be used during the workout (e.g., steps, handweights, cycle ergometers) should be clean and ready for use.

It is important to start and finish classes on time; most people are busy these days and a lack of promptness disrupts everyone's daily schedule. If exercise must be canceled because of bad weather or an unforeseen emergency, give participants plenty of advance notice whenever possible. Setting up a "telephone tree" (where one participant has the responsibility of contacting another in an emergency-type situation) to contact class members quickly may be a worthwhile endeavor for some class situations. If classes are conducted in regions of the country that experience regular bouts of inclement weather, it is advisable to have a "bad weather" policy regarding conditions when class will be canceled. Passing out the policy at the beginning of the inclement weather season and keeping the policy posted in the exercise room will keep all participants informed of potential situations in which class will be canceled. Whenever possible, it is advisable to conduct a make-up class session soon after to keep the participants engaged.

Ongoing support by the fitness instructor and others through face-to-face, telephone, or mail contact is particularly beneficial for adherence. You can encourage long-term attendance by praising participants for daily attendance and for reaching predetermined goals. Other methods of support you can incorporate are reminding the participant about the progress that has been made since joining the program, and challenging the participant to set and meet physical activity goals. Telephone and mail contacts can prompt the wayward participant as well as remind everyone about upcoming exercise "special events," such as fitness challenges or seasonally inspired, adherence-based promotions.

In general, a telephone call to a participant who has missed two consecutive classes is warranted to determine reasons for nonattendance and to provide non-judgmental support and encouragement. Newsletters that provide exercise tips, motivational strategies, and promotions for upcoming events are useful in building enthusiasm. With the advent of desktop publishing software, professional-looking newsletters can be achieved at minimal cost. To individualize the mail contacts, different newsletters can be developed for new participants and for those who are regular class attendees. Contents for the new participants can emphasize motivational tips, ways to build support for physical activity, and how to set physical activity goals. For the continuing exerciser, information about how to avoid boredom, ways to keep exercise fun, and how to strategize for high-risk situations are appropriate.

Support from family and friends is essential for adherence. This can be accomplished by encouraging participants to talk with others about goals they have set, what has been accomplished during exercise class, and rates of progression. Participants can be asked to identify someone who they will ask to support them with their physical activity program. This support can take a variety of forms; some participants may want someone to remind them to attend class, others may prefer a friend to reward them when goals are reached, and yet others may be interested in a buddy who also is an exerciser with whom they can discuss exercise-related issues. Participants should be encouraged to share their newsletters with friends and family. They can also provide story ideas and personal anecdotes that they feel would pique the interest of others. Involving others in the exercise program or providing them with knowledge of what is going on in class, as well as goals the participant has set, can encourage outside support and minimize any sabotage that might occur on the part of family members as a consequence of feeling "left out."

Traits of an Ideal Group Fitness Instructor

A group fitness instructor's attitudes, personality, and professional conduct are among the strongest motivating factors often cited for maintaining exercise adherence. Although exercise instructors are responsible for developing and administering a good class, those factors alone will not guarantee optimal adherence. Personal attributes of the exercise instructor can strongly augment his or her ability to effectively motivate participants. It is often thought that leadership is an innate trait, but leadership skills can be developed even by those not considered "born leaders." Some of the qualities of an effective, adherence-creating exercise instructor are discussed below.

Punctuality and Dependability

Instructors must assure exercise participants that each exercise class will start and end on time. A class that starts late or does not end on schedule is disruptive. Participants also want to know that their regular exercise instructor, not a parade of substitutes, will be there to greet them. Absences should be planned, substitutes scheduled in advance, and participants informed, whenever possible.

Professionalism

All participants should be treated with respect. Gossiping about other class members or staff is not only inappropriate but, if overheard from others, should not be tolerated. Professionalism extends to choice of exercise wear; although it is fine to be decked out in the latest style, be careful to avoid styles that can be perceived as being overly provocative or that may serve as a distraction.

Dedication

Part of being a professional is being dedicated to one's work. Obtaining and maintaining your group fitness instructor certification shows professionalism and dedication. Efforts should be made on a continual basis to keep exercise classes diverse, fun, and enjoyable for participants. This means going to workshops to keep up on the latest developments regarding exercise trends and finding out answers to questions participants may have on health-related topics. It is imperative to stay abreast of the latest health news and be informed of the scientific basis for health claims. Acquiring certification for new types of exercise programming, such as group indoor cycling and kickboxing classes, keeps you informed of the latest trends and also can protect against professional burn-out.

Sensitivity to the Participants

The ideal group fitness instructor recognizes that all participants are unique and come to exercise class for their own reasons. The purpose of class is not to treat all participants in the same way; instead, work with the strengths of each individual participant to maximize his or her exercise session. Interacting with participants as individuals, treating them with an open, non-judgmental manner, and expressing a willingness to listen are much appreciated.

Willingness to Plan Ahead

Participants appreciate when you provide them with advance notice of events that interfere with regular exercise class, such as holiday closures, intersession breaks, or a planned vacation. They also are grateful when you inform them of upcoming events or fitness challenges that are offered in the community. If given enough advance notice, participants may want to specifically train for an event. Helping the participants set appropriate goals to prepare for these events and counseling them if a particular event is unrealistic demonstrates interest in the participants and professionalism on your part.

Recognizing Signs of Burnout

Talking with other fitness instructors about how to prevent or work through **burnout** is invaluable. All exercise leaders will experience this phenomenon at some time or another, and getting another professional's advice will be useful. It is important to schedule regular vacations; it is amazing what a week or two away from work can do to improve one's attitude! Another strategy is to switch classes with another instructor for a time. Sometimes teaching a different class, using a different exercise format, or seeing different faces in the group can help to alleviate burnout.

Taking Responsibility

Invariably things will go wrong either with the exercise class itself or with the surroundings (e.g., broken air conditioning system). Taking responsibility for these problems and making sure that all efforts are made to correct the situation is appreciated by all. In addition, having back-up plans available when such situations arise can prove to be very useful.

Strategies That Encourage Adherence

Motivation depends on a participant's personal resources, abilities, and strengths, as well as external factors and circumstances. By assuming otherwise — that only innate personal factors influence adherence — an exercise instructor may "write off" a participant rather than try to teach skills that will help the participant develop into a regular exerciser.

Rather than placing the blame for non-adherence on the participant, you must view motivation as a joint responsibility shared with the participant. It is also helpful to view the process as a dynamic one; alternative strategies may be needed for different clients at different stages in the exercise program.

Several strategies have proven successful in motivating participants to regularly attend exercise class. The following strategies can easily be integrated into any type of exercise class and will help to motivate participants to become regular exercisers. (Some strategies, however, may not be applicable to your specific program, so determine which strategies are appropriate for a given situation and subsequently apply them in an individualized manner.) After you have developed a particular strategic plan for adherence, reassess it often to determine its continued feasibility and effectiveness.

Formulate Reasonable Participant Expectations

Early on, find out each participant's expectations from the exercise class and help them formulate reasonable goals.

Expectations must be realistic to avoid disappointment. Although regular exercise provides many benefits, it is not a panacea, and the participant must be informed of what benefits can be expected from the type of exercise being performed in the class. For instance, if a participant expects dramatic weight loss as a result of attending exercise class, he or she will be disappointed if this does not occur. It is preferable to advise the participant that, without a concomitant decrease in caloric intake, actual loss of body fat from physical training is likely to be negligible.

More realistic expectations would be weight loss on the order of one-half pound per week (.23 kg/week) (if typical caloric intake is reduced), trimmer legs or thighs over time, making new friends in class, or an increased sense of well-being after completing an exercise session.

Set Exercise Goals

When an individual joins an exercise class or program, take the time to develop realistic, flexible, individualized, short-term goals with that person. This can be accomplished by setting up a short interview with a new participant shortly after he or she joins the class. If it is not possible to arrange a specific time for this, have an experienced participant lead the cool-down phase of class and talk to the new participant during that time. Goals that are realistic are important in order to avoid injury and maintain interest.

Although you should help the participant formulate goals, the goals should be set, as much as possible, by the participant. Short-term goals determined for each exercise session in conjunction with longer-term monthly goals allow for flexibility on a daily basis without jeopardizing the longer-term goals.

Goals can be specific to the exercise process, such as attending a certain number of classes in the coming weeks, supplementing class exercise with exercise at home, or reaching a predetermined target heart rate during class by a certain date. They also can be related to some benefits not normally associated with exercise, such as making new friends or developing a new social network. It is useful to encourage goals related to enjoyment and pleasure from exercise rather than only tangible goals such as weight loss. Remind participants about their goals periodically during workouts and publicly praise those who have accomplished theirs. If goals are listed and displayed on a chart or are in participant files, they can easily be reviewed and evaluated regularly (e.g., twice a month). When goals are met, assist the participant in making new ones.

If it appears that the participant is unlikely to reach a specific goal, encourage a revised, more realistic goal. This will reduce the likelihood of disappointment or loss of interest associated with not meeting the goal, or potential physical injury that may occur when trying to "catch up" to reach a goal (such as performing too much exercise in too short a time). If a goal cannot be met, brainstorm with the participant reasons why the goal was not met in order to plan more realistic goals in the future. To avoid any potential embarrassment, this should not be done publicly, but rather by talking with the participant during the warm-up or cool-down phase of the exercise class. You can regularly use this format to talk individually with participants and provide personalized instructions.

Figure 7.2. Sample Exercise Contract
This is an example of an exercise contract that can be used to formalize an individual's commitment to exercise. It specifies short-term goals, rewards to be received when goals are met, and responsibilities of each party.

My Responsibilities

1. To attend 10 out of 12 exercise classes during the next four weeks.

2. To exercise out of class for at least 30 minutes one time each week during the next four weeks.

3. For any exercise class I have to miss due to illness or other unavoidable reasons, I will:

   a. Plan to make up the session by (specify): _____

4. To reward myself at the end of each week that I meet my exercise goals by (example, going to the movies, meeting a friend to shop, buying a new CD) (specify): _____

My Group Fitness Instructor's Responsibilities

1. To lead all classes, except when ill, unless advance notice is given.

2. To give me individual feedback regarding my progress.

3. To help me set new goals if the I ones set are unrealistic.

This contract will be evaluated on: _____
Date

_____
Participant Signature

_____
Group Fitness Instructor Signature

Consider formalizing the commitment to exercise with participants through written or oral contracts. A contract is often a written agreement signed by the participant and you (and others, if appropriate) that clearly itemizes the exercise goals and the rewards associated with achieving those goals. Contracts can increase the participant's commitment to the exercise program by defining the specific relationship between exercise goals and positive outcomes contingent on meeting those goals. They also involve the participant with the planning of the exercise program, thereby providing a sense of ownership of the program (Figure 7. 2).

Exercise contracts should contain input from both you and the participant. Prepare the contract together during a brief meeting before or after class or have a discussion during a warm-up or cool-down period, as previously described. Responsibilities each has in meeting the terms of the contract can be itemized at this time. Requirements for class attendance or additional home-exercise workouts and completion of exercise logs are often specified in contracts. Make certain that the participant has the skills necessary to meet the terms of the contract; beginning with modest goals is one way to ensure this. Precautions should be written into the contract to ensure that the participant does not engage in unhealthy practices to meet contract requirements (e.g., extended exercising over several days to meet a time-based goal or starvation tactics to meet a weight goal).

Exercise goals should be written in a manner so they can be objectively measured, thereby eliminating any questions regarding goal attainment. For example, a goal that specifies attendance requirements over one month (e.g., attend 10 out of 12 possible monthly classes) is preferable to one that states "every attempt will be made to attend as many classes as possible during the month." Make certain that the reward contracted for is delivered after the goal has been met. If the reward is an incentive, such as a T-shirt, ensure that enough are in stock so they can promptly be distributed.

Give Regular, Positive Feedback

As often as possible, provide participants with ample, ongoing, positive reinforcement, and individual praise. Feedback that is specific and relevant to the participant is known to be a powerful reinforcer. Studies have shown that personalized feedback about progress throughout the exercise session is more successful than feedback delivered in a more general manner (Martin et al., 1984). Specific feedback can include information regarding the number of exercise sessions attended during the month, sessions during which target exercise heart rate or RPE is met, and progress made on becoming proficient in an aerobic exercise routine. Feedback also can be oriented toward the exercise behavior itself, such as routine logging of exercise activity. A log sheet can be developed and kept at the exercise facility in which participants can keep a

record of resting heart rate, exercise heart rate, RPE, and feelings before and after the exercise session each time they attend class (Figure 7.3). Recording information only takes a few minutes and can be accomplished immediately after class. Reviewing log sheets at regular intervals (perhaps monthly) provides participants with important feedback (e.g., how resting heart rate has decreased over time, how many sessions were attended during the previous month, improved sense of energy or well-being after exercise). Log sheets also provide participants with information about the intensity of their exercise sessions, letting them know if they are working too hard or need to pick up the intensity in order to obtain fitness benefits.

Incentives, such as T-shirts and visors, can be provided to the participant when certain goals are met. Extrinsic rewards can be particularly important in the early stages of exercise adoption. Incentive-based goals should be set that can be realistically achieved by the majority of participants. Prizes based on attendance rather than large increases in performance are often preferred by participants and can motivate those experiencing less-than-optimal success in reaching physiological goals. Fitness "challenges" can provide rewards for different levels of participation by offering alternative prizes for a variety of achievements. It is important to be creative to ensure that the challenges are attractive to both the beginner and the long-term exerciser. One successful incentive strategy is having participants deposit a sum of money at the beginning of the program, a certain amount of which is forfeited if weekly contract goals are not met. Robinson et al. (1992) found that the group using a deposit strategy had 97% adherence to the exercise program

Figure 7.3 Sample Exercise Log
This is an example of an exercise log in which individuals record their daily exercise. This can be kept at the exercise facility for the individual to fill out before or after class, or can be given to class members to take home and record. Examine these records on a regular basis (e.g., twice a month) to check for progress.

	Sunday	Monday	Tuesday	Wednesday	Thursday	Friday	Saturday
Date							
Type of exercise							
Number of minutes							
Resting heart rate							
Exercise heart rate							
RPE							
Feelings before class							
Feelings after class							

over 6 months compared to 19% adherence in a comparable group that did not use this motivational strategy.

Public monitoring of attendance as a means of providing feedback and receiving achievement awards is useful for motivating participants. Posting attendance charts in the exercise room rewards the high attendee with a public display of adherence and may motivate the less-than-optimal adherer to attend class on a more regular basis. A chart with a group theme, such as "Exercise Around the World," can be devised in which daily attendance of each group member is worth a certain number of miles. When the group "reaches" predetermined countries, awards can be given that are representative of that country to all class participants. This strategy encourages group support and rewards the high attendee as well as the participant who attends class less often. It also may provide increased motivation to the wayward participant who receives a reward for being part of the group.

Make Exercise Sessions Easy, Interesting, and Fun

As previously mentioned, aspects of the exercise session itself are related to adherence and motivational issues. The exercise routine should be easy to follow; one means of accomplishing this is to break it up into achievable parts so the participant can successfully perform the routine.

Sure ways to guarantee dropouts are to have an exercise routine that is so complicated that participants cannot follow it or one so intense that participants are exhausted at the end of class. It is helpful to provide ample, positive reinforcement or support while participants are learning the routine and getting accustomed to your style as well as the personality of the class. Varying the routine regularly and providing different types of music that suit the tastes of the class can be useful. Ask participants what type of music they prefer and prepare routines to match their interests.

Poll participants to assess the enjoyment factor of the exercise program on a regular basis, perhaps through the use of the RPE scale or a simple enjoyment assessment scale. Participants should generally be exercising in an RPE range between 12 and 16. If participants are working in too high an RPE range, they may not be enjoying the exercise; rather, they may be working hard just to keep up with the instructor.

Exercise enjoyment also can be assessed orally during the exercise session with a 6-point rating scale, with one equaling "extremely unenjoyable" and six equaling "extremely enjoyable." You can determine which parts of the exercise class are most favorable to participants by asking about their enjoyment level throughout different points during class. Look at the faces of participants — if they are struggling and not having a good time during class, it will be obvious. Another option is to develop a brief anonymous written survey to assess enjoyment level of the class and satisfaction with different aspects of the exercise program. Survey responses can be saved in your personal files and used as documentation of exercise leader skills.

If it is evident that some participants are working excessively, lower the intensity of the routine for a while until the over-workers can "catch their breath" and get back into their exercise comfort zone. As previously mentioned, if the class is of varying abilities, visually provide both a lower-intensity and higher-intensity version of the routine.

The importance of a cheerful, friendly group fitness instructor cannot be overemphasized. The participants may enjoy coming to class just to see a friendly face and receive praise for what they accomplish in class. So, leave your personal problems in the locker room and greet your class with a smile!

Acknowledge Exercise Discomforts

Teach participants how to tell the difference between the transient discomforts associated with exercise and what discomforts are potentially a sign of injury or more serious problems. Newcomers to exercise may not be used to the feeling of increased breathing, heart rate, and sweating associated with exercise. They must be reassured that these are normal responses and should be expected.

Participants must be informed of potential injuries that may arise and be able to recognize a symptom that warrants attention. Any sudden, sharp pain that does not dissipate or a muscle soreness that does not lessen after a few days may be a sign of injury and should be examined by a health professional. Similarly, participants must know the signs and symptoms of a heart attack, particularly when the exercisers are of middle and older ages. A dull, aching discomfort in the chest, neck, jaw, or arms associated with excessive or clammy skin that is not relieved with rest may be signs of a heart attack; proper medical authorities should be contacted immediately.

It is helpful to ask participants individually how they are feeling and if they are experiencing any unusual discomforts; often these are not offered voluntarily and potential injuries may not be discovered without prompting from the group fitness instructor. Personal advice to take it easy for a class or two until a minor ache or pain lessens and follow-up during successive classes let the

Table 7.1
Support for Exercise

There are several types of support that can help individuals adopt and maintain an exercise program. Individuals can evaluate which types of support that are useful to them personally, and then identify individuals who can provide that type of support. If support is not readily available, individuals can specifically ask friends and colleagues to support them in specific ways as they make exercise-related goals.

Types of Support	Ways Support Can Be Received	Who can provide me this type of support? (fill in)
Emotional providers	Sympathetic to struggles with starting to exercise	
Affection providers	Comfort and reassurance when goals are not met Reward givers when goals are met	
Challengers	Challenge to make goals and achieve them	
Listeners	Sounding board for communicating experiences associated with exercise	
Appraisers	Feedback on goal achievements	
Role models/partners	Exercise partner, set and work on goals together	
Experts	Information associated with exercise	

participant know you care and are looking out for the participant's best interests.

Use Exercise Reminders, Cues, and Prompts

Encourage participants to develop prompts or cues in their home or work environments that will promote regular class attendance, such as scheduling exercise in a daily appointment book and laying out exercise gear the night before exercise class.

Posters placed at participants' homes or work environments that depict individuals enjoying exercise may be beneficial in encouraging attendance. Newsletters can include clever flyers that remind participants of upcoming special events or fitness challenges. A variety of prompts at work, home, and the exercise location can help to keep participants thinking about exercise.

Encourage an Extensive Social Support System

Develop a buddy system among participants so they can call each other to make sure they attend class and have an additional support person to discuss progress and goals. Additional social support for exercise can be encouraged by having participants ask friends or relatives to pitch in by reminding them to attend their exercise classes. Ask participants to identify what types of support are helpful and motivating to them personally, and then ask them to identify individuals who can provide that specific type of support. Table 7.1 lists different types of support and provides examples of how that type of support can be used to encourage exercise attendance. Support does not have to be face-to-face; telephone and mail contacts are additional avenues of support that can be utilized. As previously described, newsletters are a useful means for keeping participants informed of class activities, and they add to a sense of belonging. Telephone contacts initiated after one or two missed classes that let the lapsing participant know he or she was missed may encourage a return to class.

If a new participant is married, you may consider asking if the participant's spouse would be willing to also join the class. Wallace and colleagues (1995) found that adults who joined an exercise program along with a spouse had higher attendance compared with married participants whose spouse did not join the program.

Develop Group Camaraderie

It is particularly important for class members to feel a sense of cohesiveness. This tends to occur spontaneously; however, it also can be facilitated by you if the group does not appear to "gel" on its own. Simple introductions of a new class member, along with a unique "tidbit" about each member, helps everyone become familiar with each other. During exercise warm-up and cool-down, each participant can share an interesting aspect of his or her past, or provide details of a fun weekend activity. Letting participants talk about themselves when class time permits encourages the personality of each to shine. Providing interesting, little-known facts about each participant in a newsletter also is beneficial. The social support and reinforcement for exercise developed through group membership is powerful and should be not be overlooked.

By the same token, you must be aware of individual behaviors that threaten to undermine positive group dynamics. Most groups have chronic complainers or generally disruptive individuals. These individuals must be dealt with early to avoid the tendency for them to take charge of the group or monopolize your time. When dealing with a chronic complainer, listen attentively and acknowledge that you understand the participant's complaint, then agree on a solution with the participant and follow through to make any needed changes. The participant should be informed when the issue has been resolved, and you should acknowledge with the participant that there is no reason to discuss it further.

The disruptive individual should not be given too much attention (since that is probably what he or she wants). If lack of attention does not change the individual's behavior, then you must speak to the individual privately to discuss the interruptions and possible reasons for the disruptive behavior.

Emphasize Positive Aspects of Exercise

Participants just starting to exercise should be encouraged to generally disregard minor exercise discomforts, recognize their own self-defeating thoughts, and counteract them with positive thoughts. Encourage participants to think "good thoughts," such as how refreshing it feels to move about freely, how encouraging other class members are, and so on, while performing the exercise routine. Comment on positive aspects of the routine throughout; "here comes the fun part," "looking great," and similar comments keep the participants focused on the positive. Martin et al. (1984) found that those who were told to attend to environmental surroundings and enjoy the outdoors during a class-based running program had greater attendance and were more likely to continue exercising after the formal program ended compared to those who concentrated on increasing their performance during the exercise sessions. Pleasant thoughts that focus on enjoyment of movement and how accomplished the participants will feel when exercise class is over will help the class time move by quickly and enjoyably. For participants who have been exercising regularly and have specific performance goals, you can help them visualize the sense of satisfaction they will get when those goals are met. This can serve as a positive motivator when the exercise intensity necessary to meet goals may be intense and somewhat uncomfortable for the participant.

Help Participants Develop Intrinsic Rewards

After the exercise behavior is part of the participant's routine, it is often useful to supplement class rewards and support with a natural reward system that is provided outside of exercise class. Positive feedback on exercise habits provided from family, friends, and co-workers transfers some of the positive feedback received during exercise class to other environments, as well as provides additional avenues of social support. Encourage the participant to develop a natural reward system that focuses on increased feelings of self-esteem, a sense of accomplishment, and increased energy levels instead of merely external rewards. Natural reinforcers add to a sense of personal identification of being an exerciser and will help participants continue to exercise even when they cannot make it to class.

Prepare Participants for Inevitable Missed Classes

It is important to realize that the participant will not be able to attend classes at some point in a program. Although the participant may be unable to make it to class during vacations, holidays, or times of increased work or family pressures, they may still be able to continue a home-based exercise program and should be encouraged to do so. Confidence for exercising in different settings can be built by encouraging partici-

pants to add at least one day of exercise outside of class time, preferably using a different mode of exercise (such as brisk walking, swimming, or any other type of exercise the participant enjoys). This will give participants experience with an exercise alternative that will be beneficial when they must miss a scheduled class. Ask participants about exercise performed outside of class and praise them when it has been accomplished. When the participant successfully exercises on his or her own, confidence for continuing exercise in general is being built.

Exercising with family or co-workers is ideal for out-of-class exercise sessions. If the participant cannot find someone to exercise with, you can encourage other class members to meet him or her in an alternative exercise setting. Not only does this add an additional mode of social support for exercise, it also provides participants with an opportunity to problem-solve any difficulties encountered with exercise. Additional days of exercise can be included in the exercise contract, and exercise logs of these sessions can be kept to document these sessions. During times when participants are extremely busy, remind them that a shorter workout than normal is still beneficial and will keep them regularly exercising. DeBusk and colleagues (1990) showed that three 10-minute workouts performed throughout the day were just as effective in increasing fitness levels as 30-minute bouts performed at the same time. Although your primary responsibility is to encourage class attendance, supporting the concept of at least one out-of-class exercise session will ultimately help the participants' overall exercise achievement.

Classes may not be offered in some instances. For example, if classes are provided as part of a university environment, there may be a break in classes due to semester breaks or holidays. By advising participants in advance, they can prepare for these breaks. Using the skills mentioned in the previous paragraph will be beneficial during these times. You also can try to arrange exercise alternatives with other exercise classes at different locations in the community so participants can continue exercising in a similar format.

Prepare Participants for Changes in Instructors

A change in instructors is usually quite disruptive for participants. Unfortunately, little is typically done to prepare participants for this change. Planned change in leadership because of pregnancy leave, travel, or a permanent relocation can be smooth if participants are prepared for the change well ahead of time. If possible, advance introductions of the new exercise instructor are beneficial. Having the regular and new instructor team teach several exercise classes can help prevent fears of a change in format after the regular exercise instructor departs. There will undoubtedly be times of illness, so substitutes should be planned for and arranged in advance. It would be a bonus if you could introduce the substitutes to the participants so when they need to be used, participants are already familiar with them.

Train to Prevent Exercise Defeatism

Prepare participants for the eventual missed class. How slips are handled determines if they will be temporary or permanent. Let participants know that missing a class is a realistic probability. If participants can predict and prepare for lapses in their exercise program, their occurrences will not likely be as disruptive. Certain times make exercise class attendance unlikely (family crises, holidays, illness, and extra pressure or deadlines at work). When these can be anticipated and seen as being temporary rather than a breakdown in the success of the exercise program, adherence is more likely to be maintained. Lapses should be viewed as a challenge to overcome rather than as a failure.

Participants can be made aware of the defeatist attitude that accompanies the belief that once an exercise program is disrupted, total relapse or dropout is inevitable. Although breaking the adherence rule does place the participant at a higher risk for dropping out, it is not inevitable. If exercise is viewed by participants as a process in which there will undoubtedly be times that they will be less active than others, they will not consider themselves nonexercisers whenever a class is missed. Rather, they will catch the next available class or exercise on their own when time permits. Participants also can be encouraged to avoid "high-risk" situations (such as going to a "happy hour" before exercise class) that test their resolve to exercise. Encourage participants to surround themselves with cues that support the exercise behavior. A simple telephone call after one or two missed sessions may bring the participant back to class if he or she understands that missing class is not a sign of failure.

Emphasize an Overall Healthy Lifestyle

Exercise is only one of a number of lifestyle-related activities that participants engage in throughout the week. It is often assumed that those who regularly exercise also practice other healthy behaviors; unfortunately, this is often not the case. Diets of exercisers are generally not any different from the American diet and several studies have been unable to find a decreased smoking prevalence among exercisers (Blair et al., 1990). You have an excellent opportunity to provide accurate information and to encourage the development of additional healthy lifestyle behaviors. Questions regarding diet, weight control, and other behaviors will undoubtedly be asked; by being well-versed in these topics, you can offer sound information with scientific basis. Displaying posters that emphasize aspects of healthy lifestyles, such as the Food Guide Pyramid, can remind participants that physical activity is just one of many healthful behaviors.

Finally, you are viewed as a model for a healthy lifestyle and should try to live up to the participants' expectations. Encourage by example; do not smoke or abuse alcohol, and maintain a prudent, healthy diet and normal body weight.

Exercise and Body Image

Cultural norms for attractiveness are often centered on "ideal body types." In the United States, this ideal body type has, in recent times, been associated with extreme thinness, particularly in women. While this body type may photograph well for fashion magazines, it is not ideal for most women and is most likely an unattainable and potentially unhealthy goal for many. When women perceive that their bodies are being compared to this unrealistic "ideal," many become dissatisfied with their body shape and fret over any extra pounds in undesirable places.

High levels of physical activity have been associated with a preoccupation with weight and body shape. These unhealthy attitudes may put some individuals, particularly teenage and young adult women, at risk for developing **eating disorders**, such as anorexia nervosa and bulimia, as well as **addictions** to exercise or overexercise.

By being aware of this phenomenon, you can encourage participants to accept their own body shapes. Remind participants that everyone has his or her own unique body shape and no amount of exercise is going to change that basic shape. Avoid pointing out specific exercises to "fix" certain body parts since it may lead to a preoccupation or dissatisfaction with that body part. It is better for participants to focus on the enjoyment of moving and the overall good feelings associated with exercise.

While you want to encourage regular exercise participation, a small number of individuals may take the exercise habit to the extreme and exhibit signs of exercise **dependence** or addiction. Exercise dependence has been defined in a variety of ways; a good definition is when the commitment to exercise assumes a higher priority than commitments to family, work, or interpersonal relations (Morgan, 1979).

Excessive exercise may be associated with body image distortions or even more serious disorders, such as anorexia nervosa and bulimia, where excessive exercise is used as an additional method to lose weight or to "purge" calories that have recently been consumed (Brownell & Foreyt, 1986).

You can look for signs of exercise dependence/addiction in participants, including continuing to exercise in spite of injuries or illness, extreme levels of thinness, problems in interpersonal relationships, and feelings of extreme guilt, irritability, or depression when unable to exercise. If you suspect a participant is exercising to excess or may have an eating disorder, the matter should be dealt with using forethought and sensitivity. Express concern over what you have observed and ask the participant directly about his or her exercise and eating habits. Chances are that if a disorder exists, the participant has already been confronted about the situation. Be sensitive and understanding, offering support as well as suggesting that professional guidance be sought. It is helpful if several names and telephone numbers of qualified professionals are available to provide to the participant in need.

Summary

Dropout rates for those beginning an aerobics program can reach 50% or more after only six months. Instead of placing the blame for nonadherence on the participant, you must view motivation as a shared responsibility and work with the participant to develop a successful motivational strategy. Extra assistance should be provided to the participant who has been identified to be at high risk for dropout.

Motivation is a dynamic process, and by applying a variety of strategies and reviewing and refining these strategies regularly, achievement of regular exercise can be attained for most participants. Motivational techniques include structuring appropriate expectations and goals, identifying short-term benefits and providing specific feedback, teaching problem-solving skills, serving as a positive role model, and training participants to manage their own reward systems.

Additionally, the convenience and attractiveness of the exercise setting, enjoyability of the exercise class, supportiveness of the exercise environment, as well as personal factors specific to both the exercise instructor and the participant, are also factored into the exercise adherence equation. Understanding and applying the principles of adherence and motivation described in this chapter will help you develop into a more effective teacher and health professional.

References

Borg, G.A.V. (1982). Psychosocial bases of perceived exertion. *Medicine & Science in Sports & Exercise,* 14, 377–381

Blair, S.N., Kohl, H.W. III, & Brill, P.A. (1990). Behavioral adaptations to physical activity. In Bouchard, C., Shephard, R.J., Stephens, T., Stephens, J.R., & McPherson, B.D., (eds.). *Exercise, Fitness, and Health. A Consensus of Current Knowledge.* Champaign, Ill.: Human Kinetics.

Brownell, K.D. & Foreyt, J.P. (eds.). (1986). *Handbook of Eating Disorders.* New York: Basic Books, Inc.

DeBusk, R.F., Stenestrand, U., Sheehan, M., & Haskell, W.L. (1990). Training effects of long versus short bouts of exercise in healthy subjects. *American Journal of Cardiology,* 65, 1010–1013.

Martin, J.E., Dubbert, P.M., Katell, A.D., Thompson, J.K., Raczynski, J.R., Lake, M., Smith, P.O., Webster, J.S., Sikora, T., & Cohen, R.E. (1984). Behavioral control of exercise in sedentary adults: Studies 1 through 6. *Journal of Consulting & Clinical Psychology,* 52, 795–811.

Morgan, W.P. (1979). Negative addiction in runners. *Physician & Sportsmedicine,* 7, 57–70.

Robinson, J.I., Rogers, M.A., Carlson, J.J.,

Mavis, B.E., Stachnik, T., Stoffelmayr, B., Sprague, H.A., McGrew, C.R., & Van Huss, W.D. (1992). Effects of a 6-month incentive-based exercise program on adherence and work capacity. *Medicine & Science in Sports & Exercise,* 24, 85 – 93.

Wallace, J.P., Raglin, J.S., & Jastremski, C.A. (1995). Twelve month adherence of adults who joined a fitness program with a spouse vs. without a spouse. *Journal of Sports Medicine & Physical Fitness,* 35, 206 – 213.

Suggested Reading

American College of Sports Medicine. (1995). *ACSM's Guidelines for Exercise Testing and Prescription.* 5th ed. Baltimore: Williams & Wilkins.

Dishman, R.K., (ed.). (1994). *Advances in Exercise Adherence.* Champaign, Ill.: Human Kinetics.

King, A.C., Blair, S.N., Bild, D.F,, Dishman, R.K., Dubbert, P.M., Marcus, B.H., Oldridge, N.B., Paffenbarger, R.S., Jr, Powell, K.E., & Yeager, K.K. (1992). Determination of physical activity and interventions in adults. *Medicine & Science in Sports & Exercise,* 24, S221 – S236.

Sallis, J.F. & Owen, N. (1998). *Physical Activity and Behavioral Medicine.* Thousand Oaks: Sage.

U.S. Department of Health and Human Services. (1996). *Physical Activity and Health: A Report of the Surgeon General.* Atlanta, Ga.: U.S. Department of Health and Human Services, Centers for Disease Control and Prevention, National Center for Chronic Disease Prevention and Health Promotion.

Chapter 8

In This Chapter:

James H. Rimmer, Ph.D., is an associate professor in the Department of Disability and Human Development at the University of Illinois at Chicago. Dr. Rimmer is currently directing a federally funded Center on Health Promotion Research for Persons with Disabilities to examine the effects of exercise and health promotion on persons with stroke, arthritis, diabetes, and spinal cord injury. He is also the director of the National Center on Physical Activity and Disability, which is a grant funded by the Centers for Disease Control and Prevention. For the past 20 years, Dr. Rimmer has been developing exercise programs for persons with disabilities. He is the author of the textbook, *Fitness and Rehabilitation Programs for Special Populations*, and has written more than 40 journal articles on various topics related to physical activity and disability.

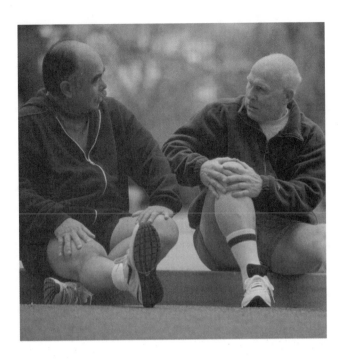

Disabilities and Health
Limitations

Until recently, many fitness professionals considered the words health and disability to be on opposite ends of the spectrum. How could a person be considered healthy if he or she already had a disability? Today that viewpoint is slowly changing, and the benefits of physical activity that have been touted by fitness organizations and policymakers for the general population are now being directed at persons with chronic diseases and disabilities.

Joining a fitness center is a viable way for persons with disabilities and health limitations to maintain their physical function after rehabilitation, and offers them the opportunity to improve their overall health in a supervised setting where, if necessary, they can get immediate assistance from a fitness professional.

People with disabilities are often faced with a higher incidence of secondary conditions (e.g., **obesity**, pressure sores, infections, **osteoporosis**), which cause further disability, and in many cases a loss of physical independence. This loss of independence often leads to depression, which causes further disease and disability (Rimmer, 1999).

This downward spiral takes a heavy physical and psychological toll on people with disabilities and often creates a life of permanent dependence on others for daily care (Figure 8.1).

People with disabilities are slowly becoming aware of the importance of maintaining an active lifestyle. They are starting to realize that as they age, exercise becomes more and more important in preserving, and in some cases restoring, their physical independence. Whereas a few years ago joining a local fitness center to maintain one's health was not even a thought among the millions of people with disabilities, particularly those with severe disabilities, today's new generation is starting to feel more comfortable using fitness centers to improve their health. The Americans with Disabilities Act has shed new light on the importance of making fitness facilities architecturally and programmatically accessible to persons with disabili-

ties, and this has raised a new awareness in the fitness community that persons with disabilities have a right to equal access to their facilities.

As we enter a new millennium, fitness professionals are being offered an exciting opportunity to reach out to people with disabilities. As managed care organizations continue their cost-saving strategies by downsizing the rehabilitation industry, there is a window of opportunity for fitness professionals to become part of the paradigm for improving the health of people with disabilities who will need community-based settings to restore, maintain, and improve their overall function. What better place to do this than in a local fitness center a few blocks from home? The purpose of this chapter is to provide you with an overview of the major disabilities and health limitations that require a modified exercise program.

Figure 8.1
Downward spiral of disability and dependence

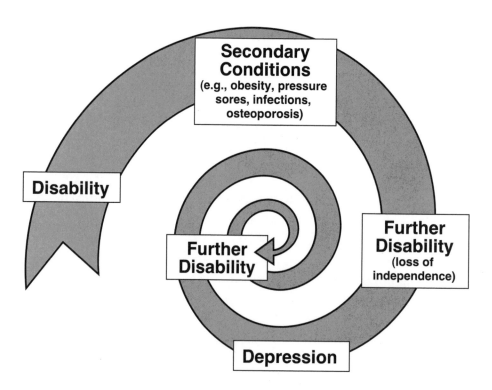

Obesity

The most prevalent health disorder in our society is obesity. Most experts agree that 25% to 40% of the population over the age of 30 can be defined as having excess body fat (U. S. Surgeon General's Report, 1996).

In large scale studies consisting of thousands of people, **body mass index (BMI)** is used to calculate the number of Americans who are **overweight**. The formula for computing BMI is weight (kg)/height^2 (m).[1] According to the National Center for Health Statistics, a BMI greater or equal to 27.3 in women and 27.8 in men is considered to be overweight, and a BMI over 30 is generally defined as obese (Expert Panel, 1998). Obesity is associated with many other medical conditions, including hypertension, **type 2 diabetes**, **osteoarthritis**, heart disease, and **low back pain** (Han et al., 1997; Rice et al., 1993).

Exercise is one of the three major cornerstones of treatment for obesity. The other two components, which are not discussed in this chapter, are diet and behavior modification (Rimmer, 1994). Since diet alone results in a loss of lean muscle tissue, the only long-term mechanism for maintaining weight loss is to increase daily energy expenditure.

Exercise Guidelines for Obesity

1. A major strategy for getting persons who are excessively overweight to develop lifelong exercise habits is to make the activity as enjoyable and pain-free as possible. Exercising with an excess amount of body fat presents a major challenge because of the additional stress that is placed on joints and muscles, particu-

---

[1] *One kg is equal to 2.2 lbs., and one m is equal to 39.37 in.*

larly in clients who are severely overweight. Additionally, these clients are often in extremely poor condition. The key to a successful program is to identify the right combination of activities that do not lead to pain or discomfort. Finding the appropriate comfort level must be done on an individual basis. Do not assume that because clients may come to you with suggested activities that they know what is best for their body type.

2. The number one priority with this clientele is to keep the activity at an intensity level that does not cause pain and soreness. Many persons who are severely overweight already have joint pain from simply performing daily activities. By using a variety of activities that involve both the arms and legs together, the stress load on the joints will be displaced over four limbs as opposed to two. Do not place heavy emphasis on the intensity level of the activity. Emphasize low-intensity, high-duration activities. It is more important for the client to move more and to enjoy the feeling of being physically active.

3. Since weight maintenance is a lifelong process, clients should understand the caloric balance equation: energy input = energy output. If this balance tilts toward the energy input side, there will be an excess of calories taken in and those not used will be stored as fat. Therefore, a daily dose of physical activity is needed to offset the calories that are being consumed. This does not necessarily mean that they have to attend the fitness center seven days a week, but does suggest that if they are going to eat every day, then they should exercise every day. A daily dose of physical activity

can be performed at home or at work by using a variety of activities that can even include housework and gardening.

4. Since arthritis is a highly prevalent condition among persons who are overweight (Rimmer, 1994), protecting the joints is paramount. Cross-training programs should be employed that involve various types of exercise routines for 10 minutes or less. More and more products are coming on the market that place a reduced load on the knee and hip joints. The elliptical trainer, stationary bike, and recumbent stepper (performed in a sitting position) are very popular among severely overweight clientele. Some clients may use two or three machines for a duration of 10 minutes on each machine. Additionally, water-based activities are excellent for obese clients who also have arthritis because of the reduced weightbearing effects of the water. Many clients, however, will not want to join an aquatics program because of their reluctance to wear a swim suit.

5. One of the areas that is often forgotten when developing exercise programs for clientele who are overweight is seat comfort. Many bicycle seats are too small or have too hard a surface for this clientele. In some cases it may be necessary to construct a special seat for severely overweight clients (300 lbs [135 kg] or more). It is also important to make sure that the seat position is adjusted in such a way that a person's stomach does not impair their ability to pedal the bike. Some overweight clients like to have their seat adjusted a little higher than normal to prevent their midsection from getting in the

way of the pedaling rotation. This usually requires the knee to be in full extension in order to pedal without obstruction.

6. Resistance training should also be performed for 10 to 15 minutes a day, three days a week. This can be done with weights or elastic bands. Weight training improves body image and increases lean body mass, which makes this activity a nice complement to the cardiovascular training component and adds variety to the program. Additionally, resistance training improves strength and makes activities of daily living such as walking up a flight of steps easier to manage.

Diabetes

Diabetes is one of the most debilitating conditions in our society, and is often linked to a number of chronic diseases and disabilities including heart disease, stroke, amputations, blindness, kidney failure, autonomic **neuropathy** (affects heart rate [HR]), and peripheral neuropathy (affects sensation in distal extremities) (Franz & Nordstrom, 1991). There are two types of diabetes: type 1 and type 2. **Type 1 diabetes** is caused by a destruction of pancreatic cells that produce the body's **insulin**. Type 2 diabetes results from insulin resistance combined with defective insulin secretion.[2]

---

[2] *The old categories for classifying diabetes that were established in 1979 included the terms insulin-dependent diabetes mellitus (IDDM, type I) and non-insulin-dependent diabetes mellitus (NIDDM, type II). These terms are no longer used since they created confusion among the general community. Many people thought that if you were taking insulin, you automatically had type 1 diabetes. The roman numerals (I, II) were dropped to avoid confusion.*

Diabetes is a broadly applied term used to denote a complex group of syndromes that result in a disturbance in the utilization of glucose. Type 1 diabetes is a much more serious condition and can result in death if not treated properly. The person must take regular amounts of insulin in order to sustain a safe amount of glucose in the blood. When insulin is not taken, blood glucose, which normally ranges between 80 to 120 mg/dL, can reach a 1,000 mg/dL or higher and cause the person to go into a diabetic coma or die.

Persons with type 2 diabetes are not dependent on insulin injections, but in many cases they are prescribed to assist glucose uptake in the body. Some clients will only be on oral hypoglycemic agents (pills), and a third group will be on a combination of insulin and pills. All of these conditions depend on the function of the liver and pancreas, the two major organs involved in glucose regulation.

Between 80% and 90% of persons with type 2 diabetes are also overweight or obese (Rimmer, 1994). Exercise can have a significant effect on lowering blood glucose and is an essential component of treatment for persons with type 1 and type 2 diabetes. However, because glucose is needed to perform exercise, persons with diabetes can easily run into trouble if their baseline blood glucose level is too high or too low.

Exercise Guidelines for Persons with Diabetes

1. The most important aspect of the exercise program for persons with diabetes is maintaining the proper balance of food and insulin dosage. If too many calories are ingested before exercise or too little insulin is taken, blood glucose can reach a high enough level where exercise will actually cause a further increase in blood glu-

cose levels because of the breakdown of fatty acids and glycogen (the storage form of glucose).

2. Most diabetes experts recommend that blood glucose levels should be lower than 250 or 300 mg/dL before exercise is initiated (Albright, 1997; American College of Sports Medicine, 1997). High blood glucose values often occur when a person forgets to take his or her insulin or has eaten significantly more calories than usual and there is not enough insulin available to assist the glucose in being metabolized by the body. Check with the client's physician to determine which dosage (250 or 300 mg/dL) should be used for delaying activity.

3. Persons with diabetes should carry a portable **glucometer** with them. This device is inexpensive and can be used to check blood glucose before and after exercise. Persons with diabetes should check their blood glucose level a few minutes before starting their exercise program. If the blood glucose level is between 120 and 300 mg/dL, they are permitted to exercise.

4. Another common problem in persons with diabetes is a condition known as **hypoglycemia**. Hypoglycemia is defined as a blood glucose level less than 60 mg/dL, and occurs when there is not enough glucose in the bloodstream. Most experts agree that this is an even more dangerous situation than **hyperglycemia** (high blood glucose) because it can happen very quickly and can lead to an **insulin reaction**. This is often a greater problem in persons who have type 1 diabetes. If some form of food is not ingested immediately, the person could go into **insulin shock** and die. Table 8.1 lists the early and

Table 8.1
Symptoms and Treatment of
Insulin Reaction (Hypoglycemia)

Early Symptoms	Late Symptoms
Anxiety, uneasiness	Double vision
Irritability	Sweating, palpitations
Extreme hunger	Nausea
Confusion	Loss of motor coordination
Headaches	Pale, moist skin
Insomnia	Strong, rapid pulse
	Convulsions
	Loss of consciousness
	Coma

Treating a Client Who Is Having an Insulin Reaction

1. Stop the activity immediately.
2. Have the person sit down and check blood glucose level.
3. Have the client drink orange juice or some other rapidly absorbing carbohydrate.
4. Allow the client to sit quietly and wait for a response.
5. When the client feels better, check blood glucose level again.
6. If the blood glucose level is above 100 mg/dL and the client feels better, resume activity.
7. Check blood glucose level after 15 to 30 minutes to reassure that levels are within a safe range.
8. Do not allow the client to leave the facility until blood glucose levels are within a normal range.
9. If client does not improve, seek medical attention immediately.

Rimmer, JH. (1994).

late symptoms of an insulin reaction and how to treat one if it does occur. Fitness professionals should keep rapidly absorbed carbohydrates on site (e.g., orange juice or other fruit drinks) in case of an emergency.

5. Blood glucose should also be measured after exercise to make sure the client does not become hypoglycemic. In persons with recently diagnosed diabetes, it will take a few sessions to learn how to maintain a normal balance of glucose and insulin before and after exercise.

6. Fitness professionals should know if clients with diabetes have secondary conditions that may will have to be considered in the exercise program (e.g., foot ulcers,

visual or kidney problems, hypertension). For example, if a client has a foot ulcer, high-impact or weightbearing exercise is contraindicated. If a person has diabetic retinopathy (damage to the retina) or hypertension, heavy resistance training is unsafe. It is important to know the complete medical history of the client and develop the exercise program based on individual needs and limitations.

7. Aerobic exercise that involves repetitive submaximal contractions of major muscle groups, such as swimming, cycling, and brisk walking, are recommended for persons with diabetes. These activities are less jarring than jogging, racquet sports, basketball, and high-impact aerobics.

8. The intensity, frequency, and duration of exercise should be based on the age, medical status, and motivational level of the client. Here is a good example of the importance of this information. A client with type 2 diabetes wanted to run on a treadmill. In doing so, she elevated her heart rate to over 85% of her age-predicted maximum heart rate. Since she had other secondary conditions of concern (e.g., hypertension, retinopathy, kidney complications), she was only permitted to exercise between 50% and 65% of her target heart rate as prescribed by her physician.

9. Since it is difficult to maintain an optimal balance of glucose and insulin, exercise should be performed daily. This does not necessarily mean that the client has to come to the fitness center on a daily basis. There are many other activities that can be done at home. Having the "best of both worlds" may involve a three-day-a-week structured program in the fitness center and a four-day-a-week program of general activity, including walking, gardening,

or stationary cycling. The key is to get a regular "dose" of activity daily.

10. The duration of activity will also depend on the client's comfort level, with a goal of 30 to 60 minutes. Individuals with higher tolerance levels for exercise, and who are more motivated, will generally prefer to exercise between 45 to 60 minutes.

11. Avoid exercise in the late evening. A person can have a nocturnal insulin reaction (an insulin reaction during sleep) if they exercise too close to bedtime and are low in carbohydrates. Since the person is unaware that they are having an insulin reaction, they could go into a coma and die.

General guidelines and safety tips for persons with diabetes are listed in Table 8.2.

Respiratory and Pulmonary Disorders

Asthma

Chronic obstructive pulmonary disease (**COPD**) is the fifth leading cause of death in the United States (O'Donnell et al., 1993). The three majors types of COPD are **asthma**, **chronic bronchitis**, and **emphysema**.

Asthma is the leading cause of respiratory problems in this country. It is considered a multifactorial disease because it is linked to several potential causes, which include heredity, infections, allergies, socioeconomic status (incidence is higher in low-income groups), psychosocial, and environmental factors. In the United States alone, there are close to 15 million people who have asthma (Centers for Disease Control and Prevention, 1996).

The majority of persons with asthma have a reduction in breathing capacity during and, more commonly, after exercise (Rimmer, 1994). This is called **exercise-induced asthma** (**EIA**). In addition to EIA,

Table 8.2
General Guidelines and Safety Tips
for Persons with Diabetes

1. Regulating blood glucose levels requires optimal timing of exercise periods in relation to meals and insulin dosage.

2. Aim for keeping blood glucose levels between 100 and 200 mg/dL one to two hours after a meal.

3. Exercise can have a significant effect on insulin reduction (Franz & Nordstrom, 1991). Some experts note that insulin may need to be reduced by 10% to 50% when starting an exercise program (Wallberg-Henriksson, 1992).

4. If blood glucose levels are lower than 100 mg/dL, have the person consume a rapidly absorbing carbohydrate to increase blood glucose.

5. If blood glucose is greater than 300 mg/dL before exercise (some doctors may recommend that exercise not be initiated at blood glucose levels greater than 250 mg/dL), make sure that insulin or the oral hypoglycemic agent has been taken. In some circumstances, clients with a high blood glucose level (> 300 mg/dL) may lower it to a safe enough level to exercise by drinking water.

6. No client should be allowed to exercise if their blood glucose level does not fall to a safe range before exercise.

7. Teach clients to check their feet periodically to avoid foot ulcers. If an ulcer is found, have the person consult with their physician immediately for proper treatment. Foot ulcers can worsen and cause major problems if left untreated.

8. Check blood glucose at the end of the exercise session to make sure that the person does not become hypoglycemic. This could happen very quickly, particularly after high intensity or long duration activities or when the person is not accustomed to understanding how their body reacts to exercise.

9. Make sure the client is well hydrated and drinking water frequently during the exercise class.

other conditions that may trigger an asthma attack are cold temperatures, stress, and air pollution (Blumenthal, 1996). Exercise is beneficial for persons with asthma provided the program is tailored to the individual's needs (Emtner et al., 1996). Most doctors now recommend exercise to child and adult asthma sufferers because of the physiological and psychological benefits derived from physical activity.

Exercise Guidelines for Asthma

1. It is important to make sure that the exercise program is coordinated with the timing of the asthma medication. Based on input from the client's physician, you must know when the medicine has to be taken to avoid an asthma episode during exercise. This will depend on the type of medication that is taken. Medicines used in inhalers work within a few minutes, while medicines taken in oral form may take up to 30 minutes to reach full capacity.

2. Encourage the client to use a **peak flow meter** to monitor the flow of air through the lungs. This simple plastic device can often determine if an asthma attack will occur or is occurring during or after exercise. The person simply blows into the meter and records the score. When peak flow drops more than 20% from normal values, activity should be reduced on that day. Peak flow meters can be purchased at any pharmacy for approximately $20 to $30. Steps for managing an asthma attack are shown in Table 8.3.

3. Light warm-ups may be very helpful in reducing the risk of an asthma attack. The client should perform a light cardiovascular activity at 40% – 50% of target heart rate for five to 10 minutes. This will help prepare the pulmonary system for more vigorous activity.

4. In persons with severe asthma as noted by their physician, short bouts of exercise may reduce the incidence of an asthma attack. For example, three sets of four- to six-minute aerobic exercise routines with a five-minute rest interval between sets will allow the respiratory system to gradually adjust to the workload.

Table 8.3
Steps for Managing an Asthma Attack

The time to treat an asthma episode is when the symptoms (e.g., coughing, wheezing, chest tightness, difficulty breathing) first appear.

Attack-management Steps
1. Rest and relax.
2. Use medicines (inhaler) prescribed for attack.
3. Drink warm liquids.

Rest and Relax
- At the first sign of breathing difficulties, the person should STOP and rest for at least 10 minutes.
- Make the person feel comfortable and relaxed.

Take Medication
- Make sure the prescribed medicine is available and that the person understands how to correctly take the medicine (inhalers require practice).

Drink Warm Liquid
- Drink slowly.
- Do not ingest cold drinks.

Emergency Care
- If you have any doubts about the severity of the attack, get medical help immediately.
- If the person's lips or fingernails are turning blue or if he or she exhibits shallow breathing and is focusing all attention on breathing, get medical help immediately.

---

5. Exercise intensity should lie within the client's comfort zone. Young individuals with asthma may be able to exercise at very high intensity levels provided they take their medication before exercise. However, older individuals may have greater difficulty exercising at moderately high (60% – 75% of target heart rate range) intensity levels. This will depend on the client's functional capacity and the severity of the asthma. Use the rating of perceived exertion (RPE) scale (see Figure 4.4) and peak flow readings along with heart rate to monitor the intensity of the exercise. A sample exercise program for persons with asthma is shown in Table 8.4.

6. Persons with exercise-induced asthma should always carry their inhaler with

Table 8.4
A Sample Exercise Program for Persons with Asthma

Duration	*Intensity*	*Frequency*	*Modality (cont.)*
In the early stages of the program, some individuals will respond more positively to short workouts with brief rest intervals.	Begin at a low intensity and gradually increase as the person's fitness level improves.	Frequency should range between three and seven days a week depending on the interest and motivational level of the client.	Stationary cycling, brisk walking (performed indoors on high pollution, high pollen, or cold days), and circuit training (with adequate rest intervals) should be safe activities.
At certain times of the year (e.g., cold weather, high pollution), duration may have to be reduced to avoid an asthma episode.	Intensity should be fall between 50% and 75% of age-predicted maximum heart rate (MHR).	*Modality* Swimming is highly recommended for persons with asthma since the temperature and humidity of the air above water seem to protect the person from an asthma episode. The one exception is with individuals who are allergic to chlorine and other chemicals that are used in pools.	Anaerobic activities such as weight training and softball should not cause problems.
	If using interval-training techniques, the rest period should be short enough or long enough depending on the individual's fitness level to lower the heart rate to 40% – 50% of age-predicted MHR before initiating the next exercise bout.		High-intensity activities such as running, soccer, and basketball may cause the most problems.
	Always check peak expiratory flow rate (PEFR) before starting the exercise session. If PEFR drops below 20% of normal values, reduce intensity level and monitor the client carefully for dyspnea and fatigue.		

them. If an asthma episode occurs, a **beta-adrenergic agent** (found in inhalers) is the only way to reverse the symptoms of a full-blown attack. Make sure that the inhaler is with the person at all times.

7. Since cold air is a major trigger of asthma attacks, when exercising outdoors the client may be advised to wear a scarf or surgical mask over the nose and mouth to warm the inspired air and reduce heat loss.

8. After a cold or the flu, persons with asthma are more susceptible to breathing problems during exercise. The client should be monitored closely after an illness and should be encouraged to start back very slowly by reducing the duration and intensity of the exercise.

Bronchitis and Emphysema

Despite the small reduction in the incidence of smoking in this nation, bronchitis and emphysema remain nagging problems in our society. Both conditions cause severe problems in breathing capacity. Damaged lung tissue reduces the delivery of oxygen to working muscles. As pulmonary function declines, breathlessness and exercise intolerance become hallmark symptoms of these diseases.

Exercise is considered to be an essential component of treatment for persons with bronchitis and emphysema. The primary aim of the exercise program is to reduce breathlessness and improve exercise tolerance. Exercise intensity should be based on RPE, which seems to be a more reliable indicator than heart rate in this clientele

(O'Donnell et al., 1993). Individuals who are in the advanced stages of the disease may require supplemental oxygen during exercise. If you do not feel comfortable working with this clientele, a respiratory therapist or physical therapist should be consulted.

Exercise Guidelines for Bronchitis and Emphysema

1. The more impaired a client with COPD is the greater the emphasis on interval-training techniques. In some clients with very low exercise tolerance levels, it may be necessary to exercise for 30 to 60 seconds and then rest for 30 to 60 seconds. As the person improves his or her fitness level, these numbers can be altered to accommodate a higher intensity level. For example, as the person's conditioning level improves, you might increase exercise time to two minutes with a 30-second rest interval.

2. The exercise program should address the interest level and capabilities of the client with prescribed endurance activities that vary little in oxygen cost. A relatively constant intensity may help prevent **dyspnea** (difficulty breathing), which is the number-one problem with exercise. Examples of low-variability exercises include walking, recumbent stepping, and stationary cycling. High-variability exercises include walking up and down inclines, calisthenics, dancing, and sports such as basketball and racquet sports.

3. Low-intensity weight training is relatively safe for persons with COPD. The person should feel comfortable lifting the weight and should not hyperventilate or become breathless. Avoid spikes in breathing rate by making sure that the weight is not too heavy and the person is not holding his or her breath.

4. Although warm-up and cool-down activities are important components of an exercise program for all individuals, they are particularly important for persons with COPD. The goal of the exercise program is to gradually increase heart rate so that the lungs can slowly adjust to the increased workload. If strenuous exercise is started too quickly, there is a higher likelihood of respiratory distress. In addition, make sure the warm-up includes exercises of decreasing intensity (e.g., walking or cycling at a progressively slower rate).

5. Teach clients to decrease their breathing frequency and to increase the amount of air they take into their lungs with each breath. Many clients with COPD take shallow breaths and do not get enough oxygen into the pulmonary system, which ultimately leads to dyspnea and fatigue. **Diaphragmatic breathing** and pursed-lip breathing can be used to help patients improve their breathing capacity. Table 8.5 explains the technique for teaching and performing these two very important techniques.

Table 8.5
Diaphragmatic and Pursed-lip Breathing Technique

Diaphragmatic Breathing
1. Have the client lie down on his/her back.
2. Have the client place one hand on the abdomen and one hand on the chest.
3. Teach the client to inspire with maximal outward movement of the abdomen.
4. Once the client is comfortable in the supine position, perform the technique in sitting and standing positions.

Pursed-lip Breathing
1. This can be performed separately or during diaphragmatic breathing exercises.
2. Teach the client to slowly exhale against a slight resistance created by lightly pursing the lips. The resistance has the potential to increase oxygen saturation.

Joint and Bone Disorders

As the average lifespan approaches 80 years of age, joint and bone disorders will become pandemic in our society. Baby boomers who are starting to enter older adulthood will, in a few short years, dramatically increase the number of people who have arthritis and/or osteoporosis. Fitness professionals will have to be integrally involved in finding ways to develop exercise programs that will allow individuals with these conditions to continue to maintain an active lifestyle.

Arthritis

The two major types of arthritis are osteoarthritis and **rheumatoid arthritis**. Osteoarthritis is often referred to as the wear-and-tear type, while rheumatoid arthritis is considered a whole body autoimmune disease, which implies that the body's own immune system attacks healthy tissue. Both types have the same joint-destroying properties and similar treatment strategies, which include exercise.

Most persons with arthritis experience some degree of pain. The pain has often been described as a nagging dull toothache. While some clients will be able to tolerate high levels of pain, others will be unwilling to perform any exercise that causes discomfort. The exercise program must be tailored to the individual's pain threshold if he or she is likely to continue with the program.

Exercise Guidelines for Arthritis

1. Most persons with arthritis can benefit from an exercise program (Ettinger et al., 1997). The fitness program must not place excessive loads around damaged joints. For persons who have been sedentary for a long while, starting slowly is very important.

2. The immediate goal of exercise is to increase muscle strength in order to maintain or improve joint stability. By strengthening muscles around damaged joints, there is a greater displacement of the stress load away from the joint and into the muscle.

3. Swimming is an ideal activity because of the lower stress loads on the joints due to the buoyancy of the water. However, many older adults do not like the time and energy that it takes to prepare for an aquatics class, particularly if it is difficult to dress and undress because of joint stiffness and pain. Others may not know how to swim or may feel self-conscious in a swim suit.

4. The emphasis of the exercise program for persons with arthritis is to mitigate pain during activity. Low-impact, non-weightbearing activities are recommended. The client must understand that they will probably have to learn to tolerate some amount of pain or discomfort with any movement, but as long as the pain does not linger for longer than two hours after exercise or return 24 to 48 hours after exercise, it is considered an acceptable activity. Pain can be minimized in a number of ways, including braces or straps, ice and/or heat before and after exercise, isolating the damaged joint during exercise, using water-based exercises, and not overusing the damaged joint. Consult with a physical therapist to learn more about pain management during activity.

5. Exercise machines that allow the person to use all four limbs simultaneously seem to have the most benefit for persons with

arthritis since the stress load is evenly displaced throughout all the limbs. Machines that require the use of all four limbs include some recumbent steppers and stationary bikes, which are performed while sitting, and elliptical machines and cross-country ski machines, which are performed while standing (this last machine may require some practice time to perform correctly).

6. In circumstances where the client is unable to use a certain leg or arm because of pain, the person can exercise with two or three limbs while resting the damaged joint. If both legs are affected, the person can use just the arms to perform a cardiovascular workout.

7. One machine that has either been too difficult to use or causes too much pain in many clients with arthritis is the stairclimber. This machine excessively loads the knee, hip joints, and spine and often results in pain in persons with arthritis. Other weightbearing activities that may cause pain include treadmill running and high-impact aerobics classes. Individuals with arthritis are advised to stay away from these activities. General exercise guidelines for persons with arthritis are listed in Table 8.6.

Osteoporosis

Osteoporosis is a disease that drains the bones of their mineral content and increases their susceptibility to fractures. In the later stages of the disease, bones often become brittle enough to fracture at the slightest tap of the wrist, or a rib could fracture from a cough or sneeze. In severe cases, the vertebra can become as thin as eggshells, leading to compression fractures and resulting in a stooped posture.

Table 8.6
Exercise Guidelines for
Persons with Arthritis

1. Any exercise that causes pain during exercise, 2 hours after exercise, or 24 to 48 hours after exercise should be discontinued.

2. Find alternative ways to exercise muscles around painful joints. For example, straight leg exercises are a good way to strengthen the leg muscles around a painful knee.

3. Warm-up and cool-down sessions are essential aspects of most exercise programs, but are especially important for persons with arthritis due to joint stiffness.

4. Resistance training activities should be conducted, but exercises that cause pain to a particular joint should be replaced with isometric strength exercises.

5. If conducting pool exercise, try to maintain water temperature between 85° and 90° F (29° and 32° C).

6. Use smooth, repetitive motions in all activities.

7. Keep the exercise intensity level below the discomfort threshold.

8. Be aware that in persons with rheumatoid arthritis, acute flareups can occur. Exercise may not be advisable until the flareup subsides.

9. Clients with osteoarthritis often perform better in the morning, while clients with rheumatoid arthritis may be better off exercising several hours after being awake.

Osteoporosis is often referred to as the silent killer because in the majority of cases there are no signs of the disease until the person fractures a hip and complications ensue. In the early stages of the disease, there are often no symptoms. However, as a person reaches their 60s and 70s, signs of osteoporosis may develop. As the bones in the spine lose their mineral content, a hunching over occurs, which is referred to as **kyphosis** or **dowager's hump**. This is often accompanied by pain and psychological distress (Rimmer, 1999).

Reduced weightbearing due to disuse or immobilization leads to progressive thinning and eventual loss of bone mineral. Studies on astronauts found significant bone loss from being suspended in a gravity-free environment (Kaplan, 1995). Likewise, studies have demonstrated that individuals who were confined to bed for several weeks at a time were also shown to have accelerated bone loss.

Exercise Guidelines for Osteoporosis

1. Before developing the exercise program, you should know if any of your older male clients (men over 65) or postmenopausal women have been diagnosed with osteoporosis. Since the vast majority of older individuals have never been tested for osteoporosis, it is important for you to go through the following checklist to determine if a member should be screened by their physician.

- Is there a family history of osteoporosis?
- Did the person go through early menopause?
- Has she had a hysterectomy?
- Does he or she smoke?
- Does he or she have a low calcium intake?
- Are there any signs of osteoporosis (previous fracture, stooped posture)?
- Is he or she taking any medication that may increase bone loss (e.g., prednisone)?

   If the client responds yes to any of these questions, it is suggested that the person be screened by their physician for osteoporosis. By knowing that a client may be at risk for osteoporosis, you are assuring that the exercise program will be tailored to the individual's needs and that the program will be as safe as possible.

2. For clients who have been diagnosed with osteoporosis and/or have signs of the disease (e.g., dowager's hump, previous fracture), resistance exercises should be approved by their physician. For safety reasons, it is always best to progress slowly using light weights for the first month of the program. As the person increases in strength, progress to heavier weights if there is no pain in the area that you are strengthening. Use six to 12 repetitions and perform one to three sets depending on the client's comfort level. For clients with advanced osteoporosis (as noted by their physician), use elastic bands in the early stages of the program. Some weight machines start at too high a resistance and are difficult to get into and out for some older, frail clients. After two to three months, progress to heavier bands or light weights. Individuals with advanced osteoporosis will require more time to adapt to a resistance-training program and must progress at a much slower rate than a healthy older adult to avoid injury.

3. Resistance exercises should be performed two to three days a week. Avoid exercises near or over the spine if pain is present. If pain is not present, target the muscles around the spine by performing shoulder retraction exercises and shoulder raises. Make sure the movements are performed slowly and do not cause pain. These exercises will also help improve posture (many older adults become round-shouldered as they age), and will potentially "load" the vertebra enough to increase or maintain their density.

4. In younger individuals (<50 years) who do not have advanced osteoporosis, use explosive-type exercises to improve bone density. This may be the most effective way to increase bone mass. Many experts have noted that bones must be

stressed to a minimal threshold value in order to attain significant gains in bone mass (Frost, 1997). If the stress threshold is not high enough, the potential for bone development is greatly reduced. One study found that exercises such as step aerobics and jumping down from a box or platform approximately 12 – 15 inches high significantly increased bone mineral density in healthy sedentary women between the ages of 35 and 45 years (Heinonen, 1996). However, one very important caveat is that there is a higher risk of injury when performing these types of exercises. Older persons and postmenopausal women interested in participating in a high-impact step class, should be asked to sign a waiver that explains the risk of injury when performing these types of exercises.

5. When developing explosive step exercises, start with one step and gradually add steps as the person becomes more conditioned. Emphasize to your clients that they should limit these classes to two to three days a week because of their high stress load and potential for injury. Monitor your clients very closely to make sure there is no soreness or pain after each class.

6. Although most of the studies on exercise and osteoporosis have indicated that resistance training and explosive-type exercises have achieved the greatest results in bone density, older persons with osteoporosis often become deconditioned from a lack of activity. This deconditioned state often leads to higher levels of inactivity and spirals the person into further disease and disability. If a person is in the advanced stages of osteoporosis (as noted by their physician), it is best to perform cardiovascular exercises from a seated position for part of the class time. A recumbent stepper is an excellent machine that allows frail clients to perform safe cardiovascular exercise. The person sits in a large seat and moves the arms and legs simultaneously. Many older adults prefer this machine over a stationary bike or standing machine (e.g., treadmill) because it is relatively easy to use and has a comfortable seat.

7. Older persons with osteoporosis may have difficulty performing repetitive exercises that use the same muscle groups for extended periods of time. Therefore, circuit-training programs that require short periods of work using various muscle groups are recommended.

8. In addition to circuit-training programs, interval-training activities that require brief periods of work followed by a rest interval may also be beneficial for deconditioned clients with advanced osteoporosis. For example, riding a stationary bike for one minute followed by a 30-second rest interval may delay fatigue and allow the person to sustain longer periods of activity. Other cardiovascular activities can be used to improve functional performance provided they do not incur pain or result in premature fatigue. Although swimming and pool exercises are excellent modalities for improving cardiovascular endurance, they are not recommended for improving bone density. Water is a non-gravity environment and does not seem to place enough of a stress load on bone tissue to increase its mass (Bravo et al., 1997). General safety guidelines for developing an exercise program for persons with osteoporosis are shown in Table 8.7.

Table 8.7
Safety Concerns when Developing an Exercise Program for Persons with Osteoporosis

- Always obtain physician consent before developing the exercise program.
- Screen your client before developing the program. Consult with his or her physician on developing resistance exercises at the site where a fracture may have occurred.
- Avoid jarring or high-load exercises in persons with advanced osteoporosis.
- Avoid back exercises in clients who have localized pain in this region and show signs of kyphosis.
- When performing standing exercises with older clients who have a high risk of injury from a fall or fracture, or who have fallen previously, make sure there is something to hold on to at all times (e.g., ballet barre, parallel bars, chair).
- Reevaluate your program if there are any signs of pain or fatigue during or after an exercise session in the osteoporosis zones (hip, back, or wrist).

Physical Disabilities

People with physical disabilities have limited or no use of their arms, legs, or both the arms and legs. The major conditions include **spinal cord injury**, **spina bifida**, **cerebral palsy**, and amputations. A description of each of these conditions is given below.

Spinal cord injuries are traumatic injuries that damage or sever the spinal cord. They typically occur from a car or motorcycle accident, diving injury, or gun shot or stab wound. Individuals with spinal cord injuries are usually classified as having one of two conditions: paraplegia — paralysis or weakness in the legs but not the arms — or quadriplegia — paralysis or weakness in both the arms and the legs.

Spina bifida is caused by spinal cord damage sustained at birth. This condition results in paraplegia. Individuals who have spina bifida have physical characteristics similar to clients with traumatic spinal cord injuries.

Cerebral palsy results from an injury to the brain before, during, or after birth. This injury often results in spasticity, or tight muscles, which makes it difficult for clients to move in a smooth, fluid manner. Some individuals will end up with paraplegia, others with a more serious form of cerebral palsy will have quadriplegia, and a third group will have hemiplegia, which is weakness or paralysis on either the right or left side of the body (very similar to stroke).

Amputations are classified under three headings: traumatic, elective, and acquired. A traumatic amputation is caused by an accident or injury. An elective amputation occurs when a limb must be removed to prevent the spread of infection or disease and is usually secondary to infection (diabetes is the most common reason) or cancer. An acquired amputation occurs when an individual is born without a limb.

Exercise Guidelines for Persons with Physical Disabilities

1. According to the Americans with Disabilities Act, fitness centers must be architecturally barrier-free so that persons with physical disabilities can participate in the same kinds of programs offered to nondisabled members. This means that both the structure of the facility and the programs that are offered must be accessible to persons with disabilities. For example, at least one bathroom and water fountain must be accessible to people who use wheelchairs. Corridors should be free of obstacles that could interfere with a wheelchair or present a hazard to someone using a walker, cane, or braces.

2. Before performing a fitness evaluation on someone with a physical disability, check to see if they have been recently evaluated by a physical therapist. Many individuals who have sustained a spinal cord

injury or an amputation will have received a comprehensive physical therapy evaluation during their time at a rehabilitation hospital or center.

3. In many instances, persons with physical disabilities have coexisting secondary conditions (e.g., bladder dysfunction, spasticity, joint problems) that must be taken into consideration when preparing the exercise program. These conditions may require a modification in the program depending on their incidence and severity.

4. Persons who use a wheelchair to ambulate will often present some important variations to the exercise prescription. Refer to Table 8.8 for exercise guidelines for wheelchair users.

Multiple Sclerosis

Multiple sclerosis is one of the most common neuromuscular disorders. It is classified as a progressive disease, which means that the symptoms have a tendency to worsen as the person ages. A wide variety of complications can occur from multiple sclerosis, including gait disturbances and bladder and bowel problems. The disease often consists of flare-ups (called exacerbations) and periods of stability (remission). In the usual course of the disease, exacerbations occur every few years. The progression of the disease varies from person to person.

Exercise Guidelines for Persons with Multiple Sclerosis

1. Be aware that the symptoms of multiple sclerosis may get progressively worse over time. The treatment strategy aims to slow the progression of the disease. People with multiple sclerosis should make exercise

Table 8.8
Exercise Guidelines for Persons Using Wheelchairs

1. Most clients with quadriplegia (little or no use of the arms and legs) and high-level paraplegia (an injury sustained to the spinal cord at the sixth thoracic vertebra or higher) will not be able to achieve heart rates higher than 120 to 130 beats per minute due to the damage sustained to their sympathetic nervous system. Consequently, these clients should use rating of perceived exertion to gauge exercise intensity.

2. Clients with low-level paraplegia (an injury occurring at the seventh thoracic vertebrae or lower) should be able to achieve a similar training intensity as clients of the same age and sex who have no disability. However, since the person is using smaller muscle groups in the arms to perform the exercise, there are circulatory limitations that prevent the person from achieving the same maximum heart rate as when performing leg exercise. There is also an earlier onset of fatigue when performing arms-only exercise.

3. Whenever possible, check blood pressure to make sure that it is within the normal range for the client. Blood pressure has a tendency to fluctuate in persons with quadriplegia and high-level paraplegia because of autonomic nervous system dysfunction resulting from their injuries.

4. Always make sure that the client has voided the bladder before exercise. In some individuals with spinal cord injury, a condition known as autonomic dysreflexia can occur from a full bladder or infection. This can increase blood pressure to dangerously high levels before exercise is even initiated. Seek medical emergency care immediately if this condition is present.

5. An upper-arm ergometer is an excellent cardiovascular training modality for persons who are nonambulatory.

6. Strength-training equipment may need adaptations to meet the needs of this clientele. Special straps and gloves are available through manufacturers of adaptive equipment that allow the feet and hands to be attached to the equipment.

an integral part of their daily regimen. As long as activities are not too strenuous, exercise should not be harmful.

2. Balance is often compromised in persons with multiple sclerosis. Take every precaution to make the exercise setting as safe as possible in order to minimize the risk of falling. Provide chairs or a portable ballet barre that the person can hold onto for stability while performing exercises in the standing position.

3. As balance worsens, the risk of falls increases. When and if balance worsens, develop activities that can be performed in a sitting position. Change from free weights to machines to eliminate the risk of a weight being dropped on a client's foot. Stationary bikes, recumbent steppers, and upper-arm ergometers can be used to enhance cardiovascular fitness in a seated position. When balance is very poor, use a recumbent bike for further stability.

4. Because clients with multiple sclerosis often experience a great deal of spasticity (tightness) as their condition progresses, make sure that flexibility exercise are a major component of the program.

5. Since clients with multiple sclerosis often have difficulty initiating a movement in the advanced stages of the disease, allow them the extra time to begin and complete each movement.

6. Swimming is one of the best activities for clients with multiple sclerosis, provided the water temperature remains below 80°F (27°C). Warm water will cause premature fatigue in this clientele.

7. Since overheating can cause a temporary loss of function, make sure the facility is well ventilated and the room temperature is at a comfortable level. Exercise should be discouraged in warm, humid environments.

8. Individuals with multiple sclerosis often lose control of their bladder in the later stages of the disease. Make sure the bladder is voided before and after exercise. Be prepared for possible accidents by having the appropriate cleaning materials available (e.g., bleach), and make sure that the client understands that you are aware that a possible accident can occur.

Coronary Heart Disease

Coronary heart disease is a multifaceted disorder that varies greatly from person to person. Since the purpose of this chapter is to discuss conditions that fitness professionals will be exposed to in their own setting, patients with advanced coronary heart disease will not be discussed here, as they would not be advised to exercise in these settings. It would be more appropriate to recommend an outpatient cardiac rehabilitation program. General exercise guidelines for clients with known coronary heart disease are shown in Table 8.9.

Exercise Guidelines for Coronary Heart Disease

1. If a client has been approved by a physician to exercise in a less supervised setting such as a fitness center, the major goal is to avoid high-intensity exercise that has a greater likelihood of precipitating a coronary event. The exercise program for persons with known coronary heart disease should include an advanced warm-up that consists of low-intensity

---

Table 8.9
General Exercise Guidelines for Clients with Known Coronary Heart Disease

1. Avoid extremes of heat and cold that can place a greater stress on the heart.

2. Use heart-rate monitors to regulate exercise intensity, and avoid activities that cause large fluctuations in heart rate.

3. Stay within the blood pressure and target heart rate zones established by the client's physician.

4. Report all symptoms, especially light-headedness, chest pain, or dizziness, to the client's physician.

5. Make sure that heart rate and blood pressure return to resting levels before the client leaves the exercise setting.

6. If a client complains of chest pain before, during, or after exercise, contact emergency medical services.

---

exercise such as light walking or riding a stationary bike with little or no resistance, several different stretching exercises particularly in the chest region if a person has had open-heart surgery, and some mild breathing exercises that could be part of a yoga or postural relaxation class. An advanced warm-up session may determine if any chest discomfort or dizziness is present before initiating higher-intensity exercise.

2. RPE should be taught to clients with known coronary heart disease. Some clients may have a pacemaker or be on beta blockers, which blunt the heart rate response and will not give an accurate indication of exercise intensity. Try to associate a certain RPE value with the person's heart rate. Although the heart rate will be lower in persons who are on beta blockers, the value should correlate fairly well with heart rate.

3. Persons who have had a stroke or cerebrovascular accident (CVA) often also suffer from coronary heart disease (Warden-Tamparo & Lewis, 1989). Strokes are caused from years of living with high blood pressure and high cholesterol, often precipitated by an unhealthy lifestyle (e.g., poor eating habits, lack of physical activity, obesity). The term brain attack has been used to associate the circumstances of having a stroke with a heart attack.

   The two major types of stroke are hemorrhagic and ischemic. **Hemorrhagic strokes** (a ruptured blood vessel in the brain) are usually more life threatening than **ischemic strokes**. Ischemic strokes are much more common and involve a reduced blood supply to the brain.

4. Since stroke is sometimes accompanied by memory loss, it is important to make sure the client has taken his or medication before starting the exercise program. Clients should carry their medication with them at all times in case they forget to take it before leaving their home. This will allow them to take their medicine while at the fitness center and not have to miss a day of exercise. Since many people with strokes have hypertension, exercise should be postponed until blood pressure is under good control.

5. As a precautionary measure, the client should complete a detailed evaluation of how they feel before each exercise session. This includes whether or not they have taken their medication, generally feel good, have no signs of fatigue or chest discomfort, have gotten a good night's sleep, have eaten a light breakfast or meal earlier in the day, resting blood pressure is within their normal range, and adequate fluid intake has occurred, especially in clients who are taking diuretics to control blood pressure. If all of these responses are positive, the client can begin the exercise program. At the end of the exercise session, the client should have blood pressure and heart rate checked before leaving the setting to make sure that resting values have been restored.

Summary

Today there are 54 million Americans with disabilities, and this number is expected to increase substantially as the baby boomers reach retirement age. In the next millennium, persons with disabilities will have a better understanding of the importance of maintaining a physically active lifestyle, and will want, perhaps even demand, the same quantity and quality of programs afforded to the nondisabled community. Fitness professionals must be knowledgeable of the specific exercise guidelines for the various disabling conditions. The key to a successful program is for you to understand what type of modifications needs to be made to the exercise prescription in order to accommodate the client's specific limitations in movement and function. A competent fitness professional must possess the skills requisite for adapting and modifying exercise programs to meet the unique needs of each individual client, regardless of age or disability.

References

Albright, A.L. (1997). Diabetes. In Durstine, J.L. (ed.), *ACSM's Exercise Management for Persons with Chronic Diseases and Disabilities*, pp. 94 – 100. Champaign, Ill.: Human Kinetics.

American College of Sports Medicine and American Diabetes Association. (1997). Diabetes mellitus and exercise. *Medicine & Science in Sports & Exercise*, 29, 12, i – vi.

Blumenthal, M.N. (1990). Sports-aggravated allergies. How to treat and prevent the symptoms. *The Physician & Sportsmedicine*, 18, 12, 52 – 66.

Bravo, G., Gauthier, P., Roy, P., Payette, H., & Gaulin, P. (1997). A weight-bearing, water-based exercise program for osteopenic women: Its impact on bone, functional fitness, and well-being. *Archives of Physical Medicine & Rehabilitation*, 78, 1375 – 1380.

Centers for Disease Control and Prevention. (1996). Asthma mortality and hospitalization among children and young adults — United States, 1980 – 1993. *Journal of the American Medical Association*, 275, 20, 1535 – 1536.

Emtner, M., Herala, M., & Stalenheim, G. (1996). High-intensity physical training in adults with asthma. A 10-week rehabilitation program. *Chest*, 109, 323 – 330.

Ettinger, W.H., Burns, R., Messier, S.P., Applegate, W., Rejeski, W.J., & Morgan, T. (1997). A randomized trial comparing aerobic exercise and resistance exercise with a health education program in older adults with knee osteoarthritis. *Journal of the American Medical Association*, 277, 1, 25 – 31.

Expert Panel. (1998). Executive summary of the clinical guidelines on the identification, evaluation, and treatment of overweight and obesity in adults. *Archives of Internal Medicine*, 158, 1855 – 1867.

Franz, M.J., & Nordstrom, J. (1991). Athletes: Juggling insulin, food intake, and activity. In Franz, M.J., Etzwiler, D.D., Joynes, J.O., & Hollander, P.M. (eds.), *Learning to Live Well with Diabetes*, pp. 363 – 373. Minneapolis: DCI.

Friedman, R.B. (1988). Helping the patient fight fat. *Postgraduate Medicine*, 83, 106 – 111.

Frost, H.M. (1997). Why do marathon runners have less bone than weight lifters? A vital biomechanical view and explanation. *Bone*, 20, 183 – 189.

Han, T.S., Schouten, J.S.A.G., Lean, M.E.J., & Seidell, J.C. (1997). The prevalence of low back pain and associations with body fatness, fat distribution and height. *International Journal of Obesity*, 21, 600 – 607.

Heinonen, A. (1996). Randomised controlled trial of effect of high-impact exercise on selected risk factors for osteoporotic fractures. *Lancet*, 348, 1343 – 1347.

Kaplan, F.S. (1995). Prevention and management of osteoporosis. *Clinical Symposia*, 47, 1 – 32.

Kavanagh, T. (1994). Cardiac rehabilitation. In Goldberg, L., & Elliot, D.L. (eds.), *Exercise for Prevention and Treatment of Illness*, pp. 41 – 79. Philadelphia: F. A. Davis.

O'Donnell, D.E., Webb, K.A., & McGuire, M.A. (1993). Older patients with COPD: Benefits of exercise training. *Geriatrics*, 48, 1, 59 – 66.

Rice, T., Borecki, I.B., Bouchard, C., & Rao, D.C. (1993). Segregation analysis of fat mass and other body composition measures derived from underwater weighing. *American Journal of Human Genetics*, 52, 967 – 973.

Rimmer, J.H. (1994). *Fitness and rehabilitation programs for special populations*. Dubuque, Iowa: WCB McGraw-Hill.

Rimmer, J.H. (1999). Programming for clients with osteoporosis. *IDEA Health and Fitness Source*, 17, 6, 46 – 55.

U. S. Surgeon General's Report. (1996). *Physical Activity and Health. A Report of the Surgeon General Executive Summary*. Washington, D.C.: U. S. Department of Health and Human Services.

Wallberg-Henriksson, H.(1992). Exercise and diabetes mellitus. In Holloszy, J.O. (ed.), *Exercise & Sport Sciences Reviews*, Vol. 20, 339 – 368. Baltimore: Williams & Wilkins.

Warden-Tamparo, C. & Lewis, M.A. (1989). *Diseases of the Human Body*. Philadelphia: F. A. Davis.

Suggested Reading

Durstine, J.L. (ed.). (1997). *ACSM's Exercise Management for Persons with Chronic Diseases and Disabilities*. Champaign, Ill.: Human Kinetics.

Franklin, B.A., Gordon, S., & Timmis, G.C. (1989). *Exercise in Modern Medicine*. Baltimore, Md.: Williams & Wilkins.

McNeil, J.M. (1997). *Americans with Disabilities: 1994 – 95*. U. S. Bureau of the Census. (Current Population Reports, P70-61). Washington, D.C.: U. S. Government Printing Office.

Miller, P.D. (1995). *Fitness Programming and Physical Disability*. Champaign, Ill.: Human Kinetics.

National Spinal Cord Injury Association. www.spinalcord.org.

Rimmer, J.H. (1997). Programming for clients with disabilities. Exercise guidelines for special medical populations. *IDEA Today*, 15, 5, 26 – 35.

Rimmer, J.H. (1998). Common health challenges faced by older adults. In Cotton, R.T. (ed.), *Exercise for Older Adults. ACE's Guide for Fitness Professionals*. Champaign, Ill.: Human Kinetics.

Rimmer, J.H. (1999). Health promotion for persons with disabilities: The emerging paradigm shift from disability prevention to prevention of secondary conditions in persons with disabilities. *Physical Therapy*, 79, 5, 495 – 502.

Chapter 9

In This Chapter:

Lenita Anthony, M.A., is the program director at the University of California of San Diego, Extension for the Professional Certificate in Exercise Science. She is a frequent presenter at industry events and has authored numerous articles for fitness publications. Anthony is certified by ACE and ACSM.

Camilla Callaway, M.Ed., owns and operates a personal training facility in Columbus, Georgia. Working with Denver's Swedish Medical Center and Katie Beck's "Mothers in Motion," Callaway has trained instructors, taught prenatal classes, educated moms-to-be throughout the Colorado region, and facilitated classes at the IDEA International Convention. She has been a volunteer with various committees with the American Council on Exercise, and serves as an ACE media spokesperson.

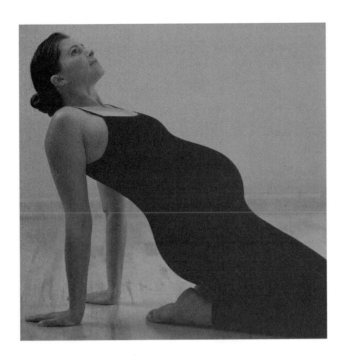

Exercise and
Pregnancy

By Lenita Anthony and Camilla Callaway

The number of women who exercise during their pregnancy has increased steadily in recent years. Cross-sectional surveys have reported that the percentage is as high as 42% (Zhang, 1996). In 1996, approximately 38% of women of reproductive age engaged in regular sustained exercise, but public health goals are to raise that number to 90% by the year 2000 (ACSM, 1996). This means more pregnant women will be seeking the instruction of knowledgeable fitness professionals. These students will need good information and guidance regarding exercise, and instructors need to be aware of the unique physical and physiological changes that occur during pregnancy.

These adaptations require continual exercise modifications to ensure exercise effectiveness and safety. Each woman enters pregnancy with different abilities and different goals and attitudes toward exercise. While broad, general guidelines apply to the pregnant population as a whole, they are not specific enough to design an exercise program around without taking into account the individual to which they are being applied.

Research on exercise and pregnancy over the last several years has taught us that the "right" exercise program for a pregnant woman should be based on many factors, pregnancy being only one of them. Equally important to consider are the pregnant exerciser's goals, experience, state of training, apprehensions, expectations, and motivation. In other words, "one size" will not fit all when it comes to prenatal exercise programs.

The objective of the American Council on Exercise is for group fitness instructors to be knowledgeable about the special needs of pregnant women and to provide classes that are well-designed, effective, challenging, and, above all, safe. Accordingly, the main purpose of this chapter is to enable you to develop such exercise programs for pregnant students and to educate you on important issues regarding exercise and prenatal conditions.

Benefits

Many benefits are associated with exercise during pregnancy. Research has shown that women who exercise during pregnancy, on the whole, experience fewer problems with constipation, swollen extremities, leg cramps, varicose veins, insomnia, fatigue, musculoskeletal discomforts, and excessive weight gain. Exercise during pregnancy can improve posture, reduce backaches, facilitate circulation, reduce pelvic and rectal pressure, and increase energy levels (Sternfeld, 1992). Exercise may also assist in controlling gestational diabetes (Clapp et al., 1992, 1995; Artal, 1992). Pregnant women who exercise can often maintain or even increase their cardiovascular fitness, as well as muscular strength and flexibility. Exercise enhances a sense of well being, increases confidence in body image, and helps to ease the negative feelings that often accompany pregnancy, weight gain, and preconceptions of labor and delivery. There are also recent data to show that exercising women have less problematic labors and deliveries, including a 30% decrease in the duration of active labor, a 75% decrease in the incidence of maternal exhaustion, and a 75% decrease in the need for operative intervention (forceps or cesarean section) (Clapp, 1995). Additionally, pregnant exercisers who gradually resumed postpartum had a higher $\dot{V}O_2$ max than nonpregnant women on a consistent training program over the same period of time (Clapp & Capeless, 1991).

Contraindications

The safety of the mother and **fetus** is the primary concern in any exercise program during pregnancy. Medical supervision of an exercise program throughout pregnancy is imperative. Each pregnant participant should be evaluated by her primary care physician and advised regarding her personal prenatal exercise program before participation in any group exercise class. The student's physician is the most appropriate person to evaluate her fitness status in relation to her pregnancy. It is advisable to require a signed physician consent-to-exercise form before the student can begin an exercise program. It is inappropriate for an instructor to assume the responsibility of prescribing a prenatal exercise program without physician approval. The first trimester is most crucial in the formation of the fetus; therefore, prenatal healthcare and education should start immediately. Early education on pregnancy and exercise could be handled with a prenatal information packet available for newly pregnant students. Suggested contents for this packet is the American College of Obstetricians and Gynecologist (ACOG) recommendations for pregnant and **postpartum** exercisers (1994) (Table 9.1). ACOG **contraindications,** both relative and absolute, warrant the participant's concern and consultation with her physician.

ACOG's relative contraindications include the following: chronic hypertension or active thyroid, cardiac, vascular, or pulmonary disease should be evaluated carefully in order to determine whether an exercise program is appropriate (ACOG, 1994).

ACOG's absolute contraindications include the following: pregnancy-induced hypertension, preterm rupture of membranes, preterm labor during the prior or current pregnancy or both, incompetent cervix/cerclage, persistent second- or third-trimester bleeding, and intrauterine growth retardation. The pregnant participant should also be made aware of the warning symptoms that indicate the need to cease exercise and consult her physician immediately. The list includes pain of any kind, uterine contractions occurring every 15 minutes or less, vaginal bleeding or amniotic fluid leakage, dizziness or faintness, shortness of breath, palpitations or **tachycardia**, persistent nausea or vomiting, back pain, pubic or hip pain, difficulty walking, general edema (swelling), numbness in any body part, visual disturbances, or decreased fetal activity (Artal et al., 1991).

Physiological Adaptations to Pregnancy

Of the myriad physiological changes that occur during pregnancy, perhaps those that have the most impact on exercise program design are those related to the cardiovascular system, the respiratory system, and the musculoskeletal system. While the adaptations listed below are by no means the only ones, the group fitness instructor who understands them will have a foundation of knowledge that allows more effective work with this special group.

Cardiovascular System

When instructors prepare beginner students for aerobics classes, they often inform them of the short-term effects of exercise. They discuss how the body will heat up and feel hotter, that since they are using more oxygen their breathing rate will increase, and that their heart rate will rise to help move the much-needed oxygen and nutrients to the working muscles via the blood or circulatory system. This simplistic statement could also describe the body's response to pregnancy; pregnancy and exercise elicit many similar physiological responses. During an exercise session, heart rate, respiratory rate, oxygen consumption, metabolic rate, cardiac output, stroke volume, and body temperature all increase; pregnancy mimics these responses. A pregnant woman's body is in a constant state of work; the acute physiological responses of a low level of exercise are constantly present. It is not an exaggeration to say that the pregnant woman is performing a certain amount of exercise, even when she is at rest.

The cardiovascular system, the respiratory system, and the reproductive system must each adapt to the level of function required to grow a new life in 40 weeks. These adaptations include a gradual climb in resting heart rate, which reaches a peak of 15 beats per minute (bpm) over prepregnancy rates near the third trimester. Left

Table 9.1
ACOG Guidelines for Exercise During Pregnancy and Postpartum

Recommendations for Exercise in Pregnancy and Postpartum

There are no data in humans to indicate that pregnant women should limit exercise intensity and lower target heart rates because of potential adverse effects. For women who do not have any additional risk factors for adverse maternal or perinatal outcome, the following recommendations may be made:

1. During pregnancy, women can continue to exercise and derive health benefits even from mild-to-moderate exercise routines. Regular exercise (at least three times per week) is preferable to intermittent activity.

2. Women should avoid exercise in the supine position after the first trimester. Such a position is associated with decreased cardiac output in most pregnant women; because the remaining cardiac output will be preferentially distributed away from splanchnic beds (including the uterus) during vigorous exercise, such regimens are best avoided during pregnancy. Prolonged periods of motionless standing should also be avoided.

3. Women should be aware of the decreased oxygen available for aerobic exercise during pregnancy. They should be encouraged to modify the intensity of their exercise according to maternal symptoms. Pregnant women should stop exercising when fatigued and not exercise to exhaustion. Weightbearing exercises may, under some circumstances, be continued at intensities similar to those prior to pregnancy throughout pregnancy. Nonweightbearing exercises such as cycling or swimming will minimize the risk of injury and facilitate the continuation of exercise during pregnancy.

4. Morphologic changes in pregnancy should serve as a relative contraindication to types of exercise in which loss of balance could be detrimental to maternal or fetal well-being, especially in the third trimester. Further, any type of exercise involving the potential for even mild abdominal trauma should be avoided.

5. Pregnancy requires an additional 300 kcals per day in order to maintain metabolic homeostasis. Thus, women who exercise during pregnancy should be particularly careful to ensure an adequate diet.

6. Pregnant women who exercise in the first trimester should augment heat dissipation by ensuring adequate hydration, appropriate clothing, and optimal environmental surroundings during exercise.

7. Many of the physiological and morphological changes of pregnancy persist 4 - 6 weeks postpartum. Thus, prepregnancy exercise routines should be resumed gradually based on a woman's physical capability.

Contraindications to Exercise

The aforementioned recommendations are intended for women who do not have any additional risk factors for adverse maternal or perinatal outcome. A number of medical or obstetric conditions may lead the obstetrician to recommend modifications of these principles. The following conditions should be considered contraindications to exercise during pregnancy:
- Pregnancy-induced hypertension
- Preterm rupture of membranes
- Preterm labor during the prior or current pregnancy or both
- Incompetent cervix/cerclage
- Persistent second- or third-trimester bleeding
- Intrauterine growth retardation

In addition, women with certain other medical or obstetric conditions, including chronic hypertension or active thyroid, cardiac, vascular or pulmonary disease, should be evaluated carefully in order to determine whether an exercise program is appropriate.

Source: ACOG (1994). Reprinted from *Exercise During Pregnancy and the Postpartum Period* with permission from American College of Obstetricians and Gynecologists.

ventricular volume and stroke volume increase 40%. Resting cardiac output and blood volume are 40% higher by the third trimester (Artal, 1992; Clapp, 1995). Resting oxygen consumption also climbs and reaches a level near term approximately 20% to 30% above prepregnancy levels (Wolfe, 1989; Artal, 1992).

These physiological changes have implications for the exercise program. Because the heart is already working at a higher capacity to pump the increased blood volume throughout the body, there is a decrease in **cardiac reserve**. The oxygen cost of weightbearing activity is also greater, due to increases in body weight. All of these factors combine to decrease maximum work capacity as pregnancy advances. Prenatal exercisers should gradually yet progressively reduce the volume of work done in exercise so as to complement the increased work load under which their body is functioning as they advance through their pregnancy.

Respiratory System

Pregnant women ventilate 50% more air per minute than nonpregnant women. This occurs through a 40% – 50% increase in tidal volume, or the amount of air in each breath. Although many pregnant women feel it is difficult to get a deep breath, maximum breathing capacity is actually maintained or increased over prepregnancy values. Respiratory rate does not change significantly. As the baby grows, the uterus pushes the diaphragm farther up into the chest cavity. The pregnant woman has to use more oxygen during inspiration as the diaphragm contracts to push the uterus downward. This increase in the oxygen cost of breathing also means less oxygen is available to the working muscles. The rib cage often flares and widens to help compensate for the decrease in lung space caused by the growing fetus.

Musculoskeletal System

To facilitate the expansion of the uterine cavity, increased amounts of the hormones **relaxin** and **progesterone** are released during the first trimester. These hormones act to soften the ligaments surrounding the joints of the pelvis (hips and lumbosacral spine), increasing mobility and joint laxity. A gentle but effective expansion occurs, providing the necessary space. This effect continues through the postpartum lactating period, when relaxin levels have been reduced.

The by-product of this hormonally induced joint laxity is a decrease in joint stability, which may leave the affected joints more susceptible to injury. Whether or not joint laxity occurs in the neck, shoulders, and peripheral joints is still controversial. If it does, the pregnant woman may have a greater chance of injuries resulting from overstretching, ligamentous tears, or sprains. However, existing research does not demonstrate an increased incidence of exercise-related joint injury among pregnant women (Clapp et al., 1995; Karzel & Friedman 1991; Schauberger et al., 1996). Researchers speculate that this is because pregnant women take greater precautions and are more careful during exercise. Whether or not relaxin has any effect on joints like the knees, common sense tells us that the increased mechanical stress of a 25 – 40 pound weight gain is cause to use caution with high-impact activities.

As weight is gained and hormonal influences on the hips and low back deepen, postural alignment is altered. The pelvis tilts anteriorly, changing the center of gravity and increasing the lordotic curve of the lumbar spine. The upper back is also realigned due to the increased weight of the breast tissue. The chest and shoulders are pulled forward and inward, increasing the kyphotic curve of the thoracic spine. A forward neck often accompanies these postural deviations and an extreme exaggeration of the vertebral column's normal "S" curve results. This is known as a kyphotic lordotic postural alignment and is further explained in Chapter 2 (Artal et al., 1990; Jacobson, 1991). Postural realignments induced by the anterior weight gain of pregnancy, and the attendant muscular imbalances created, could predispose women to upper or lower back pain. These conditions are addressed more fully later in this chapter.

Additional Concerns

Blood returning to the heart from the body is known as venous return. Due to the increase in blood volume and sensitivities to postural positions, venous return may be impaired or disturbed during pregnancy. **Supine hypotension** is an example of such a disturbance. In the supine position (lying on the back), the weight of the uterus presses against blood vessels, especially the inferior vena cava. This pressure occludes the vessels, causing a restriction in blood flow, which may, in turn, cause a reduction in cardiac output, blood pressure, and blood flow to the fetus. If the fetus is subjected to repeated periods of **hypoxia** due to prolonged and/or repetitive supine exercise, there is the potential for developmental disorders to occur. Students should be advised to avoid exercise in the supine position after the first trimester (ACOG, 1994).

Instructors often have to remind pregnant women that they are supposed to gain weight during pregnancy. Exercise should not be used as a means to prevent a healthy, normal weight gain during pregnancy. Average pregnancy weight gains are between about 27 and 34 pounds; body fat increases an average of 4% to 5% (Artal, 1992; Clark, 1992). Prevention of normal weight gain may be detrimental since weight gains are predictive of fetal birth weight. Nutritional diets should be encouraged to provide for the baby's growth and development and appropriate weight gains.

Fetal Risks Associated with Exercise

The research available at this time includes no evidence to show that regular exercise during a normal, healthy pregnancy is associated with any adverse fetal outcomes. However, there are several areas of theoretical concern, of which you should be aware. These include the effects of exercise on uterine-placental blood flow, carbohydrate utilization, and **thermoregulation**. The following section will address the basis for these concerns and the practical application for the group exercise setting.

The first concern is the potential conflict between the circulatory demands of exercise and those of pregnancy. During exercise, the oxygen transport system analyzes the actions taking place and reacts to provide for the higher level of activity. Blood flow is preferentially redistributed to the heart, skin, and working muscles and shunted away from the renal, gastrointestinal, and reproductive organs. The concern is that this may result in a decreased oxygen supply (hypoxia) and/or decreased nutrient supply to the fetus. If the fetus is subjected to repetitive, sustained bouts of hypoxia brought on by exercise, developmental abnormalities could occur.

Research has shown the fetus can adjust safely to reductions of blood flow resulting from moderate exercise bouts (Uzendski, 1989; ACSM, 1996). Several adaptations have been identified that protect the fetus and compensate for the decrease in visceral blood flow during exercise. These adaptations include an increased hemoglobin level, exercise-induced **hemoconcentration** that provides a higher percentage of oxygen to a lower level of blood volume, an improved ability for oxygen to be released from the hemoglobin present and a postexercise increase in blood flow to the fetus to compensate for the reduced flow during exercise (Schick-Boschetto & Rose, 1991). Also, cardiac output in the fetus is redistributed to favor vital organs such as the heart, brain, and adrenal gland. Women who exercise regularly in early to midpregnancy experience a more rapid growth of the **placenta** and have improved placental function. At any rate of uterine blood flow, oxygen and nutrient delivery to the baby will be higher in the woman who exercises than in the one who does not (Clapp & Rizk, 1992; Jackson et al., 1995).

The second area of concern is that of carbohydrate utilization. Maternal blood glucose is the fetus' primary energy source. Several studies have shown maternal blood glucose to drop significantly following vigorous exercise in late gestation. This has been cause for concern, since low maternal blood glucose could compromise fetal energy supply. If this scenario were repeated regularly (as with physical conditioning), intrauterine growth retardation, lower birth weight, or other developmental problems might result. Several studies have reported lower birth weights in women who continued heavy exercise through pregnancy. This weight discrepancy was primarily attributed to a decrease in subcutaneous fat in the newborn (Clapp & Capeless, 1990). Intrauterine growth retardation, or other short- or long-term effects on newborns of this decreased fat, has not been documented (ACOG, 1994; Clapp et al., 1999).

Other studies have found no difference in birth weight among exercising mothers, particularly when the mothers received nutritional counseling. Clapp and Rizk (1992)

studied placental weight in recreational athletes and found that it was significantly greater than the controls at 16, 20, and 24 weeks. The athletes who remained active but decreased or modified their activities in late pregnancy had the highest birth weight and placental weight, while the athletes who maintained or increased their exercise in late pregnancy had birth weights lower than the controls. This study suggests that exercise through midpregnancy may stimulate placental growth, allowing for better delivery of oxygen and nutrients to the baby. However, high-volume exercise in late pregnancy, when fetal and maternal energy requirements are high, may reduce fetal and placental weight (Clapp, 1992).

The group fitness instructor working with pre-natal exercisers should be aware of the nutritional demands of pregnancy and reinforce good dietary habits. The metabolic needs of pregnancy add approximately 300 kcals/day. The energy requirements of exercise must be factored in on top of this. Pregnant women have lower fasting blood glucose levels than nonpregnant women and also utilize carbohydrate during exercise at a greater rate (ACOG, 1994). They are therefore more likely to become **hypoglycemic**, both during exercise and at rest. Pregnant women should be reminded to have a pre-exercise snack and to eat frequent small meals throughout the day. Help pregnant students recognize the signs of hypoglycemia, such as weakness, dizziness, fatigue, and nausea. Suggest to those performing high levels of exercise that their exercise volume should start to taper from mid to late pregnancy. Finally, maternal weight gain and fetal growth (measured at her doctor at regular prenatal visits) should be within normal limits.

The third area of concern is that of fetal **hyperthermia** (overheating). Hyperthermia is known to be **teratogenic** (that is, capable of causing birth defects) (McMurray & Katz, 1990). Febrile illness in the first trimester has been associated with neural tube defects. Retrospective studies searching for a common factor in neural development defects found that heat (such as would be seen in fetal hyperthermia) was a major cause. However, there is no demonstrated increase in neural tube defects or other birth defects in women who participate in even vigorous exercise during early pregnancy (ACOG, 1994; Clapp & Little, 1995).

Normal fetal temperature is slightly higher than that of the mother. Fetal temperature is contingent on maternal temperature, fetal metabolic rate, and uterine blood flow, with the greatest effect stemming from maternal temperature. Fetal thermoregulation depends on the mother's ability to cool herself. Very high-intensity exercise, or exercise in a hot, humid environment, has the potential to raise maternal core temperature above the baby's and reverse the temperature gradient. This could cause the baby to take on heat from the mother.

Maternal resting core temperatures are slightly higher than prepregnancy levels, but exercise temperatures in pregnant women do not mirror this increase. Peak rectal temperature in pregnant women after exercise at 64% of $\dot{V}O_2$ max has been shown to decrease by 0.3°C by eight weeks and continues to drop at a rate of 0.1°C per month through the 37th week (Clapp, 1991; ACOG, 1996).

It appears that pregnant women have physiological adaptations that enhance thermoregulation during exercise. These adaptations include a downward shift in the sweating threshold (allowing evaporative heat loss at a lower body temperature), better skin-to-environment heat transfer due to increased skin blood flow during pregnancy, and increased heat loss through the respiratory tract (due to increased ventilation in pregnancy).

While these compensatory mechanisms serve to protect the fetus from heat stress, caution should nevertheless be taken to avoid overheating when working with this population. Remember that early pregnancy (the first trimester) is the most critical phase regarding heat sensitivity and fetal development. Students should be advised to (1) exercise in a cool, well-ventilated, low-humidity environment, (2) drink plenty of cool water to avoid **dehydration**, and (3) avoid very high-intensity activities.

Musculoskeletal System Imbalances and Dysfunctions

An understanding of these alterations to the musculoskeletal system will enable you to wisely choose and modify various exercises for the benefit of your pregnant students. The following are some of the most commonly encountered complaints in prenatal exercisers.

Muscle Imbalances

When posture is not in the ideal alignment, muscle imbalances are likely to arise. The common muscle imbalances identified in pregnancy are either "tight" (scapula protractors, levator scapula, thoracolumbar area, hip flexors, tensor fascia lata, piriformis, hamstrings, adductors, and calves) or "weak" (scapula retractors, low lumbar paravertebral, gluteus maximus and medius, abdominals, and quadriceps) (Wilder, 1988).

Muscle imbalances play a dominant role in choosing exercises for class. Prenatal classes should be designed to reduce these muscle imbalances. The reduction will, in turn, help reduce the postural deviations. When dealing with muscle imbalances, it is more effective to first relax the tightened muscles through stretches and mobility exercises and then follow with strengthening exercises for the weaker muscle groups.

When students are unable to perform certain exercises because of discomfort or irritation, you should react to the short-term situation by modifying exercises to reduce such difficulties. When discomfort or irritations persist, the student must realize that she may need to cease the activity in order to rest the area and to prevent further aggravation. In all cases, the student should communicate concerns to her physician. In severe cases in which discomfort becomes chronic, consulting a physical therapist specializing in prenatal care should be considered.

Dysfunctions and Irritations

The following section provides a summary of common dysfunctions and irritations, including backache, **pelvic floor** weakness, **diastasis recti**, ligament strain, pubic pain, sacroiliac joint dysfunction, **sciatica**, nerve compression syndromes, overuse syndromes, and muscle cramps. While suggestions for exercise modifications are touched on, detailed exercises are found later in this chapter.

Backache

The most frequent complaint during pregnancy is backache. About one half of pregnant women develop pain in the low back area. Proper body mechanics, exercise, massage, relaxation, and physical therapy can help reduce and in some cases prevent low back pain.

As noted previously, postural realignments during pregnancy contribute heavily to the incidence of backache. An exaggeratedly curved lower back, rounded upper back, and a forward head characterize the typical posture of a pregnant woman.

Exercises appropriate for this situation should focus on reducing the improper alignment. Mobility and stretching exercises should emphasize relaxing and lengthening the back extensors, hip flexors, shoulder protractors, shoulder internal rotators, and neck flexors. Strengthening exercises focused on the abdominals, gluteals, and scapula retractors will reinforce their ability to support proper alignment.

Gentle reminders to students are helpful in maintaining proper alignment throughout each section of class. To practice maintaining a neutral pelvis, instruct students to strengthen the muscles that tilt the pelvis posteriorly (i.e., the abdominal and gluteal muscle groups). The gluteal muscles should be pulled downward and together with an upward pull of the abdominals. This motion should reduce the anterior pelvic tilt position.

Various cues, such as heads up, shoulders back, buttocks tight, belly buttons up, or abdominals hugging baby may communicate alignment to students. Even a simple question, "How does that low back feel?," may stimulate better posture. Posture breaks during class for pelvic tilts and other back exercises can increase comfort.

Aside from postural alterations that bring on back pain, other factors that may contribute to the condition are increases in relaxin, hypermobility of the sacroiliac joint, improper body mechanics, **vascular disturbances** (a particular cause of nighttime back pain), **transient osteoporosis** from dietary calcium deficiency and psychosocial stress (Hummel-Berry, 1990).

Pelvic Floor Weakness.

The five layers of muscle and fascia attached to the bony ring of the pelvis are commonly referred to as the pelvic floor. From superficial to deep layers, they are as follows: the superficial outlet muscles, urogenital triangle, pelvic diaphragm or levator ani muscles, smooth muscle diaphragm, and endopelvic diaphragm. They support the pelvic organs like a sling to withstand all the increases in pressure that occur in the abdominal and pelvic cavity and provide **sphincter** control for the three **perineal** openings (Noble, 1995).

There are fascial connections between the levator ani muscles, the sacroiliac ligaments, the hip rotator muscles, and the hamstrings. This connection allows weaknesses of the pelvic floor muscles to refer stress to these areas. Pelvic floor weaknesses can cause the pelvic alignment to falter and thus irritate the sacroiliac joint and the hip joint (Wilder, 1988). It is crucial that these muscles function competently. In addition, prolapse of the bladder, uterus or rectum may develop if muscles become too weak to support the pelvic organs. Finally, urinary **incontinence** can often be initiated during pregnancy because of pelvic floor weakness.

Kegel exercises are designed to strengthen the pelvic floor and ensure its proficient function. The benefits of strengthening the pelvic floor are providing support for the heavy pelvic organs; preventing prolapse of the bladder, uterus, and rectum; supporting pelvic alignment; reinforcing sphincter con-

trol; enhancing circulation through a congested area of the vascular system; and providing a healthy environment for the healing process after labor and delivery (Dunbar, 1992).

Diastasis Recti

This is the partial or complete separation of the rectus abdominis muscle. Diastasis recti occurs as the linea alba widens and finally gives way to the mechanical stress of an advancing pregnancy (Wilder, 1988). The linea alba, a tendinous fiber that merges the abdominal muscles with the fascia, extends from the xiphoid process to the **symphysis pubis** (see Chapter 2). Some separation is a normal part of every pregnancy.

Proficient prenatal instructors may test for diastasis recti. The most common test is performed by placing two fingers horizontally on the suspected location of the diastasis recti while the student lies supine with knees bent. Have her perform a curl-up. If the fingers are able to penetrate at the location there is probably a split. The abdominal muscles can be felt to the side of the split. The degree of separation is measured according to the number of fingerwidths of the split. One to two fingerwidths is considered normal. If the separation is greater than three fingerwidths, avoid exercises that place direct stress on this area (Noble, 1995). Focus on abdominal compression exercises and using the abdominals to help maintain neutral spinal alignment with all activities. Abdominal curl-ups can be performed in a semirecumbent position rather than supine.

Diastasis recti is most common during the third trimester and immediately postpartum and is attributed to the following influences:
1. *Maternal hormones.* Relaxin, **estrogen**, and progesterone encourage the connective tis-

sue to become less supportive. There is a loosening effect on the abdominal fascia and a reduction of the cohesion between the collagen fibers.

2. *Mechanical stress within the abdominal cavity.* This varies according to fetus size and number, placenta size, the amount of amniotic fluid, the number of previous pregnancies, and the amount of weight gain. The abdominal musculature is designed to function in a vertical direction, shortening and lengthening, but pregnancy demands that the abdominal wall expand horizontally, and it is not normally elastic in the transverse direction. This situation causes mechanical stress that can end in functional failure for the abdominal wall. After a slow deformation of the soft tissue, the separation is often caused by a sudden action, made with improper body mechanics.

3. *Weak abdominal muscles.* A correlation exists between diastasis recti and weak abdominal muscles. Women with strong abdominal musculature are considered more prepared to resist this condition (Boissonnault & Blaschak, 1988). Other predisposing factors include heredity, obesity, multiple-birth pregnancy, a large baby, excess uterine fluid and a lax abdominal wall from former pregnancies.

Abdominal exercises that may introduce susceptibility in those prone to diastasis are those that put direct pressure on the linea alba from within, due to uterine resistance, and from without, due to gravitational resistance.

Round, Inguinal, and Broad Ligament Irritations

The round, inguinal, and **broad ligaments** are the ligaments most commonly irritated or strained during pregnancy. The **inguinal ligament** is formed as the fascia of the internal oblique, the external oblique, and transverse abdominis muscles blend together at their lower margin. It runs between the pubic tubercle and the anterior superior iliac spine. As the abdominal wall expands, the inguinal ligament is also stretched. It continues to be stretched throughout the pregnancy, slowly adapting with the abdominal wall expansion. This constant state of tension can easily turn into a spasm with an increase in abdominal pressure such as results from a cough, sneeze, or laugh.

Workouts must be attuned to the current state of ligamentous tension. On days when the student feels vulnerable, the intensity of the workout and strain put on the ligament should be reduced. Sensitivity is common with abdominal exercises and inner and outer thigh exercises. When performing abdominal exercises try to relieve the tension by keeping the knee and hip joints bent and the curling height low. With hip abduction and adduction the knee and hip joints should again be slightly bent. This places the inguinal ligament in a more relaxed position and also reduces the leverage of the leg. Avoid quick shifts of body position, especially changing from right to left side-lying positions. Prepare the body to change positions by warming joints with pelvic tilts, maintaining proper alignment, and using the arms to help lift the body from the floor.

The round and broad ligaments directly support the uterus within the pelvic cavity. The **round ligament** connects to both sides of the uterine fundus and extends forward through the inguinal canal and terminates in the labia majora (Figure 9.1). The round ligament may be irritated with extreme stretches above the head, rapid twisting movements, or jackknifing off the floor or bed. The use of proper mechanics for lying

Figure 9.1

Round and broad ligaments.

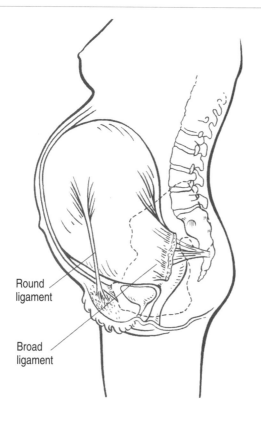

Round ligament

Broad ligament

Figure 9.2a-c

Proper body mechanics for rising from the side-lying position to the sitting position

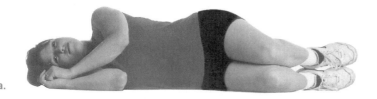

a.

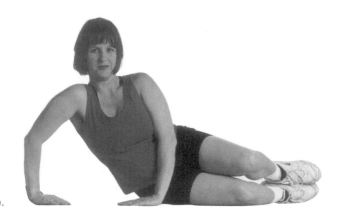

b.

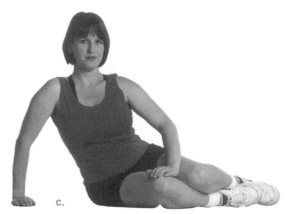

c.

down and rising will also prevent, strain on the round ligament (Figure 9.2). In the exercise arena, women may experience discomfort when the round ligament is jostled from jogging or jumping. A unilateral, standing hip hike held for five seconds and repeated for several repetitions can decrease the discomfort of, or even prevent, round ligament pain. To perform this exercise, have the student elevate one illiac crest by shifting the weight to one leg, unloading the other leg, and lifting it slightly off the floor. The knee should be straight. Adequate warm-up for the inguinal ligament, the round ligament, and the abdominal wall may also include torso range-of-motion activities, pelvic tilts, and an effleurage massage. (An effleurage massage is a very light, stroking movement, done here by placing the fingertips on the pubis and sliding them upward along the linea alba, then sliding them down both sides of the abdominal wall near the round ligament, gently rubbing along the inguinal ligament, and meeting at the pubis to begin the circular motion again.)

The largest ligament supporting the ovaries, as well as the uterine tubes, uterus, and vagina, is the broad ligament. It connects the lateral margins of the uterus to the posterior pelvic walls. The pull it receives from the enlarged uterus can cause a severely arched and aching low back. Relaxation of this ligament can be aided with performance of pelvic tilts, the cat stretch, trunk flexion exercises, self-massage of the low back, and torso range-of-motion movements. All of these help to relieve tension in the broad ligament as well as in the extensor muscles of the back. Encourage students to avoid exaggerating the arch of the low back, to maintain good postural alignment, and to use good body mechanics.

Pubic Pain

As the growth of the fetus demands more space, the pelvis accommodates by expanding. The loosened ligaments that allow this necessary expansion also allow increased motion. The irritation of the pubic symphysis caused by the increased motion at the joint is called symphysitis (Wilder, 1988).

This irritation may be worsened by exercise. Ice (RICE technique) may be used to relieve immediate irritation (see Chapter 10 for RICE guidelines). A physician consultation is advised and physical therapy may be ordered. Pelvic belts, which compress the pelvis and minimize motion in the symphysis pubis and sacroiliac joint, may be prescribed. Partial symphyseal separations and complete dislocations are possible during pregnancy as are pubic stress fractures. They usually result from delivery and, therefore, are of more concern for postnatal students.

When pubic pain occurs with students, efforts to alleviate irritation will determine the choice of activity and exercise. Exercises using hip adduction and abduction and, to a lesser extent, hip extension can cause further irritation of the pubis. The relationship of the tendons to the hip joints during hip abduction, adduction, and extension may cause

Figure 9.2d-f
Proper body mechanics for getting up from the floor

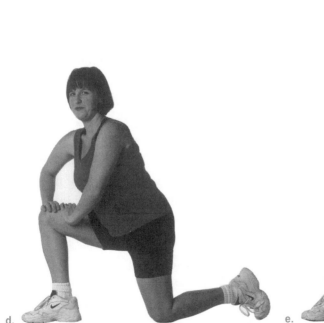

d.

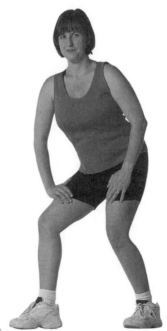

e.

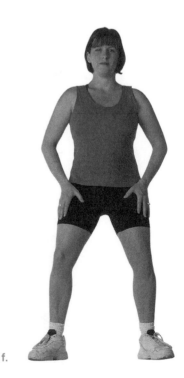

f.

excessive movement of the pubis, which intensifies the pain. Appropriate modifications are to reduce hip joint exercises to a level of tolerance or to avoid pain completely. Perform standing hip abduction and extension exercises to reduce symphysis pubis irritation. Reduce the impact and weightbearing aspects of aerobic activities and suggest aqua aerobics, swimming, or stationary biking as alternative exercises. Shoe quality is important to mention to these students; walking or jogging in worn out shoes can worsen joint irritations.

Sacroiliac Joint Dysfunction

Fifty percent of all back pain is related to lumbosacral pain (Hummel-Berry, 1990). During pregnancy, the sacroiliac joint functions to resist the anterior pelvic tilt that is accentuated by the increase in lumbar lordosis caused by the uterine growth and weight gain. To facilitate the passage of the fetus through the pelvis, relaxin is released and softens the normally rigid ligaments of the sacroiliac joint and symphysis pubis. Postural adjustments, which pull the pelvis anteriorly, in conjunction with the hormonal relaxation effect ultimately combine to force the sacroiliac ligaments to give, to stretch, and, possibly, to become hypermobile (Daly, 1991).

Symptoms of sacroiliac dysfunction include pain during the following activities: prolonged sitting, standing, or walking; climbing stairs; standing, with weight on one leg; or twisting activities (Lile & Hagar, 1991). The pain is usually unilateral (on one side) and in some cases radiates to the buttocks, lower abdomen, anterior medial thigh, groin, or posterior thigh (Daly et al., 1991). Students may complain of having pain in the sacroiliac area when they stand up out of a chair or when they

get out of bed. The pain is felt at the sacroiliac joint, then radiates into the buttocks, but it does not radiate down the leg as is characteristic of sciatica.

Exercises should be chosen to add strength and support to the sacroiliac area and to facilitate pelvic stability. If the lumbosacral angle (the angle between the lumbar vertebrae and the sacrum) is reduced, pain will usually be reduced. The gluteal muscles add the most direct support, but endurance exercises for the abdominals are also helpful. Abdominal endurance assists in preventing the anterior pelvic tilt that is straining the sacroiliac joint and ligament. Suggestions for class include accentuating proper postural alignment, using abdominal compression exercises throughout class, and using standing hip extension and abduction exercises. All of the preceding actions should incorporate pelvic stability (refer to hip exercises in floor-work section of this chapter). Participants with severe cases of dysfunction should be advised to see their physician.

Sciatica

Pressure placed on the sciatic nerve due to the position of the fetus or postural structures can produce nerve irritation that is extremely painful. A woman experiencing pain that radiates from her buttocks down to her legs is probably experiencing sciatic nerve irritation. Exercise can do little to relieve this situation. Students should be advised to note the activities that preceded the irritation and either to avoid those activities in the future or review the body mechanics used during the aggravating activity. Pelvic tilts may offer some immediate relief by shifting the irritating pressure away from the nerve. After experiencing a sciatic nerve irritation, the gluteal muscles and hamstrings will respond by tightening. Gently stretching these muscles can help to relax them out of this protective response.

Nerve Compression Syndromes

More than 80% of pregnant women have some degree of swelling during their pregnancy. Soft tissue swelling may decrease the available space in relatively constrained anatomical areas. The result of this constriction and fluid retention can be nerve compression syndromes or, less commonly, compartment syndromes. Nerve compression syndrome is possible in many areas that have a compressed nerve compartment. The most prevalent nerve problem during pregnancy is carpal tunnel syndrome. It results from compression of the median nerve within the wrist. Complaints of numbness and tingling sensations in the thumb and index and middle fingers are characteristic. Avoid loading the wrists in hyperextension, grasping objects tightly, and repetitive flexion/extension of the wrist. Keep the wrist joint in its neutral position as much as possible. A related nerve compression syndrome is tarsal tunnel syndrome or posterior tibial nerve syndrome, which involves cramping and compression of the calf. The characteristic complaint is numbness from the inside of the ankle to the medial plantar aspect of the foot. Thoracic outlet syndrome results from compression and aggravation of the brachial plexus. Tingling and numbing sensations may be felt down the arms and hands. Postural deviations with internally rotated shoulders can aggravate the situation. Exercises to encourage external rotation of the shoulder and stretches to reduce internal rotation of the shoulder should be added to the workout regime to balance the muscles. A bra that supports

the weight of the breast tissue may help to reduce upper back strain.

Encourage your students to avoid long periods of standing and sitting throughout their day. Taking short breaks at work to walk around or sitting with the feet elevated can help to improve circulation and reduce swelling. Prolonged standing should be avoided, as it can cause significant reductions in venous return and cardiac output. Advise students to lie when possible on their left side with feet slightly elevated; for example, side-lying on a sofa with their feet elevated on the sofa arm. This position is the most efficient at facilitating venous return and reducing fluid retention. Drinking plenty of water and reducing salt intake may also prevent excessive fluid retention. Severe swelling and fluid retention can indicate other medical conditions related to pregnancy besides contributing to nerve compression and should be reported immediately to the primary physician.

Overuse Syndromes

Weight gain, postural changes, and hormonal influences create a perfect environment for producing overuse syndromes. Many common overuse syndromes associated with exercise are intensified by these adaptations of pregnancy. Chondromalacia, a gradual degeneration of the articular cartilage that lines the back surface of the patella, can become irritated and inflamed because of the stress placed on the knee joint due to poor alignment. Pain can become incapacitating. Classes should include strengthening exercises for the quadriceps muscles to add support to the knee joints, and extra attention should be given to maintaining proper knee alignment during these exercises. Hyperflexion of the knee when bearing weight can accentuate the aggravation. Alignment is an especially important issue in stepping activities in which the repetitive motion can easily result in improper alignment as the student becomes fatigued.

The feet often become flatter and more pronated during pregnancy due to weight gain. When the feet are not striking properly, further alignment deviations in the hips and knees can res ult. Plantar fascitis, an inflammation of the plantar fascia, the broad band of connective tissue running along the sole of the foot, may result from improper foot placement. Advise students to avoid wearing worn or unsupportive shoes.

Muscle Cramps

Awakening abruptly to a muscle cramp can be very painful and frustrating. This is not an uncommon experience for pregnant women, who often do not know how to relieve cramps. Advise students to avoid extreme pointing of the toes (plantarflexion) and wearing high heels and tight shoes. All of these may stimulate muscle cramping. To relieve a muscle cramp, put the muscle in a stretched position and hold it there until the sensation subsides. For example, with a hamstring cramp straighten the knee, for a calf cramp straighten the knee and dorsiflex the foot, and for a foot cramp dorsiflex the foot and spread the toes.

Exercise Classes and Programs for Pregnant Women

Cardiovascular Exercise

Research on pregnancy and exercise has advanced significantly in the last 10 – 12 years. ACOG published the first guidelines on exercise and pregnancy in 1985. At that time, most of the research was limited to animal subjects. The initial guidelines were justifiably conservative, reflecting the lack of information available at that time. Since 1985, studies involving the use of human subjects have given us much more information on the physiological responses (both maternal and fetal) to exercise during pregnancy. The most recent ACOG guidelines, published in 1994, reflect this increase in the body of scientific knowledge and include significant changes from the original recommendations. Notably, the recommendation to use heart rate as a means of monitoring exercise intensity has been removed (the original recommendation was to limit heart rate to 140 bpm or less). The heart rate response to exercise among pregnant women is variable. Blunted, exaggerated, and normal linear responses may all be seen at different stages during the same pregnancy. It is important to realize that these changes are not due to exercise itself but rather to the other physiological influences of pregnancy. Rate of perceived exertion (RPE) has been shown to correlate much more closely than heart rate to actual measured oxygen consumption during exercise in pregnancy. RPE is a simple yet effective way for you to cue intensity. Since it is a subjective rating, it allows for the large variances in exercise capacity that exist in a typical class setting. The original Borg RPE scale (6 – 20) or the modified Borg scale (0 – 10) may be used. The numbers corresponding to "fairly light" to "somewhat hard" are the recommended range during pregnancy (Pivarnik et al., 1991; White, 1992; Clapp et al., 1999).

The ACOG guidelines state: "There are no data to indicate that pregnant women should limit exercise intensity and lower target heart rates because of potential adverse effects."

However, you must keep in mind that there may be other reasons to limit exercise intensity. The 1994 ACOG recommendations also removed specific limitations on exercise duration, reflecting the tremendous individual differences that exist in pregnant women's abilities. ACOG recommends "mild to moderate" exercise but adds that highly trained women may be able to maintain higher intensities in the earlier part of pregnancy. ACOG further states that consistent exercise (three days per week or more) is preferable to intermittent activity. It is essential that you know your clients and their exercise history and cue pregnant women as to the effort appropriate for the individual. The exercise intensity and duration selected should not result in fatigue or exhaustion. Maternal symptoms are the basis for changes and modifications to the program (ACOG, 1994). ACOG's recommendations are the standard of care for exercise during pregnancy.

It takes a thoughtful and purposeful plan to teach an effective fitness class. The challenge for you is to design and choose exercises that will allow success, comfort, and safety for the pregnant student.

Whether a pregnant exercise student wishes to be integrated into an exercise class of nonpregnant women — perhaps a class she has already been in — or joins a prenatal class, it is your responsibility to be aware of any pregnant woman's new physical status and to make appropriate individualized adjustments for that student.

For instructors with large classes, the greatest challenge may be just knowing who, if anyone, is pregnant in the class. Many women well into their second trimester may not "show." While preexercise screening will identify the newcomer to exercise, it does not help the instructor identify a new pregnancy in a regular class participant. So unless an instructor actually mentions to her class from time to time her need to know about pregnancies, she may not find out about pregnancies for quite a while.

Specialized classes for pregnant women have several benefits over integrated classes. Participants can be individually monitored better for such things as strain, discomfort, and fatigue. In addition, the prenatal exercise class forms a natural support group, with discussions of many pregnancy-related issues and help in maintaining stress control, self-esteem, and body confidence. However, the experienced or highly fit pregnant woman may wish to continue to exercise in a nonspecialized group fitness environment, especially when her favorite exercise mode is not taught specifically for pregnant women. This situation may arise in early pregnancy or if is not the participant's first baby. While this should not be discouraged, you will need to give additional attention and guidance to the pregnant student in an integrated class.

In both specialized and integrated classes, there should be communication between the instructor and pregnant women on a range of subjects, including sufficiency of warm-up time, needed modifications of exercises, intensity of movements, perceived exertion, weight gain, and comfort and pain levels.

Always be mindful of conditions such as hyperthermia, hypoxia, hypoglycemia, and musculoskeletal injuries. An exercise activity should be stopped and alternatives immediately given if the student finds it awkward to perform or if it causes discomfort, pain, or embarrassment.

The aerobic exercise warm-up should gradually increase muscle temperature through general body movement and joint range-of-motion activity. Give special emphasis to stimulating those areas under mechanical stress from pregnancy — the abdomen, pelvis, back, and hips.

Conditioning Exercises

All exercises should be performed with smooth and controlled speed and a range of motion that allows the exerciser to maintain proper alignment and comfort. If any exercise stimulates discomfort it should be immediately discontinued. Special attention should be given to teaching proper body mechanics when lying down and rising from the floor (see Figure 9.2).

Neck

Neck range-of-motion activities help to reduce tension. After muscles are warmed, stretch the sternocleidomastoid, levator scapulae, and the upper trapezius to further relieve tension and reduce the forward head position associated with poor postural alignment. During this segment it is important to

keep some movement in the legs to facilitate circulation. Complete the neck stretches with an examination of proper head and neck alignment (refer to discussions related to spinal alignment in Chapter 2).

Shoulder Girdle

To correct suspected muscle imbalances, begin with a warm-up and stretch of the scapula levators, scapula protractors, and shoulder internal rotators. Balance this with scapula retraction exercises of the rhomboids, middle trapezius, and lower trapezius. Correct body placement during scapula retraction exercises can reduce the chance of low back extension; a slight lunge such as used when stretching the calf muscles is perfect. The abdominals and gluteals function as pelvic stabilizers and need to be incorporated into this workout to prevent hyperextension of the lower back. Shoulder external rotation exercises improve postural alignment by widening and opening the chest area. These also reduce constriction of the brachial plexus, a negative element associated with thoracic outlet syndrome.

Shoulder and Elbow Joint

The workout of the anterior, middle, and posterior deltoids, pectoralis major, and the latissimus dorsi may proceed as usual. Work on the biceps and triceps also does not need extensive modification. Maintaining functional ranges of motion during exercises, especially when weights are being used, will help prevent overlengthening muscles, tendons, and ligaments associated with vulnerably loose joints. Body placement and positioning, chosen for various exercise performances, should facilitate circulation and promote proper alignment. Many arm exercises can be performed in combination with

Figure 9.3
Back alignment may be facilitated by placing a towel roll just under the tailbone to slightly tilt the pelvis anteriorly

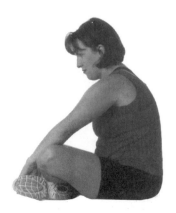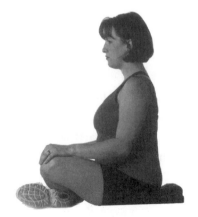

other exercises, such as standing legwork or stretches. If performed in a sitting position, back alignment may be facilitated by placing a towel roll just under the tailbone, which will tilt the pelvis slightly anteriorly and adjust for the rounded back (Figure 9.3). Sitting on the edge of a bench may be another comfortable sitting position when focused on the shoulder and elbow joint muscles.

Wrist Joint

A small amount of time should be allocated to wrist range of motion to promote circulation in a tight compartment area. Finger motion may also be performed to reduce swelling of this stagnant peripheral, circulatory area. These movements can be used during arm exercises or choreographed into the aerobic segment.

Low Back

These muscles are often tight and strained from the weight of the uterus pulling the abdominal wall and pelvis forward, resulting in the exaggerated lumbar lordosis posture. The class goal for this area is to relax these muscles to improve posture and decrease possible back pain. Range-of-motion exercises may be used to warm these muscles, followed by stretches to encourage them to lengthen and relax. Back range of motion consists of flexion, extension, lateral flexion, and rotation.

The many possible exercises and stretches include side bends, twists, standing back rolls, pelvic tilts, pelvic rotations, pelvic side lifts, cat stretches (Figure 9.4), lateral rolls, tail wags, modified press-ups, cross backs, knee-to-chest stretches, and knee rolls.

Abdominal Wall

This area, in particular, seems to be of concern to instructors. The concern is probably derived from attempting to maintain abdominal strength while avoiding supine hypotension and diastasis recti. Concern is definitely warranted since most abdominal workouts are performed in the supine position. Exercising in the supine position may induce supine hypotension syndrome and place excessive mechanical stress on the abdominal wall along the linea alba, especially in mid to late pregnancy. Positioning students in a semirecumbent position removes the constricting uterine pressure from the inferior vena cava and aorta and reduces the direct gravitational strain on the linea alba. Many of the conventional abdominal exercises may be easily modified into the semirecumbent position (Figure 9.5). For additional support to the linea alba, the abdominal wall may be splinted with crossed arms and hands (Noble, 1995). Stress to the inguinal ligament is reduced when the hip and knee joints remain flexed and rolled to

Figure 9.4
The cat stretch

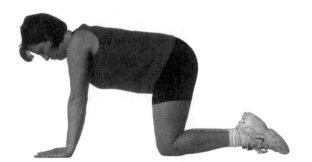 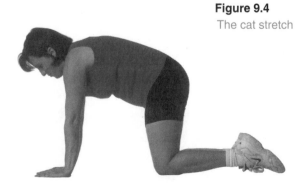

the side, as in the semirecumbent position. Besides the usual curl-up abdominal exercises, experiment with various pelvic tilt and abdominal compression exercises. This group of exercises is essential for maintaining postural alignment and pelvic stability. They may be performed in a variety of positions, from standing to the all-fours position. Abdominal compression should be combined with other exercises throughout class to help maintain proper pelvic alignment.

Pelvic Floor

Introducing Kegel exercises to students is mandatory. There are numerous routines for performing Kegel exercises. For example, begin with an isometric contraction of the pelvic floor, feel the muscles lift and tighten, hold it for a slow count of 10, then relax the muscles for another count of 10 and repeat again. Most students will have difficulty identifying and isolating these muscles if they have not performed Kegels before. Since it is impossible for you to know if students are performing them correctly, effective cues are essential. Asking students to contract the muscles they would use to stop urinary flow improves awareness and control of these muscles (Noble, 1995). Another exer-

cise is to imagine an elevator going up and down, as the pelvic floor is lifted. Stopping the elevator on each floor is a variation that requires more muscle control (Nurse Practitioner, 1985; Noble, 1995).

Kegel exercises can be placed in class along with abdominal and gluteal exercises. For example, initiate a semirecumbent curl-up, lift for 2 counts, hold for 2 counts, incorporate a Kegel during the hold for 2, then lower for 2 counts and repeat the sequence again. Suggest each student choose a cue to remind themselves to Kegel outside of class; when they brush their teeth, talk on the phone, cough, sneeze, or laugh, they can be cued to Kegel. A suggested workout program of four daily sets of 10 initially, working up to four daily sets of 25, seems reasonable.

Hip Flexors

The hip flexor muscles are often tight as a result of the prenatal posture. The fact that people tend to spend a large part of their day sitting causes them to shorten. Therefore, the emphasis in class is to stretch and relax them. Care should be taken not to hyperextend the low back when performing hip flexor stretches in the standing, kneeling, or side-lying positions.

Hip Extensors

The role of the hip extensors is to oppose the hip flexors' pull of the pelvis anteriorly and to assist the abdominals in their role of tilting the pelvis posteriorly. In assisting with the posterior pelvic tilt, it also helps alleviate the strain being placed on the sacroiliac joint. Standing may be a more comfortable position for gluteus maximus workouts, since it seems to place less stress on vulnerable areas. The common all-fours and side-lying positions often place strain on the symphysis

Figure 9.5

The semirecumbent position easily replaces the supine position for abdominal exercises.

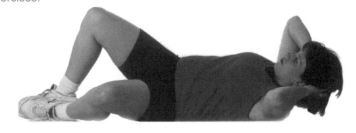

pubis, inguinal ligament, sacroiliac joint, and the lumbar spine and, therefore, may be replaced with the standing position. To facilitate support for the sacroiliac joint, hip extension exercises are used to strengthen the gluteal muscles. In order to recruit more muscle fibers from the gluteal muscle group, perform hip extensions while the hip joint is abducted, adducted, or externally rotated (Figure 9.6). Abdominal compression should be included in the exercises to assist in maintaining pelvic stability.

Hip Abduction

To promote more fiber recruitment of the gluteal muscles, perform hip abduction while the hip is extended and/or externally rotated, in addition to in the neutral position. Participants should be encouraged to perform this exercise in a standing position, as with hip extensors. This is another exercise that offers indirect muscle support to

the sacroiliac joint. Incorporating abdominal compression will assist in maintaining a stable pelvis. A towel roll may be used to support the neck and the abdominal wall, and thus maintain body alignment when lying sideways (Figure 9.7). If the inguinal ligament or the symphysis pubis is sensitive, the hip and knee joints should be flexed during hip abduction. This repositioning reduces the leverage weight and puts the inguinal ligament in a more relaxed position. If irritation still occurs, then the exercise should be deleted from the workout.

Hip Adductors

Because of the anterior tilt position of the pelvis, the tendons of the hip joint muscles are pulled slightly forward. The hip adductors, may become tensed and strained in this new alignment. During hip adduction exercises, strain may occur in nearby vulnerable areas, such as the symphysis pubis,

Figure 9.6
Standing hip exercises should be performed in conjunction with a posterior tilt of the pelvis triggered by abdominal and gluteal contractions.

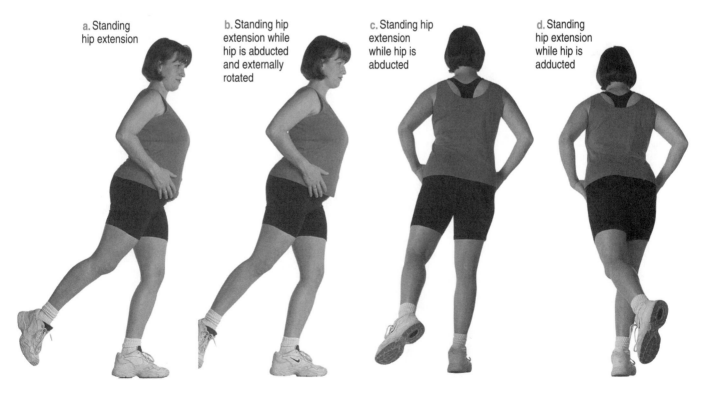

a. Standing hip extension

b. Standing hip extension while hip is abducted and externally rotated

c. Standing hip extension while hip is abducted

d. Standing hip extension while hip is adducted

Figure 9.7
A towel roll may be used to support the neck and to facilitate proper alignment.

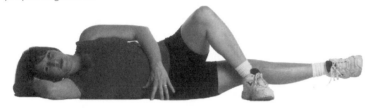

Figure 9.8
Hip adduction is performed with both the knee and hip joints bent to reduce the leverage of the leg; a towel roll is used to support the abdominal wall.

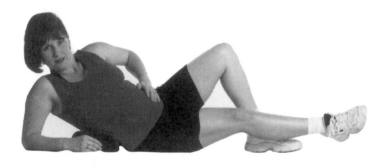

Figure 9.9
The butterfly sitting position for hip adduction

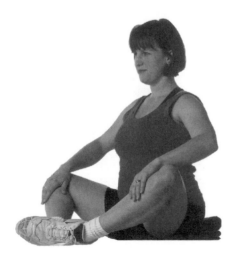

the groin area, or the inguinal ligament. If exercises cause a significant amount of stress on these areas, the student may complain of discomfort during or after class. Modifications for hip adductor work may relieve the stress. Side-lying hip adductor exercises may be conducted with minute variations, such as use of a towel roll to promote body alignment (Figure 9.8). By bending the hip and knee joints, less stress is placed on the inguinal ligament, symphysis pubis, and hip joint because of the more relaxed position and reduced leverage (Figure 9.9). If irritation becomes chronic or if the exercise feels uncomfortable, then adductor exercises should be deleted from the workout. Lateral movement such as slide training is best avoided because of the decreased stability of the pelvis during pregnancy.

Quadriceps/Knee Extension

An important muscle group to strengthen is the quadriceps. Strength in this muscle group better equips the student for the squatting and bending necessary in her daily activities. Activities such as getting out of a chair take on new dimensions with the pregnant body. The abdominal wall may limit the ability to lean forward and stand, thus legs and arms must assist more in rising. Exercises that incorporate daily activities are most helpful. They not only train the muscles but also educate students on proper body mechanics when performing simple activities with a sometimes awkward pregnant body. Pretending to be picking up a 2-year-old, taking groceries out of the car, opening lower drawers, vacuuming, or any other daily scenario may be utilized. Safety for the knee joint is the same as with all populations, but remember a greater weight is being carried. Deep knee bends or squats past 90 degrees of flexion should be avoided. Students should remain around a comfortable 45 degrees of flexion. Avoid hyperflexion of the knee while bearing weight because of the extreme pressure this places on the knee joint.

Hamstrings/Hip Extensors and Knee Flexors

The hamstrings may be tighter during pregnancy due to postural adaptations, such as the anteriorly tilted pelvis. Range-of-motion activities and stretches may be implemented to reduce tightness. The common supine hamstring stretch may be replaced with a standing or side-lying hamstring stretch to avoid discomfort and supine hypotension.

Ankle Joint

The main goals for this joint are to facilitate circulation and maintain flexibility. Warm-ups should include stimulation of the calf muscles and the anterior lower leg muscles. Ankle range-of-motion activities may help reduce swelling in the ankles by promoting venous return. Avoid extreme plantarflexion or pointing of the toes in all exercises. This can easily initiate a calf muscle cramp, which may be relieved by dorsiflexing the ankle to stretch the calf muscles. A pleasant activity for cool-down or relaxation is self-foot massage. The pregnant woman's feet are overloaded with her natural weight gain, and a massage can be very soothing.

Water Exercise

The favorite exercise modality for many pregnant women is water activities. In the water, body temperatures appear to rise less and dissipate sooner, which can help minimize the risk of hyperthermia (McMurray & Kats, 1990). However, water temperatures should feel cool or these benefits may be negated. If the water feels like bath water, it

is probably too warm (Karsenec & Grimes, 1984). Because of the hydrostatic effects of water, submaximal exercise in water is associated with a smaller **plasma** volume decrease than exercise on land, which may result in better maintenance of uterine and placental blood flow (Watson, 1991).

The pressure of water appears to lessen fluid retention and swelling, two common discomforts of pregnancy. The prone position in swimming actually facilitates optimum blood flow to the uterus, by redistributing the weight of the uterus away from the inferior vena cava and the aorta. A positive attribute of water classes is the buoyant effect of water, which increases comfort by supporting body weight and eliminating trouble with balance. This wonderful weightless feeling can be a major relief to the pregnant woman. Water exercises are easy on the musculoskeletal system, due to the reduced stress placed on the weightbearing joints and ligaments. This nonweightbearing position gives relief to those muscles bearing extra mechanical stress and pressure from the pregnancy.

Pregnant swimmers should use caution with forceful frog or whip kicks, as they may place undue stress on the unstable pubic joint. Additionally, traditional use of a kickboard may amplify the exaggerated lumbar lordosis of pregnancy and should therefore be used judiciously.

Indoor Cycling

Because cycling is nonweightbearing, many women find it a comfortable activity even in the later trimesters, when activities like walking can become awkward and difficult. As with other forms of exercise, there are some modifications and precautions that should be kept in mind when pregnant women participate in studio cycling classes. Cross-current convective cooling (fans) and adequate hydration are a must, as the potential to overheat or dehydrate is great. Fluids should be taken frequently, with a goal of drinking 6 ounces for every 15 minutes of exercise. Workload (cadence, resistance, or both) should be decreased to achieve the same relative cardiovascular overload as pregnancy progresses. The tendency to overexert in these classes may be high, and, therefore, specific, individualized instruction should be given to the pregnant rider regarding exercise intensity. Morphologic changes will affect cycling mechanics; the hips gradually externally rotate to accommodate the enlarging uterus. Increased weight on the saddle may necessitate wider, padded saddles or seat covers, in addition to padded shorts. The anterior weight gain of pregnancy coupled with the laws of gravity make maintaining neutral lumbar alignment while hinging at the hip to reach the bars difficult and fatiguing; adjust the handlebars to the most upright position and give pregnant riders frequent postural breaks. Be aware that toward the later trimesters, anterior weight gain will tend to pull a pregnant rider farther forward over the pedals during out-of-the-saddle drills, putting the knee in a position susceptible to injury. Edema (swelling) in the feet can make tight toe straps uncomfortable; cleated shoes eliminate this problem.

Strength Training

Strength training is a beneficial and safe activity during a normal, uncomplicated pregnancy if the standard safety rules of weight-lifting are adhered to. Safety suggestions include staying in control of the weights, moving through a functional range of motion, using slow, appropriate speeds for the exercise, and avoiding the Valsalva maneuver and the supine position (Work, 1989; Sinclair, 1992). Problems could arise if the student tends to jerk, swing, perform the exercise too quickly, or use poor control when she is lifting. Functional range of motion should match (not exceed) prepregnancy range to protect the joints from injury. Exercises done in the supine position should be modified after the first trimester; a semirecumbent position (inclined) is often an acceptable modification. Overhead lifting should be avoided to prevent irritation or injury to the low back due to the lessened ability of the weakened abdominals to stabilize the torso against the pull of the belly (Artal, 1992).

Strength training that is functional in nature is recommended for pregnant students. Exercises should be selected based on the physical demands a new mom will face. Extended periods of time spent carrying, lifting, nursing, and holding an infant place the postpartum student at risk for upper and lower back strain and injury. The emphasis during prenatal training is to develop the muscular strength and endurance necessary to ward off these chronic aches and pains common in new moms. Regular strength training will also help to reduce the time needed to resume normal activities of daily life without undue fatigue.

Repetitions and load will be determined based on the individual's exercise history, state of pregnancy, motivation, and other variables. Repetitions in the range of 10–15 would be appropriate for the pregnant woman who is new to strength training, while a woman who has been lifting regularly and is in the early prenatal stages may safely perform 8–12 repetitions and make very few changes, if any, in her current program. Instructors teaching group strength-training classes will need to give close and constant attention to the pregnant students' technique, biomechanics, and exercise choice, giving modifications as necessary.

Mind-Body Classes

Classes like tai chi, yoga, and pilates, among others, are seeing more pregnant participants as well. The mind-body orientation of these classes is known to facilitate relaxation and reduce stress. Most women feel that although pregnancy is a happy, exciting time for them, it is also a stressful time. Any major change in one's life, good or bad, can create stress — and a new baby certainly changes one's life. Classes such as these can be a great opportunity for effective management of stress. Other relaxation techniques, such as progressive relaxation, visualization, and breathing techniques, can easily be incorporated into the cool-down/stretch portion of any group exercise class, and will especially benefit the pre- or postnatal student. Participants should be cautioned to stretch in an average to normal range of motion in order to protect potentially hypermobile joints. Additionally, you can reassure the pregnant student that the stress or anxiety they feel is a normal part of pregnancy, and help equip them with tools they can use once the baby arrives.

Programming Suggestions and Modifications

The following suggestions and modifications may be implemented as needed to further individualize programming for the prenatal exerciser.

1. Design longer warm-ups to soothe vulnerable areas, such as the inguinal, round, and broad ligaments.
2. Demonstrate and emphasize proper alignment to be used throughout class.
3. Keep legs moving while standing to stimulate sluggish venous return.
4. Choose positions to give the student the best workout within her comfort zone while maintaining proper body alignment.
5. Supine positions may be replaced with semirecumbent positions, and prone positions with an all-fours position or an elbows-and-knees position.

Many positions may be easier with the use of towel rolls or pillows to help maintain body alignment. Changing positions often in class may facilitate circulation, but be aware that simply moving from the left side to the right side can be a strain if good body mechanics are not used. There are an infinite number of exercises for each muscle of the body. Use creativity to discover exercises to train muscles without causing discomfort for the pregnant student. Experiment with methods to challenge students appropriately.

The prenatal exerciser presents many interesting challenges to a fitness instructor. From the initial warm-up through the final cool-down, numerous factors must be considered to make an exercise program both safe and effective for the pregnant exerciser. Table 9.2 summarizes an entire prenatal class format in the form of substitute instructor guidelines.

Postnatal Exercise

Returning to exercise after delivery is like going backward through pregnancy. The situation is similar to the relationship between a warm-up and cool-down; they mirror each other, but in reverse. So all the things a woman does to prepare and endure pregnancy continue to be done

Table 9.2
Prenatal Class Format (Substitute Instructor Guidelines)

Please! *Watch each individual student* for signs of stress, strain, discomfort, fatigue, and/or disgust. Always be prepared to show modifications of exercises for each student's personal needs. The instructor must ask her if she need modifications.

Warm-up	General movements to increase muscle temperature	
	Normal joint range of motion (ROM): Neck, shoulders, wrist, pelvis, hips, knees, and ankles	
	Emphasis on back, pelvis, and hip joints	
	Stimulate postural alignment	
	Keep movements slow, controlled, comfortable	
	Gradually increase ROM	
Nonimpact Aerobics	Intensity	Perceived exertion, fairly light to somewhat hard
		Breathing rate, conversational
	Duration	Depends on each participant's fitness level and state of pregnancy
	Mode	Nonbouncy, nonjerky, rhythmical
		Contract – relax, smooth, flowing
		Large, controlled ROM of arms and legs
		Maximize traveling, minimize standing in place
		Avoid quick changes of direction
Cool Down I	Easy pumping leg movement to facilitate circulation (ankle ROM, anterior lower leg stimulated)	
	Stretches — easy positions, not to maximum tension	
Body Work	Positions	Varied to promote circulation (standing, sitting or side-lying)
	Upper Body	Deltoids, triceps, pectorals, biceps, middle and lower traps (stimulate scapular retraction and posture here and throughout class)
(Muscular strength, endurance, and flexibility)	Lower body	Quadriceps, hips (extension, abduction and adduction in controlled repetitions, keep knees and hips slightly bent to eliminate strain to commonly irritated areas)
	Abdominals	Avoid supine position in those past the first trimester
		Slow repetitions, smaller ROMs, low lift, knees and hips bent, predominately from side
		Alternative: use stability ball as incline
		Abdominal compression exercises
		Pelvic tilts with emphasis on lower abdominals
		Attention to posture with all standing activity
	Additional	Exhale during contraction, inhale as relaxing
		Remember modifications for those with diastasis recti
		Pelvic tilts as well as back ROM exercise (e.g., cat stretch) are welcomed throughout class whether standing, sitting, or lying
Cool Down II	Final stretching, low-back stretch	
	Relaxation, visualizations, deep breathing	
	Neck ROM and stretches	
	Normalize circulation for standing	

in the postpartum period to slowly return to prepregnancy status.

The first priority after delivery is to bond with one's baby. The second priority is to resume Kegel exercises as soon as possible. The pelvic floor has been traumatized during delivery by severe stretching and possibly episiotomy or tears. Kegels after delivery may be a little scary, since the incision may be felt. Postoperative nurses should assure patients that Kegels will help the healing process of the pelvic floor. Before thinking about doing intense abdominal exercises, the pelvic floor should be rehabilitated.

Postpartum Return to Exercise

The suggested time for returning to group exercise activities is after the student's postpartum doctor appointment, or six weeks after delivery. Factors that may determine postpartum return include complications of labor and delivery, uterine involution, pelvic floor healing, prepregnancy fitness levels, and self-motivation. Before this appointment, gentle walking can be resumed and gradually progressed if the student desires.

Walking will help tone and strengthen the muscles of the lower body and, to some extent, the torso. During labor and delivery, the muscles of the pelvic floor undergo considerable stress and become relaxed and weakened. Temporary urinary stress incontinence is a common problem and may make exercise like running or aerobics difficult. The low impact nature of walking helps to minimize this problem. Additionally, it has been shown that women who exercise during their pregnancy and in the early postpartum months have a shorter duration of urinary stress incontinence than those who do not (Clapp, 1998). Focusing on good spinal alignment and form while walking will allow the body to strengthen important postural muscles in the torso that have become weakened by the shift in center of gravity created by the increased size of the uterus during pregnancy.

When a student returns to group exercise classes, advise her to gradually build back up to prepregnancy exercise levels. Remind her to listen to her body, exercise comfortably hard, but not to overdo it. Goals at this time are often unrealistic. A return to prepregnancy body weight and composition will take six months to one year in most cases. An instructor can help set realistic goals and create an environment that discourages weight loss as the sole reason to exercise.

As the postpartum student rejoins your group exercise class, remember that caring for an infant is a 24-hour-a-day, seven-day-a-week commitment. Personal time often disappears, sleep is diminished, and a feeling of being overwhelmed coupled with fatigue may cause increased tension and anxiety. This can affect not only the new mom's health and well-being but her relationship to the baby and other family members as well. One out of four first-time moms experience these feelings to such a degree that postpartum depression occurs. Help new moms learn to recognize this "overwhelmed" feeling in the early stages and encourage them to create some time for self-care. This time can help them to master the necessary coping skills. Exercise has been shown to help reduce stress and to create significant gains in general psychological well being. Studies have indicated that women who engage in regular exercise programs before, during, and after pregnancy have higher levels of self-esteem, which has been linked to a reduction in symptoms of postpartum depression.

Postpartum Musculoskeletal Conditions

Many women find that the back pain they experienced during pregnancy is relieved once the baby is born. However, attention should still be placed on low back health. The weight of the uterus is no longer pressing against the abdominal wall, but the abdominal wall is now loose and nonsupportive to the low back. The use of good body mechanics is crucial during this hectic, new period. Poor body mechanics and postural adjustments, in combination with the fatigue experienced by a new mother, can easily predispose her to back pain unless these muscles are retrained and are again able to effectively stabilize the spine.

Breast weight is increased for lactation, which pulls the shoulders and scapula forward, exaggerating the thoracic kyphotic (cuddling) posture. Prior to delivery, students should be instructed on shoulder external rotation and scapula retraction exercises for the postpartum period. If the student plans to push a stroller while walking, she should make sure the handles are high or use handle extenders; handles that are too low will exacerbate thoracic kyphosis and make good spinal alignment impossible. If the handles are raised, she can focus on scapular retraction and maintenance of a neutral head and pelvis while she walks. Good breast support during postpartum exercise is essential, especially for the nursing mother. Bras that compress the breasts against the chest are preferable to those that lift but should be changed immediately after exercise to avoid discomfort or inhibition of milk production. Some women find layering two sports bras gives them better support during exercise.

Diastasis recti is of less concern after delivery than during pregnancy due to the fact that the internal mechanical stress on the abdominals (the baby) is no longer exerting force against them. However, students should still be advised to evaluate their abdominal wall for the extent of separation that exists. All students will have some separation; one to two fingers is considered normal. Although research has not shown abdominal hernias to result from postpartum crunches (Clapp, 1998), if the gap is three fingers or wider, special care and attention to strengthening is warranted. An intelligent progression from early isometric abdominal exercises to pelvic tilts and pelvic stabilization exercises to head raises and partial crunches will rapidly improve abdominal tone and facilitate closure of this gap. For students with wide separations, it is prudent to avoid abdominal exercises that involve spinal rotation. The other abdominal muscles that are indirectly attached to the rectus abdominis can exert a pull that may widen the gap as they shorten. Noble's splinting abdominal exercises are a cautious first choice for early abdominal curl-up exercises (Noble, 1995). Remind students that they should focus on using their abdominals throughout their day. Abdominal compression (pulling the navel towards the spine while slowly and forcibly exhaling) can be done whenever they think of it to help strengthen the transverse abdominals and improves kinesthetic awareness. To balance the abdominal workout, complete it with back extension and scapula retraction exercises.

Breastfeeding and Exercise

New mothers are often concerned that exercise may affect the quality or quantity of breast milk. Research has shown that regular, sustained, moderate to high intensity exercise does not impair the quality or quantity of breast milk (Dewey, 1994; Dewey & McCrory, 1994). However, in a minority of women, exercise that is anaerobic in nature (e.g., high intensity interval training) may increase lactic acid levels in breast milk enough to cause a sour taste and decrease infant suckling (Wallace et al.,1992). Only minor changes in breast milk lactic acid content appear after more typical workouts, and these small amounts do not affect infant suckling behavior (Wallace et al., 1994). If you encounter a student whose baby rejects postexercise breast milk, you can offer the student several solutions: decrease exercise intensity to prevent accumulation of lactic acid, nurse the baby before exercising, collect preexercise breast milk for later consumption (lactic acid will clear the breast milk 30 minutes – 1 hour after exercise), or pump and discard the breast milk produced during the first 30 minutes after exercise (Wallace, 1993). In sum, this is an infrequent problem, which should not prevent any lactating woman who wishes to exercise from doing so.

References

American College of Obstetricians and Gynecologists. (1994). *ACOG Technical Bulletin*, Washington, D.C.: ACOG.

American College of Sports Medicine (1990). The recommended quantity and quality of exercise for developing and maintaining cardiorespiratory and muscular fitness in healthy adults. *Medicine & Science in Sports & Exercise*, 22, 265 – 274.

Artal, R. (1992). Exercise and pregnancy. *Clinics in Sports Medicine*, 11, 2.

Artal, R. et al. (1990). Orthopedic Problems in Pregnancy. *The Physician and Sportsmedicine*, 18, 9.

Artal, M.R. et al. (1991). *Exercise in Pregnancy*, Baltimore: Williams and Wilkins.

Boissonnault, J.S. & Blaschak, M.J. (1988). Incidence of diastasis recti abdominis during the childbearing year. *Physical Therapy*, 68, 7.

Clapp, J.F. III. (1998). *Exercising Through Your Pregnancy*. Champaign, Ill.: Human Kinetics.

Clapp, J.F. III. (1990). Neonatal morphometrics after endurance exercise during pregnancy. *Journal of Obstetrics and Gynecology*.

Clapp, J.F. III et al. (1992). Exercise in Pregnancy. (S294-S300). *Medicine & Science in Sports & Exercise*, 24, 6.

Clapp, J.F. III., Lopez, B., & Harcar-Sevcik R (1999). Neonatal behavioral profile of the offspring of women who continued to exercise regularly throughout pregnancy. *American Journal of Obstetrics & Gynecology*, 180 (1 pt 1): 91 – 94

Clapp, J.F. III & Little, K.D. (1995). Effect of recreational exercise on pregnancy weight gain and subcutaneous fat deposition, *Medicine & Science in Sport & Exercise*, 27, 2, 170 – 177

Clark, N. (1992). Shower your Baby with good nutrition. *The Physician & Sportsmedicine*, 20, 5.

Daly, J.M. et al. (1991). Sacroiliac subluxation: A common, treatable cause of low-back pain in pregnancy. *Family Practice Research Journal*, 11, 2.

Dunbar, A. (1992). Why Jane stopped running. *The Journal of Obstetric and Gynecologic Physical Therapy*, 16, 3.

Hummel-Berry, K. (1990). Obstetric low back pain: Part I and Part II. *The Journal of Obstetric & Gynecologic Physical Therapy*, 14,1, 10 – 13 and 14, 2, 9 – 11.

Jacobson, H. (1991). Protecting the back during pregnancy. *AAOHN Journal*, 39, 6.

Karsenec, J. & Grimes, D. (1984). *Hydrorobics*. Leisure Press.

Karzel, R.P. & Friedman, M.C. (1991). Orthopedic injuries in pregnancy. In *Exercise and Pregnancy*, Artral, R.A., Wiswell, R.A., & Drinkwater, B.L. (eds.). Baltimore: Williams & Wilkins.

Lile, A. & Hagar, T. (1991). Survey of current physical therapy treatment for the pregnant client with lumbopelvic dysfunction. *Journal of Obstetric and Gynecologic Physical Therapy*, 15, 4.

McMurray, R.G. & Katz, V.L. (1990). Thermoregulation in pregnancy, implications for exercise. *Sports Medicine*, 10, 3.

Noble. (1995). *Essential Exercises for the Childbearing Year*, 4th ed. Boston: Houghton Mifflin Company.

Nurse Practitioner. (1985). Kegel Exercise. *Nurse Practitioner*.

Pivarnik, J.M. et al. (1991). Physiological and perceptual responses to cycle and treadmill exercise during pregnancy. *Medicine & Science in Sports & Exercise*, 23, 4.

Schauberger, C.W., Rooney, B.L., Goldsmith, L., Shenton, D., Silva, P.D., & Schaper, A . (1996). Peripheral joint laxity increases in pregnancy but does not correlate with serum relaxin levels. *American Journal of Obstetrics & Gynecology*, 174, 667 – 671.

Schick-Boschetto, B. & Rose, N.C. (1991). Exercise in Pregnancy Review. *Obstetrical and Gynecological Survey*, 47, 1.

Sinclair, M. (1992). In training for motherhood? Effects of exercise for pregnant women. *Professional Nurse.* May.

Uzendoski, A.M. et al. (1989). Short review: Maternal and fetal responses to prenatal exercise. *Journal of Applied Sport Science Research*, 3, 4.

Wallace, A.M., Boyer, D.B., Dan, & Holm, K. (1986). Aerobic exercise, maternal self-esteem, and physical discomforts during pregnancy. *Journal of Nurse Midwifery*, 31, 255 – 262.

Wallace, J.P. (1993). Breast milk and exercise studies. *ACE Certified News*, 3, 6 – 8.

Wallace, J.P., Inbar, G., & Ernsthausen, K. (1992). Infant acceptance of postexercise breast milk. *Pediatrics,* 89, 1245 – 1247.

Watson, W.J. et al. (1991). Fetal responses to maximal swimming and cycling exercise during pregnancy. *Obstetrics & Gynecology*, 77, 3.

Wilder, E. (1988). *Obstetric and Gynecologic Physical Therapy.* Edinburgh: Churchill Livingstone.

Wolfe, L.A. et al. (1989). Physiological interactions between pregnancy and aerobic exercise. *Medicine & Science in Sports & Exercise.* Supplement.

Work, J.A. (1989). Is weight training safe during pregnancy? *The Physician & Sportsmedicine*, 17, 3.

Zhang, J., & Savitz, DA. (1996). Exercise during pregnancy among US women. *Annals of Epidemiology*, 6, 1, 53 – 59.

Suggested Reading

Bursch, G.S. (1987). Interrater reliability of diastasis recti abdominis measurement. Polyform Products Inc., 67, 7.

Clapp, J.F. III. (1996). Exercise During Pregnancy in O. Bar-Or (ed), *Exercise and the Female: A Life Span Approach, Perspectives in Exercise Science and Sports Medicine.* (1996) 9, 413 – 451.

Clapp, J.F. III., Simonian S., Lopez, B., & Harcar-Sevcik R (1998). The one-year morphometric and neurodevelopment outcome of the offspring of women who continued to exercise regularly throughout pregnancy. *American Journal of Obstetrics and Gynecology*, 178, 3, 594 – 499.

Clapp, J.F. III. (1991). The changing thermal response to endurance exercise during pregnancy. *American Journal of Obstetrics & Gynecology.* Dec; 165(6 pt 1): 1684 – 1689.

Huch, R. & Erkkola, R. (1990). Pregnancy and exercise — exercise and pregnancy. A short review. *British Journal of Obstetrics and Gynecology*, 97.

Jones, R. et al. (1985). Thermoregulation during aerobic exercise in pregnancy. *Obstetrics & Gynecology*, 65, 340.

McMurray, R.G. et al. (1991). The thermoregulation of pregnant women during aerobic exercise in the water: A longitudinal approach. *European Journal of Applied Physiology*, 61.

Prentice, A. (1994) Should lactating women exercise? *Nutrition Reviews.* 52, 10, 358 – 360.

Schelkun, P.H. (1991). Exercise and breast-feeding mothers. *The Physician & Sports-medicine*, 19, 4.

Sol, N. (1991). Modifications of health conditions and special populations. In Sudy, M. (ed.), *Personal Trainer Manual: The Resource for Fitness Instructors.* San Diego: American Council on Exercise, pp. 335-356.

Wallace J.P., Inbar, G., & Ernsthausen, K. (1994). Lactate concentrations in breast milk following maximal exercise and a typical workout. *Journal of Women's Health*, 3, 91 – 96.

Wolfe, L.A., Brenner, I., & Mottola, M. (1994) Maternal exercise, fetal well-being, and pregnancy outcome in exercise and sports science reviews, *American College of Sports Medicine*, 22, 145 – 194.

Chapter 10

In This Chapter:

Christine "CC" Cunningham, M.S., A.T.C./L., C.S.C.S., is a NATABOC-certified athletic trainer and a personal trainer. She is a private consultant specializing in fitness program development and education. Cunningham is a frequent writer and industry lecturer on the issues of exercise and injury. She is a NIKE athlete and member of the ACE Advisory Committee for Clinical Exercise Specialists.

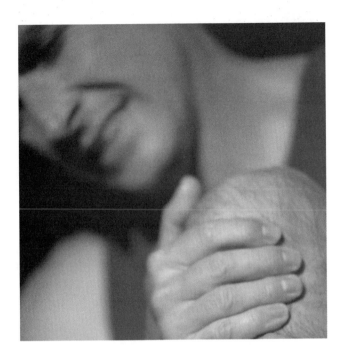

Injury Prevention and
Emergency Procedures

Christine "CC" Cunningham

Musculoskeletal injuries present complicated challenges for group fitness instructors. They are experienced by participants as well as instructors and can interfere with an individual's ability to participate. It is a difficult task to create an environment in which participants can achieve their varied fitness goals, while also addressing all the individual needs to ensure everyone's safety. The task requires knowledge of the factors associated with injuries, methods for prevention, and appropriate modifications for specific injuries. This chapter will address all of these areas, as well as guidelines for developing a facility emergency policy.

The injury-related responsibilities of group fitness instructors are to (1) prevent injury by careful preparation and carrying-out of every exercise session, (2) provide modifications for participants with injury limitations, and (3) properly handle injuries

that may occur during a class (refer to *Emergency Procedures*, later in this chapter). It is beyond the scope of the group fitness instructor to diagnose an injury or prescribe rehabilitative exercise. Execution of the previously stated responsibilities is challenging because participants attending a group exercise class have a wide variety of exercise goals, backgrounds, and physical strengths or limitations. It is your job as a group fitness instructor to instruct the participants to work within themselves and to inform them that they ultimately have control over their workout intensity. You are there for the participants' workout, not their own, and should appropriately set the intensity of the class by example. It is important to remember that the risk of a musculoskeletal injury occurring or being aggravated is always present and provide a safe environment for all participants.

New class formats are constantly being introduced into group exercise schedules. They range from yoga and martial arts to group strength training and indoor cycling. Classes are even leaving the aerobics studio and moving outdoors. Equipment being used ranges from the traditional steps to microhurdles and treadmills. There are many new risks and potential injuries emerging with each new format. Group fitness instructors must be able to manage the risks and provide modifications for participants with injury limitations. Success is dependent on understanding musculoskeletal injuries, their cause, and **contraindications** for participation.

Symptoms and Types of Musculoskeletal Injuries

Symptoms of Injury

Musculoskeletal injuries have several symptoms that define and determine their severity. These characteristics are

- Pain
- Swelling and discoloration
- Loss of range of motion
- Loss of strength
- Loss of **functional capacity** or use

These symptoms indicate the presence of an injury that should be investigated and treated. Participants should always be instructed to consult their healthcare provider if symptoms are present. At no time should you attempt to diagnose or treat the injury or symptoms. Instead, focus on providing the appropriate modifications for the participant so they can continue to participate safely.

Types of Injuries

There are two main classifications of injuries: acute and chronic. In most situations, acute refers to a rapidly occurring, new injury such as an ankle **sprain**, muscle **strain**, or broken bone. Acute injuries can be linked to a specific event that caused the injury and the symptoms are sharply defined. It is helpful to note that the term acute is also used to describe a phase of injury healing. The acute phase is when symptoms are severe, tissue damage is new, and healing has just begun.

In contrast, chronic, or overuse, injuries are usually of gradual onset, occurring from repeated stress over time without allowing adequate recovery time. Exercise starts a normal cycle of tissue stress and repair. In most situations this cycle occurs within a day or two, but it is dependent on the amount of damage caused by the stress. More stress or more intense activity causes more damage. The healing process is essential for the tissue to accommodate the stress and be able to tolerate it the next time it is introduced. Healing requires recovery time. Inadequate amounts of recovery between exercise sessions can cause the tissue damage from the stress to build up and break down the tissue. A lack of appropriate recovery time is the main cause of overuse injuries. The symptoms of a chronic injury may be less distinct and direct diagnosis may be more difficult. Examples of chronic injuries are lateral epicondylitis, **plantar fasciitis**, and **stress fractures**. Chronic injuries may linger for months and vary in their severity. It should be noted that an **acute injury** may evolve into a chronic condition if the mechanism for injury is repeated or the injury is not properly healed. It is not uncommon for group exercise participants and instructors to continue to exercise "through" injuries, causing more damage and prolonging the healing process. This is not recommended. Proper care, treatment, and rehabilitation are essential for a successful recovery from a musculoskeletal injury.

Factors Associated with Injury

There are many factors that can lead to an injury, including flooring, footwear, equipment, movement execution, and class intensity. Other factors such as teaching technique, warm-up, and cooldown are discussed in other chapters. You should be aware of all of these factors and assess each new class format for additional factors that may lead to injury to themselves or participants.

Flooring/Exercise Surface

Flooring needs to absorb shock to reduce the negative effects on the bones and joints. Repeated jarring can result in stress fractures and **tendinitis**. Hardwood flooring should be suspended to provide additional shock absorption and reduce injury risk. In addition, hardwood flooring offers good traction for dynamic movements and allows for lateral movement and pivoting. Concrete is not recommended as a surface for group exercise. It absorbs little shock and can be quite dangerous in the event of a fall. Carpeting reduces the stress on the bones and joints, but can catch the edge of shoes during dynamic lateral movements or pivoting, resulting in ankle sprains or knee injuries. Carpeting is appropriate for floorwork-based classes such as yoga or stretching.

Outdoor classes take exercise onto grass, sand, and hiking trails. Each surface offers concerns for participant safety. In general, natural surfaces offer good shock absorption, but may vary in terrain predictability and traction. Be aware of potential risks and choose the appropriate surface for the class format.

Footwear

Proper footwear will provide good cushioning, support, and flexibility. Many group exercise formats, including step, boxing, and sport conditioning classes, require that the ball of the foot absorb repetitive impact during the landing and pushing-off of dynamic movements. Footwear must provide cushion under the forefoot in addition to heel cushioning in order to reduce the possibility of injury to the foot from the repeated impact. Lateral movement demands support on the lateral aspect of the shoe to keep the foot from rolling over the base of support and spraining an ankle. Various sole designs allow for good forefoot flexibility without sacrificing traction. They provide freedom of movement without slipping during cutting, stopping, or rapid changes of direction. Forefoot flexibility is also necessary for many flexibility-based classes where full range of motion is desired.

Surface, equipment, intensity, and quality of movement determine the requirements of appropriate footwear. Be sure to evaluate the class content and adhere to any footwear guidelines indicated for different formats.

Equipment

Improper equipment set-up, fit, or use can cause injury. Class formats have adopted the use of a wide variety of equipment, from steps and tubing to bikes, hurdles, and treadmills. Each piece of equipment has specific set-up and fit requirements. Adhere to these requirements at all times in order to minimize the risk of injury. Check equipment regularly for wear and tear and replace when necessary. If equipment is manufactured in various sizes, have all sizes available to accommodate all participants.

Misuse of equipment can also cause injury. Use caution when incorporating new equipment and/or movements into a group situation for the first time. Be sure to learn the intended use, limitations, and safety precautions for all equipment. Apply these to the development of the class format and specific movements. Instructor creativity without adequate consideration for safety may lead to unintentionally dangerous situations for participants.

Movement Execution

Improper execution creates the greatest risk for injury in a group exercise class. Large instructor-to-student ratios make individual attention difficult and students can often repeat movements incorrectly numerous times without correction, leading to injury. The best defense for avoiding movement error is to use teaching progressions, provide modifications, and explain methods for self-evaluation.

Progressions should gradually build complicated movements in a step-by-step fash-

ion. Along the way, participants should be instructed on modifications for range of motion, strength, and impact. Include methods for participants to use to determine if they are ready to go on with the next step safely.

When incorporating movements from other disciplines, such as elite sport training or the martial arts, be sure to learn what progressions and evaluations are used in the traditional settings to safely teach the movement. Incorporate these techniques into the class format to reduce the risk of poor execution and the resulting injury.

Class Intensity and Frequency of Participation

Class intensity needs vary from participant to participant. Training effects are achieved at individually relative intensities, not absolute intensities. In other words, maximum intensity for each participant occurs at a different rate of work, so one intensity may be too easy for one participant and too hard for another. Intensity applies to heart rate, loading, speed of movement, and impact. A common teaching error is to assume that the intensity needed for a good workout for the instructor is the same intensity needed for all the participants. A fit and experienced instructor may direct the class in exercise at intensities too high for the less fit or experienced. This can result in participant fatigue and overexertion, increasing the risk of injury. Avoid this problem by assessing the participants prior to each class using the suggestions below. Gear the intensity of the class to the participants, not yourself.

Frequency of participation is a factor because individuals often attend class too often without allowing for adequate recovery in between. Inform participants of the appropriate frequency of participation before each class session. Promote cross-training by suggesting alternative classes that use different muscle groups or are nonimpact for days when participants should be recovering.

Overtraining is also a concern. Group fitness instructors are especially at risk for overtraining. Teaching numerous classes a day without enough recovery can lead to sleep loss, elevations in resting heart rate, and injury. Apply the alternative class approach to teaching as well.

Pre-class Evaluation

The group exercise environment makes individual participant evaluation difficult. Because instructors usually do not know who will attend class on any given day, using a health and exercise history to screen participants is not always realistic. With experience, you can become very proficient at using on-the-spot indicators to assess your class prior to each session. Whenever possible, however, utilize a preparticipation screening to assess individual needs and limitations.

There are three on-the-spot indicators that can be used to gauge potential participants' limitations and alert you to the type of exercise modifications that may need to be provided during the class. These indicators are :

1. *Age* — Older or young participants may have age-associated limitations that require the group fitness instructor to offer appropriate modification of the class content. Be sure to monitor these participants and evaluate if they are in need of modifications throughout the class.

2. *Posture* — Poor posture is associated with some muscles being short and tight while others are long and weak. This results in range of motion being limited by the short

muscles and strength or endurance being affected by the muscle weakness. This makes proper movement execution increasingly difficult and increases the importance of providing modifications.

3. *New participation* — New participants always make teaching more difficult. The more frequently an individual attends class, the less instruction they need to change moves and perform them safely. New students require increased attention and should be watched during the class.

If possible, use the warm-up to incorporate movements that could indicate which participants are in need of modifications or increased attention. Watch for range-of-motion or strength limitations and coordination or balance problems. As the class progresses, incorporate modifications for these individuals to ensure safety and participation success.

General Musculoskeletal Injuries

The following descriptions explain a few general musculoskeletal injury umbrellas. These injuries can occur at numerous sites in the body. More specific injuries are discussed later in the chapter. As a group fitness instructor, it is important to be familiar with these injuries and know enough about them to prevent their onset and provide appropriate modifications during an exercise session. The suggestions given in this chapter should only be used as guidelines for exercise modification. Diagnosis and treatment of musculoskeletal injuries is the domain of the healthcare professional. Refer all participants with complaints of injury symptoms to their healthcare provider.

Sprain

A sprain refers to an acute injury to a **ligament** caused by sudden trauma to the joint. Sprains can occur at any joint but are most common at the ankle and knee. Damage can vary from stretched ligaments to complete tears. Sprains are rated in degrees: 1st degree (mild), 2nd degree (moderate), and 3rd degree (severe). Symptoms of sprains include pain, localized swelling, discoloration, loss of motion, loss of use, and joint instability. A medical evaluation is recommended for sprains to rule out tears or associated **fractures**.

Treatment for sprains by a healthcare professional ranges from conservative, using ice and rest, to surgery. Ligaments can heal, but the healing is dependent on the degree of injury and the blood supply to the damaged ligaments. It is these factors that determine the chosen course of treatment.

Considerations for Group Exercise

- Choose exercise that does not involve the injured joint until the symptoms of sprain are minimal or no longer present.
- Gradually reintroduce activity involving the joint, since exercise introduced too early or too aggressively can increase the amount of damage.
- Avoid movement in the end ranges of motion. The instability of the joint caused by the damage to the ligament makes it more susceptible to further and recurrent injury.
- Monitor the participant for an increase or return of symptoms resulting from the activity.

Strain

A strain, often called a muscle "pull," is an injury to a muscle, usually caused by overexertion. Strains can be acute, occurring suddenly during activity or can gradually develop from repeated overuse. Symptoms of a muscle strain are pain, loss of motion, and reduced strength. Swelling and discoloration are often difficult to see depending on the location or how deep within the muscle the injury occurred. Bruising may be found below the actual injury site where it can pool close to the surface of the skin. A healthcare professional may treat a muscle strain using ice, gentle stretching and exercise. Gentle muscle activity promotes healing by assisting with circulation and reducing deep swelling.

Considerations for Group Exercise

- Participants should avoid strenuous or ballistic exercise after experiencing a muscle strain until the symptoms are minimal or no longer present.
- Gradually increase the intensity of activity.
- Incorporate additional gentle stretching of the muscle before and after exercise.
- Confine movement to the pain-free range of motion.
- Monitor the participant for an increase or return of symptoms resulting from the activity.

Tendinitis

The term tendinitis refers to the inflammation of the **tendon** or muscle-tendon junction. Tendinitis is a classic overuse injury caused by repeated stress without adequate recovery time. Symptoms of tendinitis include pain, swelling, and loss of function. There are many common locations of tendinitis, such as the patellar tendon (jumper's knee), the Achilles tendon, and the lateral epicondyle (tennis elbow). Activities consisting of high-repetition lifting or jumping, poor lifting technique, or repeated movement throughout the same range of motion can cause this condition.

Tendinitis is very difficult to treat because the symptoms often return when activity is reintroduced. A healthcare professional may use ice, stretching, and very slow, progressive loading of the tendon to allow the tissue to heal and become able to accommodate increasing stress levels. If not treated, tendinitis can lead to failure of the tendon and rupture. Surgical intervention for tendinitis is rare. Anti-inflammatory medication and injections are used most commonly. Due to the complexity of the condition, treatment for tendinitis is best directed by a healthcare professional.

Considerations for Group Exercise

- Avoid high-repetition activity or heavy loading of the tendon.
- Assess participant appropriateness for jumping, especially box jumps and other **plyometric** techniques with high loads.
- Use caution when incorporating ballistic movements, such as kicking and punching, that place high eccentric loads on the muscles and place the tendons at risk.
- Check equipment for proper fit. Repetitive movements, like cycling, can cause tendinitis if the equipment fit is wrong.
- Allow adequate recovery between sessions.
- Avoid very high repetitions in strength training and always use proper technique.
- Monitor the participant for an increase or return of symptoms resulting from the activity.

Specific Musculoskeletal Injuries

The following descriptions cover some of the most frequently seen musculoskeletal injures. There are many other injuries you will encounter as a group fitness instructor. Use these guidelines to understand prevention and modifications for activity. Do not attempt to diagnose an injury based on the symptoms given. Many injuries have similar symptoms but very different treatment and modifications for exercise. Always refer participants to their healthcare provider. In the event that the guidelines provided here are different than those provided by a physician or therapist, follow the guidelines provided by the healthcare professional. The description of each specific musculoskeletal injury presents the anatomy involved, the common treatment used by healthcare professionals during rehabilitation, and the **prognosis** for recovery. Considerations for the group fitness instructor include suggestions for modifying class content for participants who have had previous injuries and methods for preventing injury when designing a class session. It is beyond the scope of the group fitness instructor to diagnose an injury or prescribe rehabilitative exercise.

Lateral Ankle Sprain

A lateral ankle sprain occurs when the foot is inverted forcefully during weightbearing activity (Figure 10.1). Damage to the anterior talofibular ligament is most common; however, the calcaneofibular ligament can also be involved. Sprains range in severity from slight tears or stretching of the ligament to complete ruptures of one or more of the lateral ligaments (Malone & Hardaker, 1990). Lateral ankle sprains are commonly treated with **RICE** (rest, ice, compression, and elevation) and progressive exercise to return function. Surgical intervention is less common but may be used to correct chronic instability. The prognosis for a lateral ankle sprain is very positive and most individuals recover full range of motion, strength, and function to preinjury levels.

Considerations for Group Exercise

- Limit motion to a pain-free range and intensity.
- Resume activity only when released by a physician or all symptoms of the injury are gone.
- Avoid cutting, jumping, and lateral movements until full strength and **proprioception** of the ankle has returned.
- Encourage workouts that are predominantly nonimpact to minimize ankle discomfort until the ankle has fully healed.
- Load closed-chain strengthening of the lower extremity, such as squats and

lunges, according to the tolerance of the ankle joint.
- Double check that participants are wearing footwear appropriate for the class. Ankle sprains frequently occur when participants wear running shoes in classes that involve dynamic lateral movement.
- Use lateral movement cautiously on carpet or uneven surfaces.
- Monitor the participant for an increase or return of symptoms resulting from the activity.

Plantar Fasciitis

Plantar fasciitis is microtearing of the fascia at or near its attachment to the calcaneus bone (heel) and is thought to be caused by repetitive overloading of the tissue at its calcaneal attachment (Kibler et al., 1991). Common treatment for plantar fasciitis is rest, ice massage, stretching, modifications in training intensity, and strengthening of the muscles of the foot and ankle. Orthotics to correct abnormal foot mechanics and surgery are used in some cases of plantar fasciitis. Evaluation of exercise footwear to ensure proper fit and support is also recommended. Full return to preinjury range of motion, strength, and function, including athletic participation, is expected in most cases of plantar fasciitis. However, the condition may recur in some individuals.

Considerations for Group Exercise

- Encourage an extended warm-up prior to class.
- Incorporate additional stretching of the gastrocnemius, soleus, and plantar fascia.
- Avoid sudden increases in training intensity or frequency.
- Do not perform plyometric exercises such as jumping or high force loading of

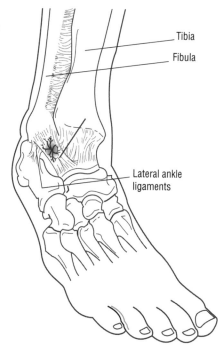

Figure 10.1
Ankle sprain

Tibia

Fibula

Lateral ankle
ligaments

the foot until full strength and range of motion have returned.

- Monitor the progression at which you increase the impact of the given activity.
- Suggest strengthening the muscles of the lower leg and foot to reduce the chance of recurrence of plantar fasciitis.
- Double check that participants are wearing footwear appropriate for the class.
- Watch for an increase or return of symptoms resulting from the activity.

Rotator Cuff Strain

A rotator cuff strain is the overstretching, overexertion, or overuse of the musculotendonus unit of one or more of the rotator cuff muscles (Kisner & Colby, 1990). Symptoms of a rotator cuff strain include pain, loss of motion, loss of strength, and loss of function. Rotator cuff strains can be acute or chronic. Rest, stretching, and slowly progressive strengthening exercises are used to return the shoulder to preinjury function. The prognosis for return to full range of motion, full strength, and full functional capacity is good following a rotator cuff strain.

Considerations for Group Exercise

- To aid shoulder stabilization, avoid loading of the shoulder joint in excess of the tolerance of the rotator cuff. Overloading might occur in the dumbbell press or pec flies, where the rotator cuff is too weak to stabilize the shoulder against the load needed to effectively stimulate the chest muscles.
- Watch for complaints of pain and altered mechanics that indicate that the load is too much for the shoulder.
- Do not fatigue the rotator cuff muscles with isolated exercise prior to executing movements that require their activity for stabilization. These include punches,

medicine ball throws, some stretching positions, and strength exercises. This is likely to exacerbate the rotator cuff strain and prolong healing.

- Monitor the participant for an increase or return of symptoms resulting from the activity.

Rotator Cuff Impingement

Rotator cuff impingement is a common overuse syndrome of the shoulder in athletes that participate in overhead sports (swimming, baseball, volleyball) or individuals who perform repetitive overhead work (carpenters, painters). It is characterized as a pinching of the rotator cuff tendon under the coracoacromial arch when the arm is abducted (Roy & Irvin, 1983) (Figure 10.2). Rotator cuff impingement is treated conservatively with rest, stretching, and gradual strengthening exercises. Other treatments for impingement include various surgical

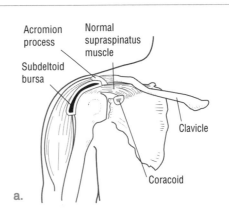

Figure 10.2

Impingement of bursa and supraspinatus under the coracoacromial arch with abduction movement:
a. with arm adducted
b. with arm abducted

techniques and anti-inflammatory injections. Each treatment is different in its approach to relieving the disorder and in the exercise guidelines. Impingement syndrome treated early, before anatomical damage has occurred, will likely return to full functional capacity, including participation in athletic competition (Jobe & Pink, 1993).

Considerations for Group Exercise

- Encourage additional stretching of the posterior cuff.
- Discourage stretching of the anterior shoulder.
- Avoid active abduction and overhead arm movements unless pain-free.
- Minimize the repetition of abduction or overhead motion, including lifts and arm swings.
- Do not do military press, triceps pull-overs, lat pull downs behind the neck, and pull ups behind the neck, as they are likely to exacerbate shoulder impingement (Litchfield et al., 1993).
- Monitor the participant for an increase or return of symptoms resulting from the activity.

Anterior Shoulder Instability

Anterior shoulder instability is a weakness in the anterior wall musculature (subscapuaris, pectoralis major, latissimus dorsi, and teres major) and/or stretching of the anterior capsule and ligaments that allows the humeral head to sublux or dislocate anteriorly (Jobe & Pink, 1993). This condition can be caused acutely from a fall or blow to the shoulder. Chronic instability is a gradual onset of muscle weakness and progressive damage of the anterior structures.

Anterior shoulder instability is treated conservatively with rest, stretching, and gradual strengthening of weak muscles. Significant anatomical damage to the anterior structures is repaired surgically. If conservative treatment is appropriate and started early, there is a high rate of return to full activity. Postsurgical prognosis is dependent upon the surgical procedure used and the adherence to rehabilitation guidelines (Jobe & Pink, 1993). Different surgical procedures result in varying losses in range of motion and function and, therefore, an exercise that is allowed after one type of repair may not be allowed after another. Always follow the guidelines for exercise provided by the healthcare provider.

Considerations for Group Exercise

- Limit motion to avoid humeral abduction with external rotation or horizontal extension. An unstable shoulder can dislocate or sublux if put in these positions.
- Be very cautious of all movements that place the shoulder in an externally rotated position, even with stretching.
- Avoid pec flies, lat pull downs behind the neck, and full range or wide grip chest press because of the stress they place on the anterior shoulder (Litchfield et al., 1993).
- Encourage stretching of the posterior cuff.
- Discourage stretching of the anterior shoulder.
- Monitor the participant for an increase or return of symptoms resulting from the activity.

Lateral Epicondylitis (Tennis Elbow)

Lateral epicondylitis, **tennis elbow**, is an overuse injury affecting the musculotendonus junction of the wrist extensor muscles at the lateral epicondyle of the humerus (Figure 10.3). Repetitive activities involving the wrist, such as playing tennis, carpentry, or pruning shrubs, result in microdamage to the tissue. The injury is associated with inadequate wrist extensor strength, power, endurance, and flexibility. The onset of lateral epicondylitis is usually gradual. Conservative treatment consists of rest, ice, gradual stretching, and strengthening of the wrist extensors. Cortisone injections and surgery are used when conservative management is not successful. Return to full activity is expected.

Considerations for Group Exercise

- Encourage stretching for all motions of the wrist. This includes flexion, extension, radial/ulnar deviation, and pronation/supination.
- Perform wrist flexion stretching before all activities that involve the wrist (i.e., punching, push-ups, and jumping rope).
- Use lighter loads for the wrist during repetitive motion to avoid overloading the tissue and causing pain during or after the exercise.
- Do not perform high repetitions of wrist exercises.
- Avoid holding hand positions for a prolonged period of time during cycling. Encourage frequent changes of position to avoid irritation.
- Monitor the participant for an increase or return of symptoms from the activity.

Anterior Cruciate Ligament Tear and Replacement

The anterior cruciate ligament (ACL) lies within the joint capsule of the knee (Figure 10.4). It attaches superiorly on the femur and inferiorly on the tibia. The ACL is instrumental in preventing the tibia from shifting forward on the femur, especially during forceful quadriceps contraction. Injuries to the ACL

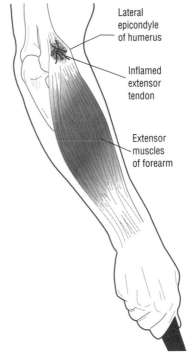

Figure 10.3
Tennis elbow

Lateral epicondyle of humerus

Inflamed extensor tendon

Extensor muscles of forearm

are commonly caused by rapid deceleration, such as a basketball player stopping suddenly, or by a direct blow to the knee causing the knee to hyperextend (Roy & Irvin, 1983). Instability of the knee, or the tendency for the tibia to shift during quadriceps contraction or weight bearing, is a concern when the integrity of the ACL is disrupted. This shifting can cause additional damage to the structures of the knee, such as the meniscus. The amount of instability is related to the extent of the damage to the ACL. ACL injuries range from a partial tear to a complete rupture of the ligament. Partial tears are frequently treated with RICE and an extensive rehabilitation program to return the knee to full range of motion and strength. Throughout rehabilitation, and all activity thereafter, the ACL is protected to prevent additional damage to the ligament, which may result in a increased instability. Reconstructive surgery is often encouraged with large tears and complete ruptures to restore the stability of the knee and avoid further damage.

Figure 10.4

Anatomy of the knee

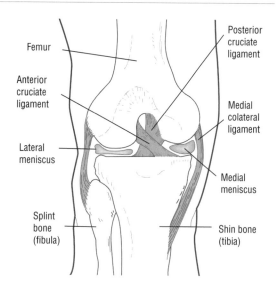

Femur

Anterior cruciate ligament

Lateral meniscus

Splint bone (fibula)

Posterior cruciate ligament

Medial colateral ligament

Medial meniscus

Shin bone (tibia)

The most common procedure for ACL reconstruction involves taking a portion of the patellar tendon out and using it as a graft to replace the torn ligament. The lengthy rehabilitation after an ACL reconstruction is a careful progression to return full range of motion, strength, proprioception, and function to the knee without damaging the graft. Range-of-motion limitations are used to avoid premature stress on the graft. One's ability to contract the quadriceps reflects the state of tissue healing and integrity of the graft during each phase of rehabilitation (Wilk & Andrews, 1992). All exercise involving the knee should be directed by a physician or therapist to avoid complications. Successful ACL reconstruction and rehabilitation results in the return to full activity, including participation in athletic competition.

Considerations for Group Exercise

- Do not allow participation in group exercise until the participant is released by a physician or therapist.
- Adhere closely to all limitations in range of motion and loading provided by the physician or therapist.

- Avoid cutting, jumping, sprinting, kicking, and pivoting unless specifically approved by a physician or therapist.
- Watch for difficulty with balance and movement execution caused by the strength and proprioception loss after the injury. Provide safe modifications for these activities.
- Encourage participation in cycling or aqua classes after an ACL injury if directed by a physician or therapist.
- Incorporate additional stretching of the lower-extremity muscles before and after class.
- Monitor the participant for an increase or return of symptoms resulting from the activity.

Patellofemoral Pain Disorders

The patellofemoral pain disorders (PFPD) may involve the patella, the femoral condyles, the quadriceps muscle, and/or patellar tendon (Figure 10.5). These components as a whole are referred to as the extensor mechanism. There are numerous conditions that affect the extensor mechanism including **chondromalacia**, patellar tendinitis, anterior knee pain, and patellofemoral malalignment (Shelton & Thigpen, 1991). The majority of PFPD are considered overuse syndromes and, thus, are associated with overload or repetitive microtrauma to the knee. Training errors, improper footwear, anatomical abnormalities, and postsurgical complications all contribute to PFPD (Rintala, 1990). There are many similarities among the conditions, which allow the exercise guidelines to be generalized. It should be noted, however, that each specific condition requires modifications that should be determined by a healthcare professional in order to assure appropriateness.

Conservative treatment of PFPD is highly effective and generally used prior to surgical treatment. If nonoperative treatment fails, surgical management may be used. Rest, ice, lower extremity strengthening emphasizing the quadriceps, lower extremity stretching, and gradual functional progressions are all used in conservative management of PFPD. Nonsteroidal anti-inflammatory medication and bracing or taping may also be included. Prognosis for recovery depends on the specific cause of PFPD.

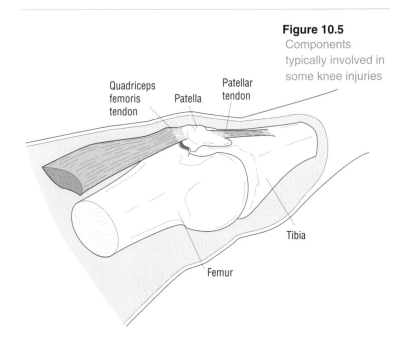

Figure 10.5
Components typically involved in some knee injuries

Quadriceps femoris tendon
Patella
Patellar tendon
Tibia
Femur

Considerations for Group Exercise

- Avoid full squats or excessive knee flexion.
- Use strengthening within a mid-range of 8 – 20 repetitions, since most PFPD disorders are sensitive to overuse.
- Encourage additional stretching of the lower extremity as full range of motion is essential for extensor mechanism function and the reduction of PFPD (Hertling & Kessler, 1996; Shelton & Thigpen, 1991; Woodall & Welsh, 1990).
- With indoor cycling, elevate the seat as high as possible without causing the pelvis to rock. This reduces the amount of knee flexion at the top of the pedal stroke.
- Avoid repeated jumping or plyometrics.
- Monitor the participant for an increase or return of symptoms from the activity.

Shin Splints

Shin splints are also known as **tibial stress syndrome**. The exact pathology involved in shin splints is not known. It is theorized that shin splints are microtearing of the attachment of the muscles of the lower leg on the tibia (Figure 10.6). Pain is the major symptom associated with shin splints. The anterior tibialis is frequently involved, but all of the muscles that attach below the knee on the anterior tibia may be affected. Shin splints are an overuse injury caused by repetitive loading of the lower leg with weak musculature. Runners frequently experience shin splints from the repetitive impact. An inability of the foot to absorb shock from weak arches can contribute to the onset of the condition. Lack of flexibility of the posterior muscles can also overload the anterior musculature, causing the microtearing. Footwear and exercise surface are major factors in the onset of shin splints. Treatment for shin splints includes ice, rest, stretching, and strengthening of the muscles of the foot and lower leg. Footwear should be evaluated and orthotics may be prescribed. With treatment and rehabilitation, shin splints can be managed to allow full return to activity.

Considerations for Group Exercise

- Avoid repetitive impact on hard surfaces.
- Do not drastically change the amount of impact in a class format, as this can lead to shin splints.

Figure 10.6

Shin splints

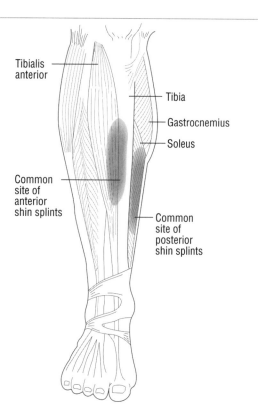

Tibialis anterior

Tibia

Gastrocnemius

Soleus

Common site of anterior shin splints

Common site of posterior shin splints

- Use shock-absorbing surfaces for all class formats involving impact.
- Encourage additional stretching of the anterior and posterior muscles of the lower leg.
- Incorporate additional warm-up before class.
- Double check that participants are wearing footwear with adequate support and cushioning in both the forefoot and heel.
- Watch indoor cyclists who do not regularly participate in weightbearing/impact class formats for signs of shin splints when taking a class with impact.
- Monitor the participant for an increase or return of symptoms from the activity.

Low Back Pain

Low back pain is one of the most difficult conditions to understand. Low back pain itself is a symptom that can be caused by a number of underlying conditions. These conditions include genetic abnormalities, muscle strains, sprains, disc herniations, and bony abnormalities. In general, symptoms of low back pain include pain, loss of motion, loss of strength, and reduced function. Each condition has contraindications and modifications specific to the injury. It is far beyond the scope of the group fitness instructor to try to determine the cause of a participant's low back pain. Refer all complaints of low back pain to a healthcare provider. The following guidelines can be used to provide modifications for movement and create a safe environment for exercise.

1. Avoid motion that causes an increase in pain. It is not always true that back extension is bad. In some cases trunk extension is preferred over flexion. In other cases, this is reversed. For example, the condition of spinal stenosis, a narrowing of the spinal canal due to aging, is a contraindication for lumbar extension. It is therefore always a good rule to offer a modification for activity that requires the trunk to move into extremes of flexion or extension. This is necessary for loaded and unloaded (stretching) movements. Rotation of the lumbar spine may also be contraindicated, especially with herniated discs. Disc compression is greatest in the seated position, so seated rotation can be a risk. Modify the movement by using a standing or **supine** position.

2. Always engage the abdominal muscles for protection of the lumbar spine during motion. The abdominal and back muscles work in concert to support and move the trunk without overloading the spine. Abdominal strength and endurance is essential and should be trained in the supine and standing positions. In standing, training involves the functional incorporation of abdominal contraction into movement so that the pelvis is stabilized throughout the movement. Always cue participants to remember to actively contract the abdominals for lumbar support. Modify movements that place high demand on abdominal support to accommodate participants who do not have the strength or coordination. Loaded squats, ballistic kicks, and end-range trunk motion are examples of high-demand activity. Failure to provide modifications can result in injury to the low back.

3. Enforce the maintenance of good posture. Poor posture can cause low back strains and sprains, as well as potentially damage the discs and bony structures. Good postural alignment has the head aligned with the ears over the shoulders. The shoulders should be pulled back to align with the hips. The back is slightly curved forward at the lumbar region with the top of the pelvis parallel to the ground. Excessive lumbar or thoracic curvature indicates poor posture and high risk of low back problems. Cueing for posture is essential and participants with poor posture may require movement modifications to reduce the risk of injury. Avoid loading of the spine with increased curvatures (e.g., **lordosis** or **kyphosis**) or poor posture.

4. Encourage stretching of the trunk and lower extremities to maintain full range of motion. Limited range of motion, especially in the hamstrings, has been associated with the onset of low back pain. It is theorized that the hamstring tension reduces the ability of the pelvis to move properly, placing more mobility demands on the intervertebral joints. This can cause sprains and strains of the low back, especially with ballistic movements. Tight hip flexors can also alter pelvic mobility and cause lordosis (increase in the lumbar curve). Flexibility is essential for proper execution of many group exercise movements. Participants without the necessary flexibility may overexert their backs, trying to execute movement. Offer modifications for movements such as kicks, leg lifts, and advanced stretching.

Emergency Policy

Despite the most vigilant attention to careful preparation of class content and in-class modifications, emergency situations will arise. Being prepared to handle the emergency appropriately is one of the responsibilities of a group fitness instructor. Since emergencies do not occur frequently, the procedures for dealing with them can be unfamiliar or forgotten if they are not attended to on a regular basis. Unfortunately, in an emergency situation, lack of familiarity with the emergency plan can result in the loss of valuable time, and possibly a life. You must review emergency policies and procedures frequently, rehearse the handling of different events, and always be prepared to act quickly to assist in any situation. Every club or exercise facility must have a written emergency plan with detailed procedures for contacting the local emergency services. If a group fitness instructor teaches at numerous locations, a copy of the existing plan for each site should be obtained and reviewed on a regular basis.

The Emergency Plan

The following information provides an outline of the necessary content for a group exercise emergency plan. Use these guidelines to develop or assess a facility's group exercise emergency plan.

> Be ready for an emergency by making the following as much a part of your job as teaching each class.
> - Review emergency policy and procedures frequently.
> - Rehearse dealing with different events.
> - Always be prepared to assist in any situation.

A group exercise emergency plan will include the following four main areas of information:

1. How to contact emergency services
2. Necessary emergency medical supplies
3. Who to alert within the facility in the event of an emergency
4. Documentation

A written version of the plan is essential to ensure that all staff members are equally informed about the plan and to allow easy review and updating of the plan as necessary.

How to Contact Emergency Services

When an emergency occurs, stay with the victim to provide first-aid and send another staff member or class participant to make the necessary phone call. The following details are needed in order for this to occur efficiently.

- *Phone numbers:* In most areas the emergency services can easily be accessed through the use of 911. However, this is not always the case and the emergency number must be provided. If an additional digit is needed to reach an outside line, this must be stated in the plan. Post all emergency phone numbers on or near each phone in the facility.
- *Phone locations:* Indicate the phone location nearest the group exercise room. If the closest phone is a pay phone, and change is needed to access the emergency

services, carry the necessary change at all times. If there is a locked door between the group exercise area and the phone, this door must be unlocked during classes or you must be provided with a key.

- *Building access information:* Once the phone call is made, the emergency services will need to know the facility address and the exact location of the group exercise area within the facility. Include this information in the written plan. Also, provide a written description of how to verbally direct the emergency personnel to the nearest accessible facility entrance.

Remember to let the emergency services individual end the phone call by hanging up first to ensure that all the information needed has been given.

Emergency Medical Supplies

All facilities should have a first-aid kit and blood clean-up supplies available for possible group exercise emergencies. Their location and contents should be indicated in the emergency plan so that all staff members are aware of where to find needed supplies.

First-aid kit: A stocked first-aid kit should be kept near the group exercise area. The following provides a list of recommended supplies:

- Assorted bandage materials
- Sterile gauze pads
- Elastic wraps
- Liquid soap
- Topical antibiotic cream
- Triangular bandages
- Splinting material
- Blood pressure cuff and stethoscope
- Penlight
- Scissors
- Paper bag

- Chemical cold packs or small plastic bags if ice is available
- Latex gloves (multiple sizes)
- Resuscitation masks

Blood clean-up supplies: For all incidents where blood or body fluids are involved, the following supplies must be provided. (For more information on dealing with blood refer to OSHA's Blood-Borne Pathogen Rule.)

- Latex gloves (multiple sizes)
- Resuscitation masks
- Liquid soap
- Mixture of water and household bleach in accordance with the Centers for Disease Control and Prevention guidelines

Who to Alert Within the Facility

In the event of an emergency, contacting emergency services and providing the necessary first-aid have priority over contacting additional staff and management. However, it is critical to make sure that the front desk and other area staff members (fitness floor, child care, etc.) are aware of the situation and can direct emergency services if they should happen to arrive in the wrong location or address other members' questions about the situation. Facility management should also be notified. Additionally, in the event that assistance is needed in handling the emergency while awaiting emergency services, the method for reaching other staff members in the facility should be included in the emergency plan.

Documentation

The emergency plan should indicate which facility forms need to be completed following an emergency situation. Include the location of these forms in the emergency plan. Separate forms should be available for incidents involving class participants or other members and for incidents involving staff.

Emergency Procedure

In the event of an emergency, quick and efficient response by the instructor can be critical to minimizing the injury or preventing death. Every situation has to be handled differently, whether it is a sprained ankle or cardiac arrest. The details of how to cope with each situation are covered in first-aid and CPR courses; hence, every instructor should be up to date with these certifications at all times. In general, however, the following procedure can be used to organize an efficient response.

1. EVALUATE

   Evaluate the victim/situation
   - assess consciousness, bleeding, and immediate danger
   - follow first-aid or CPR procedures

2. GET HELP

   Send someone to call emergency services*
   - direct someone to alert the necessary emergency service and meet them at the facility entrance
   - provide this person with a condition description (**vital signs**, bleeding, obvious injury, etc.) and indicate if a medical alert tag is found on the victim. (Do not assume that the condition on the medical alert tag is the cause of the situation; allow a medical professional to make the determination of the situation.)

3. ALERT FACILITY

   Assign someone to control the crowd and alert the other facility locations of the situation.

---

* In the event that there is not someone available to contact the emergency services, follow the guidelines established by CPR or first-aid for caring for the victim before leaving to phone for help.

4. CONTINUE VICTIM SUPPORT

Continue to provide necessary victim support until emergency personnel arrive.

5. CLEAN UP

Clean area appropriately. Restock first-aid kit.

6. DOCUMENT

Complete the necessary documentation. Review the situation with management to determine what steps, if any, could be taken to reduce the chance of the emergency occurring again.

Summary

Group fitness instructors have several responsibilities regarding musculoskeletal injuries. They must (1) prevent injury by carefully preparing and executing every exercise session, (2) provide modifications for participants with injury limitations, and (3) properly handle injuries that may occur during a class. Success is dependent on knowing the factors associated with injuries, methods for prevention, and appropriate contraindications/modifications for specific injuries.

Symptoms of many musculoskeletal injuries include pain, swelling, loss of motion and strength, and reduced functional capacity. These symptoms are present in various degrees and combinations in most injuries. Acute injuries are the result of an immediate trauma. Chronic injuries are developed gradually from repeated stress over time. Both types of injuries can be caused by any number of factors. These factors include footwear, flooring or exercise surface, equipment, movement execution, class intensity, and frequency of participation. Other factors such as teaching technique, warm-up, and cool-down are discussed in other chapters.

Three general descriptions of injuries encompass many of those seen in a group exercise setting. They are sprains, strains, and tendinitis. Sprains are acute injuries of the ligaments surrounding a joint. Strains involve the muscles and can be caused by exercise intensity overloads. Tendinitis is an overuse injury frequently seen in participants and instructors who do not incorporate appropriate recovery into their exercise schedule.

Specific musculoskeletal injuries can be described based on the structures involved and their symptoms. Every injury has different recommendations for modifying movements or class formats to avoid exacerbating the condition. Diagnosis and treatment of musculoskeletal injuries is the responsibility of a physician or other healthcare professional and is not within the scope of the group fitness instructor.

Continuously changing class formats introduces new potential for injuries in every class. Group fitness instructors cannot forget their responsibility of preventing injury through proper design and execution of the class. Providing modifications for all participants based on their needs is difficult but essential to ensure an outstanding group exercise experience for everyone.

Emergency situations can occur at any time and, therefore, a group fitness instructor has to be prepared to handle the situation appropriately. It is essential to have a written emergency plan that includes all necessary information for contacting local emergency services. Frequently review the plan for each facility and practice the procedures for coping with a variety of different emergencies. Prepare and manage each class to minimize the chance of an emergency and always be prepared to respond if one does occur.

References

Hertling, D. & Kessler, R.M. (1996). *Management of Common Musculoskeletal Disorders*, 3rd ed. Philadelphia: Lippincott.

Jobe, F.W. & Pink, M. (1993). Classification and treatment of shoulder dysfunction in the overhead athlete. *Journal of Orthopaedic and Sports Physical Therapy*, 18, 2, 427 – 432.

Kibler, W.B., Goldberg, C., & Chandler, T.J. (1991). Functional biomechanical deficits in running athletes with plantar fasciitis. *American Journal of Sports Medicine*, 19, 1, 66 – 71.

Kisner, C. & Colby. L.A. (1990). *Therapeutic Exercise: Foundations and Techniques*, 2nd ed. Philadelphia: F.A. Davis.

Litchfield, R., Hawkins, R., Dillman, C.J., Atkins, J., & Hagerman, G. (1993). Rehabilitation for the overhead athlete. *Journal of Orthopedic and Sports Physical Therapy*, 18, 2, 433 – 441.

Malone, T.R. & Hardaker, W.T. (1990). Rehabilitation of foot and ankle injuries in ballet dancers. *Journal of Orthopaedic and Sports Physical Therapy*, 11, 8, 355 – 361.

McHugh, M.P., Tyler, T.F., Gleim, G.W., & Nicholas, S.J. (1998). Preoperative indicators of motion loss and weakness following anterior cruciate ligament reconstruction. *Journal of Orthopaedic and Sports Physical Therapy*, 27, 6, 407 – 411.

Rintala, P. (1990). Patellofemoral pain syndrome and its treatment in runners. *Journal of Athletic Training*, 25, 2, 107 – 110.

Roy, S. & Irvin, R. (1983). *Sports Medicine: Prevention, Evaluation, Management, and Rehabilitation*. Englewood Cliffs, N.J.: Prentice-Hall.

Shelton, G.L. & Thigpen, L.K. (1991). Rehabilitation of patellofemoral dysfunction: a review of literature. *Journal of Orthopedic and Sports Physical Therapy*, 14, 6, 243 – 249.

Wilk, K.E. & Andrews, J.R. (1992). Current concepts in the rehabilitation of the athletic shoulder. *Journal of Orthopedic and Sports Physical Therapy*, 15, 6, 279 – 289.

Woodall, W. & Welsh, J. (1990). A biomechanical basis for rehabilitation programs involving the patellofemoral joint. *Journal of Orthopaedic and Sports Physical Therapy*, 11, 11, 535 – 542.

Recommended Reading

Alter, M. J. (1981). *Science of Flexibility*, 2nd ed. Champaign, Ill.: Human Kinetics.

Balady, G.J., Chaitman, B., Driscoll, D., Foster, C., Froelicher, E., Gordon, N., Pate, R., Rippe, J., & Bazzarre, T. (1998). Recommendations for Cardiovascular Screening, Staffing, and Emergency Policies at Health/Fitness Facilities. *Circulation*, 97, 2283 – 2293.

Brukner, P. & Khan, K. (1993). *Clinical Sports Medicine*. Sydney: McGraw-Hill.

Garrick, J.G. & Webb, D.R. (1990). *Sports Injuries: Diagnosis and Management*. Philadelphia: W.B. Saunders Co.

Kisner, C. & Colby, L.A. (1990). *Therapeutic Exercise: Foundations and Techniques*, 2nd ed. Philadelphia: F.A. Davis.

Radcliffe, J.C. & Farentinos, T.C. (1985). *Plyometrics; Explosive Power Training*. Champaign, Ill.: Human Kinetics.

Roy, S. & Irvin, R. (1983). *Sports Medicine: Prevention, Evaluation, Management, and Rehabilitation*. Englewood Cliffs, NJ: Prentice-Hall.

Tharrett, S.J. & Peterson, J.A. (eds.). (1997). *American College of Sports Medicine Health/Fitness Facility Standards and Guidelines*, 2nd ed. Champaign, Ill.: Human Kinetics.

Chapter 11

In This Chapter:

David K. Stotlar, Ed.D., is a professor in the School of Kinesiology and Physical Education at the University of Northern Colorado, where he teaches sport law, sport administration, and finance. He has served as a consultant to school districts, sports professionals, attorneys, and international sports administrators, and has been published extensively on sports law issues.

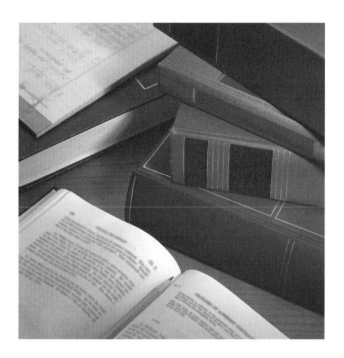

Legal and Professional
Responsibilities

By David K. Stotlar

Most people who teach or administer group fitness programs have been trained as physical educators or exercise specialists. Often their experience with the law, if any, has been limited to cases involving common sports injuries. However, the rapid expansion of the fitness industry has created new forms of legal liability. The purpose of this chapter is to explain basic legal concepts that concern group fitness instructors and to show how these concepts can be applied to reduce injuries to program participants, thus reducing the likelihood that an instructor or studio owner will be involved in a lawsuit.

Liability and Negligence

The term **liability** refers to responsibility. Legal liability concerns the responsibilities recognized by a court of law.

Every instructor who stands in front of a class faces the responsibilities of knowing capacities and setting limitations of participants before they begin an exercise program.

Studio owners and managers have the added responsibility of ensuring that the facilities and equipment are appropriate and safe. Fitness professionals cannot avoid liability any more than they can avoid assuming the responsibilities inherent in their positions. However, those liabilities may be reduced through adherence to the appropriate standard of care and the implementation of certain risk-management principles.

The responsibilities arising from the relationship between the group fitness instructor and the participant produce a legal expectation, commonly referred to as the standard of care. **Standard of care** means that the quality of services provided in a fitness setting is commensurate with current professional standards. In the case of a negligence suit, the court would ask the question, "What would a reasonable, competent and prudent group fitness instructor do in a similar situation?" An instructor or studio owner who failed to meet that standard could be found negligent by a court of law.

Negligence is usually defined as "failure to act as a reasonable and prudent person would act under similar circumstance." For the group fitness instructor, this definition has two important components. The first deals specifically with actions: "Failure to act" refers to acts of omission as well as acts of commission. In other words, an instructor can be sued for not doing something that should have been done, as well as for doing something that should not have been done. The second part of the definition of negligence pertains to the appropriateness of the action in light of the standard of care, or a "reasonable and prudent" professional standard. If other qualified instructors would have acted similarly under the same circumstances, a court would probably not find an instructor's action negligent.

To legally substantiate a charge of negligence, four elements must be shown to exist. As stated by Wong (1994), they are: (1) that the **defendant** (person being sued) had duty to protect the **plaintiff** (person filing the suit) from injury; (2) that the defendant failed to exercise that standard of care necessary to perform that duty; (3) that such failure was the proximate cause of the injury; and (4) that the damage or injury to the plaintiff did occur.

Consider this situation: A participant in an aerobics class badly sprains her ankle while following instructions for an aerobic dance routine. The movement that led to the injury consisted of prolonged and excessive hopping on one foot, something not recommended by reasonable and prudent aerobics instructors. If the participant sues the instructor for negligence, the following questions and answers might surface in court: Was it the instructor's duty to provide proper instruction? Yes. Was that duty satisfactorily performed? Probably not. Was the instructor's failure to provide safe instruction the direct cause of the injury? It probably was. Did actual damages occur? The plaintiff's doctor concluded that they did.

Areas of Responsibility

The duties assigned to fitness professionals vary from one position to another and from organization to organization. Overall, there are seven major areas of responsibility: health screening, testing and programming, instruction, supervision, facilities, equipment, and risk management. Each area poses unique questions for the professional that are important even to the beginning instructor. The American Council on Exercise (ACE) has developed a statement on ethics that is quite helpful in guiding the actions of fitness professionals (see Appendix A).

Health Screening

A fitness professional's responsibility begins when a new participant walks in the door.

Most prospective participants will be generally healthy people with the goal of improving their personal health and fitness level. Others, however, may come as part of their recovery from heart attacks or other serious health conditions. Therefore, it is imperative that instructors compile a medical history for each participant to document any existing conditions that might affect performance in an exercise program (see Chapter 4). For a complete review, consult the *AHA/ACSM Scientific Statement: Policies for Cardiovascular Screening, Staffing, and Emergency Policies at Health/Fitness Facilities*.

An instructor's responsibility does not end with collecting information. The health history and other data must be examined closely for information that affects programming decisions. Instructors have been charged with negligence for not using available information that could have prevented an injury. Every club or studio needs to establish policies and procedures to ensure that each participant's personal history and medical information are taken into account in designing an exercise program.

Fitness Testing and Exercise Programming

Many states require "medical prescriptions" to be developed by licensed medical doctors. Once the medical prescription is developed, a physical therapist is legally allowed to administer and supervise its implementation. The purpose of an exercise "prescription" is to induce a physiological response within a patient that will result in a clinical change in a given condition. As a result, fitness professionals are usually limited to providing exercise programs, not exercise prescriptions, which may be construed as medical prescriptions under these circumstances. Although the difference between the terms "program" and "prescription" may seem like a technicality, it may be important in a court of law.

Fitness testing presents similar issues. The health and fitness level of the client, the purpose of the test, and the testing methods should all be calculated before test administration. The use of relatively simple tests, such as a skinfold caliper to measure percentage body fat, would not normally pose significant legal problems. On the other hand, the use of a graded exercise test on a treadmill with a multiple-lead electrocardiogram could expose an unqualified instructor to a charge of practicing medicine without a license. Therefore, it is important that the test be recognized by a professional organization as appropriate for the intended use, be within the qualifications and training of the instructor, and that an accepted protocol (testing procedure) be followed exactly.

Instruction

To conduct a safe and effective exercise program, fitness professionals are expected to provide instruction that is both adequate and proper. Adequate instruction refers to the amount of direction given to participants before and during their exercise activity. For example, an instructor who asks a class to perform an exercise without first demonstrating how to do it properly could be found negligent if a participant performs the exercise incorrectly and is injured as a result.

Proper instruction is factually correct. In other words, an instructor may be liable for a participant's injury resulting from an exercise that was not demonstrated or was demonstrated improperly or from an unsafe exercise that should not have been included in a group fitness routine.

In the courtroom, the correctness of instruction is usually assessed by an expert witness who describes the proper procedures for conducting the activity in question. Therefore, the instructional techniques used by a group fitness instructor should be consistent with professionally recognized standards. Proper certification from a nationally recognized professional organization, as well as appropriate documentation of training (degrees, continuing education, etc.), can enhance an instructor's competence in the eyes of a court, should he or she ever be charged with negligence.

In addition to providing adequate and proper instruction, fitness professionals should also be careful not to diagnose or suggest treatment for injuries. This includes not only injuries received in the instructor's exercise class, but also those injuries acquired by other means. When participants ask for advice, it may be best to suggest they call their doctor. In general, only physicians and certain other healthcare providers are allowed to diagnose, prescribe treatment, and treat injuries. An instructor can provide first aid, but only if he or she is qualified to do so.

Simple advice for a sprained ankle once resulted in a nasty lawsuit. When a participant sprained her ankle during a fitness routine, the instructor told her to go home and ice the ankle to reduce the swelling. Because the ice made the injury feel much better, the participant kept her foot in ice water for two to three hours. As a consequence,

several of her toes had to be amputated because of frostbite.

This example may be extreme, but it serves as a valuable warning. There are several ways the instructor could have avoided this tragedy. First, the instructor could have advised the participant to see a physician. While this approach protects the instructor, it would be costly if every participant who suffered a sprained ankle had to see a doctor. Second, the instructor could have provided a more precise description of the first-aid ice treatment. The third and best approach would be a combination of the first two; the instructor would provide specific instructions (both written and verbal) on the first-aid procedures recommended by the American Red Cross and suggest that if the injury did not respond well, then the participant should seek the advice of a physician.

Supervision

The instructor is responsible for supervising all aspects of a class. The standards that apply to supervision are the same as those for instruction: adequate and proper. A prerequisite to determining adequate supervision is the ratio of participants to instructors and supervisors. A prudent instructor should allow a class to be only as large as can be competently monitored. The participant-instructor ratio will, of course, vary with activity, facility, and type of participant. An exercise class of 30 may be appropriate in a large gymnasium, but too big for an aqua class. Adequate and proper supervision may be different for a class of fit 20-year-olds than for a class of 55-year-old beginning exercisers.

General, or nonindividualized, supervision can be used when the activity can be monitored from a position in general proximity to the participants. For example, in an aerobics class a conscientious instructor can give enough attention to all participants through general but systematic observation to keep them relatively safe. On the other hand, a series of fitness tests administered to a participant before an exercise program calls for specific, or individualized, supervision. The person qualified to administer the testing must provide continuous attention in immediate proximity to the participant to ensure safety. Whether general or specific, required supervision should be based on one's own judgment of the nature of the activity and the participants involved, compared with what other prudent professionals would do under the same circumstances.

Facilities

Safety is the basic question for a fitness facility. Is the environment free from unreasonable hazards? Are all areas of the facility appropriate for the specific type of activity to be conducted in that area? For example, martial arts require a floor surface that will cushion the feet, knees, and legs from inordinate amounts of stress. Similarly, workout areas or stations of a circuit-training class should have adequate free space surrounding them to ensure that observers will not be struck by an exercising participant.

Some facilities provide locker room and shower facilities. These areas must be sanitary, the floors must be textured to reduce accidental slipping, and areas near water must be protected from electrical shock. Although group fitness instructors may not be responsible for designing and maintaining the exercise facility, any potential problem should be detected, reported, and corrected as soon as possible. Until then, appropriate

warning signs should be clearly posted to warn participants of the unsafe conditions.

In some cases, an instructor may be assigned to teach in an area that is unsafe or inappropriate for the activity. Under these circumstances, a prudent instructor would refuse to teach and would document that decision in writing to the club or studio management so that constructive action may be taken.

Equipment

For a program that uses exercise equipment, the legal concerns center primarily on selection, installation, maintenance, and repair. Equipment should meet all appropriate safety and design standards. If the equipment has been purchased from a competent manufacturer, these standards will probably be met. However, some organizations may try to save money by using homemade or inexpensive equipment. If an injury is caused by a piece of equipment that fails to perform as expected, and the injured party can show that the equipment failed to meet basic safety and design standards, the club or studio would be exposed to increased liability.

It is also important that trained technicians assemble and install all equipment. Having untrained people assemble some types of machinery may void the manufacturer's warranty and expose the program to additional risks. A schedule of regular service and repair should also be established and documented to show that the management has acted responsibly. Defective or worn parts should be replaced immediately, and equipment that is in need of repair should be removed for service.

Instructors and supervisors should instruct each participant on equipment safety. In addition, each instructor and participant should be required to examine the equipment before each use and report any problems to the person in charge.

Another equipment-related situation arises when participants ask their instructor about which shoes to wear or what exercise equipment to purchase for home use. An exercise professional should be extremely cautious when giving such recommendations. Before an instructor is qualified to give advice, he or she should have a thorough knowledge of the product lines available and the particular characteristics of each product. If this condition cannot be met, an instructor should refer the participant to a retail sporting-goods outlet. Otherwise, the instructor could be held liable for a negligent recommendation. An instructor who makes a recommendation based solely on personal experience should clearly state that it is a personal and not a professional recommendation. Instructors who are receiving money for endorsing a particular product must be particularly careful not to portray themselves as experts giving professional advice.

Risk Management

One of the duties of professionals in the fitness industry is to effectively manage risk. The process of **risk management** is more than just avoiding accidents; it encompasses a total examination of risk areas for the fitness professional. Each of the responsibilities identified above presents various levels of risk that should be assessed. The steps involved in a comprehensive risk-management review include the following:

1. Identification of risk areas
2. Evaluation of specific risks in each area

3. Selection of appropriate treatment for each risk
4. Implementation of a risk-management system
5. Evaluation of success

Risk management is an important professional duty. Too often, it is considered merely a process by which to avoid lawsuits. Professionals in the fitness industry should approach risk management as a way to provide better service to their clients. With this philosophy, risk management can become a method of conducting activities, not just a way to avoid legal trouble. The end goal is to have a safe, enjoyable experience for clients.

Guidelines

The following guidelines reflect the general areas described in preceding sections of this chapter and are intended to provide group fitness instructors with criteria necessary for reducing injuries to participants and the accompanying legal complications.

Health Screening

Each client beginning a fitness program should receive a thorough evaluation. Specific risk-management criteria may include:

- Evaluation is conducted prior to participating in exercise.
- Screening methods concur with national guidelines (ACE, ACSM, etc.).

Programming

Primary responsibilities of all fitness instructors include program design and exercise selection. Specific risk-management criteria may include the following:

- Health history is used appropriately in program design.
- Programs and tests selected are recognized by a professional organization as appropriate for the intended use.
- Programs and tests are within the qualifications and training of the group fitness instructor.
- Accepted protocols are followed exactly in all programs and procedures.

Instruction

A fitness professional must provide instruction that is both "adequate and proper." To fulfill this standard the following criteria would apply to instruction:

- Instructions or directions given to clients prior to and during activity that are sufficient and understandable.
- Conformance to "standard of care" (what a reasonable and prudent instructor would provide in the same situation).

Supervision

Group fitness instructors must perform their supervisory duties in accordance with the professionally devised and established guidelines:

- Continuous supervision is provided in immediate proximity to the client to ensure safety.
- Larger participant group is supervised from the perimeter of the exercise area to ensure all participants are in full view of the instructor.
- Specific supervision is employed when the activity merits close attention to an individual client.

Facilities

The basic issue regarding facilities centers on the safety of the premises. The cen-tral issue is whether the environment is free from unreasonable hazards. Examples of risk-management criteria include:

- Floor surface is appropriate for each activity.
- Free area around equipment is sufficient for the exercise.
- Lighting is adequate for performance of the skill and for supervision.
- Entries and exits are well marked.
  See Table 11.1.

Table 11.1
Standards of Care for Health and Fitness Facilities

---

1. A facility must be able to respond in a timely manner to any reasonably foreseeable emergency event that threatens the health and safety of facility users. Toward this end, a facility must have an appropriate emergency plan that can be executed by qualified personnel in a timely manner.

2. A facility must offer each adult member* a preactivity screening that is appropriate to the physical activities to be performed by the member.

3. Each person who has supervisory responsibility for a physical activity program or area at a facility must have demonstrable professional competence in that physical activity program or area.

4. A facility must post appropriate signage alerting users[†] to the risks involved in their use of those areas of a facility that present potential increased risk(s).

5. A facility that offers youth services or programs must provide appropriate supervision.

6. A facility must conform to all relevant laws, regulations, and published standards.

With regard to addressing the issue of to which organizations or groups should apply, it is important to note that ACSM has not attempted to define precisely what types of physical activities and programs collectively constitute a "facility." It is the position of ACSM that any business or entity that provides an opportunity for individuals to engage in activities that may be reasonably be expected to involve placing stress on one or more of the various physiological systems (cardiovascular, muscular, thermoregulatory, etc.) of a user's body must adhere to the six standards.

* A member is an individual who has entered into an agreement with a fitness facility that allows her access to a facility for a fee. The definition of adult may vary from state to state but the last would describe an individual who is capable of making an educated decision about his readiness for physical activity based on the results of a preactivity screening.

[†]Users are individuals of any age who who have access to a facility, either on an individual or a group basis. Users may or may not be under a fee-based agreement to use the facility.

Source: American College of Sports Medicine.

Equipment

In the equipment area, the legal concerns center primarily on selection, maintenance, and repair of the equipment. A risk-management plan should examine the following points:

- Equipment selected meets all safety and design standards within the industry.
- Assembly of equipment follows manufacturer's guidelines.
- A schedule of regular service and repair is established and documented.
- Caution is exercised in relation to recommending equipment.
- Homemade equipment is avoided if at all possible.

Accident Reporting

Regardless of the safety measures provided, some injuries are going to occur in the conduct of fitness activities. When someone is injured, it is necessary for the instructor to file an accident report, which should include the following information:

- Name, address, and phone number of the injured person.
- Time, date, and place of the accident.
- A brief description of the part of the body affected and nature of the injury (e.g., "cut on the right hand").
- A description and model number of any equipment involved.
- A reference to any instruction given and the type of supervision in force at the time of the injury.
- A brief, factual description of how the injury occurred (no opinions as to cause or fault).
- Names, addresses, and phone numbers of any witnesses.
- A brief statement of actions taken at time of injury (e.g., first aid given, physician referral, or ambulance called).

- Signatures of the supervisor and the injured person.

Accident reports should be kept for three to five years, depending on each state's **statute of limitations**. If the person was injured in a formal class setting, it may also be helpful to file a class outline or lesson plan with the accident report. In addition, a yearly review of injuries can be helpful in reducing accidents causing injuries to clients.

Selection of Appropriate Response for Risks

The most common approaches for the treatment of potential risks are: *avoidance, retention, reduction,* and *transfer.*

Avoidance — This simply means that the activity is judged to be too hazardous to justify its use. Some examples of this include high-risk exercises such as full squats and straight-leg sit-ups.

Retention — In some instances, instructors will simply want to budget for the situation. This might include paying for the cost of an emergency room visit for an injured client. It's much cheaper than litigation!

Reduction — Instructors should continue to compare their instruction, facilities, equipment, and procedures to national standards. Implementing changes constitutes reduction.

Transfer — This usually is accomplished through insurance. Fitness personnel and clubs should have viable programs of insurance that will cover the cost of legal defense and any claims awarded. Read the coverage carefully because company policies vary considerably. The general types of coverage that should be obtained include:

- **General liability insurance** — covers basic-trip-and-fall-type injuries.

- **Professional liability insurance** — covers claims of negligence based on professional duties.
- **Disability insurance** — would provide income protection in the event of an injury to the instructor.
- **Individual medical insurance** — provides hospitalization and major medical coverage.

Group fitness instructors and personal trainers who are independent contractors should pay special attention to their coverage. They should make sure that if they work for clubs all aspects of coverage are understood and included in the written agreements for services.

Duties also include enforcing conduct and ensuring adherence to safety guidelines. Clearly written safety guidelines for each type of activity should be posted in appropriate areas of the facility and rigidly enforced by the supervisor.

Of particular importance are the policies and procedures for emergencies. All employees should be thoroughly familiar with them and should have actual practice in carrying out an emergency plan. For example, every club or studio should conduct a "heart attack drill," requiring all staff to carry out emergency plans and procedures such as those recommended by the American Heart Association. The program manager should maintain records of these simulations.

Many group fitness instructors and supervisors are needlessly exposed to liability because they permit indiscriminate use of the facility. Supervisory personnel should restrict the facility to people who have a legitimate entitlement. Each staff member should have a list of the people scheduled to use the equipment and facilities during specific time periods, and the supervisor should allow access only to those people. This policy should be enforced with the same vigor as the safety procedures.

Implementation of a Risk-management System

Implementation is a management function. For a complete review of considerations regarding the creation and implementation of policy and staffing concerns, consult the *AHA/ACSM Scientific Statement: Policies for Cardiovascular Screening, Staffing, and Emergency Policies at Health/Fitness Facilities*. Attention must be given to all subject areas identified above. This process is normally called a safety audit and should be conducted regularly. Many professionals in the field develop safety check lists, while clubs often have professional consultants conduct safety audits. Regardless, a systematic evaluation of the risks in group fitness activities is essential for safe program operation.

Waivers and Informed Consent

The staff of many programs attempt to absolve themselves of liability by having all participants sign a liability **waiver** to release the instructor and fitness center from all liability associated with the conduct of an exercise program and any resulting injuries. In some cases, these documents have been of little value because the courts have enforced the specific wording of the waiver and not its intent. In other words, if negligence were found to be the cause of injury, and negligence of the instructor or fitness center was not specifically waived, then the waiver would not be effective. Therefore, waivers must be clearly written and include statements to the effect that the participant waives all claims to damages, even those caused by the negligence of the instructor or fitness center.

Some fitness centers use an **informed consent** form. While this document may look similar to a waiver, its purpose is different. The informed consent form is used to make the dangers of a program or test procedure known to the participant and thereby provide an additional measure of defense against lawsuits.

Obtaining informed consent is very important. It should be an automatic procedure for every person who enters the program, and it should be done before every fitness test. The American Council on Exercise suggests the following procedures:

1. Inform the participant of the exercise program or the testing procedure, with an explanation of the purpose of each. This explanation should be thorough and unbiased.

2. Inform the participant of the risks involved in the testing procedure or program, along with the possible discomforts.

3. Inform the participant of the benefits expected from the testing procedure or program.

4. Inform the participant of any alternative programs or tests that may be more advantageous to him or her.

5. Solicit questions regarding the testing procedures or exercise program, and give unbiased answers to these inquiries.

6. Inform the participant that he or she is free, at any time, to withdraw consent and discontinue participation.

7. Obtain the written consent of each participant.

For extensive guidance on many of the issues, you may want to consult IHRSA's *Standard Facilitation Guide,* which provides specific standards, sample forms, and sug-

gested policies and procedures that could be used in risk-management implementation.

Basic Defenses Against Negligence Claims

It is important for instructors to know and understand that they are not without protection under the law. Several defenses are available for use by fitness professionals as defendants in litigation in fitness-related personal injury cases.

Assumption of Risk

This defense is used to show that the client voluntarily accepted dangers known to exist with participation in the activity. The two most important aspects of this definition are "voluntary" and "known danger." If the client does not voluntarily engage in a program or test, this defense cannot normally be used. Also, if the participant was not informed of the specific risks associated with the program or test, then he or she cannot be held to have assumed them. The best way to prove that a client was knowledgeable of the risks involved is to utilize the informed consent and **assumption-of-risk** documents described earlier.

Contributory Negligence

This defense means that the plaintiff played some role in his or her own injury. Although this legal doctrine is viable in only a few states (check applicable state law), it provides a total bar to recovery for any damages. An example might consist of a client exceeding the designated maximum heart rate in a prescribed exercise program. A salient factor would also be whether an instructor was there to monitor the client, or if the client was exercising alone and following program guidelines.

Comparative Negligence

In this defense, the relative fault of both the plaintiff and the defendant are measured to see who was most at fault for the injury. The result is an apportionment of guilt and any subsequent award for damages. The court (or jury) determines the percentage of responsibility of each party and then prorates the award. This can be useful if a client is somewhat to blame for his or her own injury.

Act of God

Although this defense is not often used in fitness and sport law cases, it may be of interest. It involves injury caused by unforeseeable acts of nature. The foreseeability aspect is the most crucial. If, during an exercise session, an earthquake opened the floor and a client were engulfed, it may be applicable.

Other Legal Considerations

Group fitness instructors are providers of a special service. As a result, professionals in this field must be familiar with the special aspects of the law that are most frequently encountered in the conduct of their business.

Contracts

Fitness personnel must have an adequate knowledge of legal **contracts** to perform their tasks, to get paid, and to avoid costly legal battles with clients and/or clubs. Some instructors will want to work as individuals, not affiliated with one particular club, while others may want to be employed by a club or fitness center, yet specialize in one-on-one instruction.

Whatever the nature of the work arrangement, an instructor must be aware of the essentials of contract law. Basic contract law

indicates that the following elements are necessary to form a binding contract:
- *An offer and acceptance* — mutual agreement to terms
- *Consideration* — an exchange of items of value
- *Legality* — acceptable form and subject under the law
- *Capacity* — such as majority age and mental competency

The general considerations that should be addressed in contracts for use with clients, as well as contracts between exercise professionals and clubs for which they intend to work, should include the following:
- Identification of the parties (trainer and client/club)
- Description of the services to be performed (fitness training and consultation)
- Compensation ($X.00 per hour, day, month, or class, and payment method)
- Confidential relationship (agreement by each party not to divulge personal or business information gained through the relationship)
- Business status (confirmation of employment status)
- Term and termination (express definition of the length on the contract and the conditions under which termination is allowed by either party)

Employment Status

As noted above, another prominent concern for many fitness professionals deals with employment status: **independent contractor** versus employee. Both of these terms can apply to those who work in a fitness center. However, only the independent contractor status applies to self-employed personal trainers working independently from a club.

However, most clubs still require independent contractors hired by the club to follow club rules.

Clients who hire a personal trainer do not intend, for the most part, to hire that person as an employee, but prefer to lease their services for a brief period of time. Hence, most self-employed personal trainers are independent contractors and not employees of their clients.

In some instances, owners of fitness centers or clubs have used the term independent contractor for employees. Club owners are often motivated to hire independent contractors in place of regular employees because the company does not have to train, provide medical or other benefits, arrange for social security withholding, or pay into worker's compensation or unemployment funds for independent contractors. Club owners also find an advantage in having independent contractors because it is more complicated, from a legal standpoint, to fire existing employees than it is to simply renew contracts with independent contractors.

A legal dichotomy exists between regular employees and independent contractors. Most commonly, the courts have considered 10 questions or "tests" to determine if the business relationship in question between a club and a fitness professional is that of a regular employee or an independent contractor. These tests are:

1. The extent of control that, by agreement, the employer can exercise over the details of the work. The existence of a right to control is indicative of an employer-employee relationship.
2. The method of payment, whether by time or by the job. Generally, those persons scheduled to be paid on a regular basis at an hourly or weekly rate have been con-

sidered employees. Conversely, those paid in a single payment for services rendered have more easily qualified as independent contractors.

3. The length of time for which the person is employed. Individuals hired for short periods of time (a few days or weeks) have more often been seen as independent contractors, whereas employment periods that extended upward of a full year have been ruled as establishing an employer-employee relationship.
4. The skill required for the provision of services. When the worker needs no training because of the specialized or technical skills that the employer intends to utilize, the independent contractor status has prevailed. On the other hand, if an employer provides training to a recently hired individual, that person will more than likely be judged to be an employee.
5. Whether the person employed is in a distinct business or occupation. If a worker offers services to other employers or clients, a status of independent contractor would probably be found. If, however, the worker only intended to provide services for one employer, and failed to offer the services to others as an independent business, the employee status could be found.
6. Whether the employer of the worker provides the equipment. If independent contractor status is desired, group fitness instructors will have a better chance getting it if they provide their own equipment.
7. Whether the work is a part of the normal business of the employer. Court rulings have favored classifying individuals as regular employees when services rendered are integral to the business of the employer. Supplemental, special, or one-

time services are more likely to be provided by independent contractors.

8. Whether the work is traditionally performed by a specialist in similar businesses. Employers and employees must examine their field of business to gain an understanding of current practices and align themselves with the prevailing trends.

9. Intent of the parties involved in the arrangement. The courts will attempt to enforce intent of the parties at the time the agreement was executed. If a professional thought that he or she were hired as an independent contractor, as did the club, it would influence the court's determination. Therefore, a clear understanding of the arrangement is a must.

10. Whether the employer is engaged in a business. The intent here is to protect clients from being construed as employers when a personal trainer is hired to perform work of a "private" nature. This is most common when one-on-one trainers sell their services to private citizens rather than to clubs or corporations.

The process of determining employment status is marked by careful analysis of the facts and the weighing of interpretations on both sides of the issue. All of the issues addressed above have been used in court cases dealing with this matter, each with varying degrees of authority. It is, therefore, imperative that all fitness professionals and club owners understand and examine these factors when initiating agreements.

For more specific information on the legal aspects surrounding the independent contractor versus employee issue, you may want to consult the guidelines published by the Internal Revenue Service.

Copyright Law

One of an exercise instructor's major legal responsibilities is compliance with **copyright** law. All forms of commercially produced creative expression are protected by copyright law, but music is the area most pertinent to exercise instructors.

Simply stated, almost all musical compositions that one can hear on the radio or television or buy in the music store are owned by artists and studios and are protected by federal copyright law. Whether an instructor makes a tape from various songs on the radio or from tapes he or she has purchased does not matter; the instructor who uses that tape in a for-profit exercise class — legally speaking, a **public performance** — is in violation of copyright law.

Performance Licenses

To be able to use copyrighted music in an exercise class, one must obtain a performance license from one of the two major **performing rights societies,** the **American Society of Composers, Authors and Publishers (ASCAP)** or **Broadcast Music, Inc. (BMI)**. These organizations vigorously enforce copyrighted law for their memberships and will not hesitate to sue a health club, studio, or freelance instructor who plays copyrighted music without a license.

Accordingly, most clubs and studios obtain a **blanket license** for their instructors. The license fees for the clubs are determined either by the number of students who attend classes each week, by the number of speakers used in the club, or by whether the club has a single- or multi-floor layout.

Instructors who teach as independent contractors at several locations may have to obtain their own licenses. They should check with the clubs where they teach to see if each club's blanket license covers their classes. If freelance instructors teach at several different locations with their own tapes, they will have to obtain their own performance licenses.

Given that the fees for either getting licenses or paying damages for copyright infringement may be prohibitive, independent instructors, in particular, may want to consider other options. One is to create rhythm tapes of their own using a drum machine, an electronic instrument that can range in sophistication from toy to professional recording device. A professional model is not needed, however, to make an appealing rhythm tape. A local musical instrument store owner or salesperson could probably steer the instructor to someone who could help create such a tape.

Other options include buying tapes expressly made for fitness and aerobic exercise classes, which the copyright holder expressly permits to be used in a class, or asking exercise class students to bring their own recordings for the workouts, in effect using them for the clients' own noncommercial use.

Obtaining Copyright Protection

Some group fitness instructors may want to obtain copyright protection for certain aspects of their work. The following are several examples of what an instructor may want to copyright:

Pantomimes and choreographic work — If an instructor creates more than a simple routine, and publicly distributes (through a dance notation system), performs, or displays the choreography, it can be copyrighted.

Books, videos, films — If a choreographed work by an instructor is sold to a **publisher**, video distributor, or movie studio, that business entity will own the copyright for the material and the instructor will be compensated with either or both an advance and a certain portion of the proceeds (royalties). Through negotiation with the producing or distributing company, the instructor may be able to retain certain rights to the material.

Compilations *of exercise routines* — If an instructor makes an original sequence of routines, it may be protected by copyright and licensed to others for a book, video, film, or other presentation form.

Graphic materials — If an instructor creates pictures, charts, diagrams, informational handouts, or other graphic materials for instructional aids or promotional material, these too may be copyrighted.

For copyright information or applications, write to:

> Register of Copyrights
> United States Copyright Office
> Library of Congress
> Washington, D.C. 20559

Liability Insurance

Every group fitness instructor will want to assess his or her liability insurance needs. An instructor employed at a club should inquire about the general liability policy and any other liability insurance the owner might have.

Independent contractors may not be covered by a club's general policy and, if not, should ask the club if they can be added by special endorsement.

Many nonprofit groups, such as churches and recreation centers, may not have coverage that includes their contract instructors. The instructors at these venues should have their own general liability coverage.

General liability coverage will cover an accident where a student trips over a loose floorboard or falls and breaks an arm. What about a student hurting herself in a routine that she says was improperly demonstrated? For this kind of claim, instructors would be wise to have professional liability insurance.

Since professional standards in the exercise field are becoming the norm, the expectations of students (and courts, as well) are rising to include all facets of exercise-class management, from screening participants correctly to adequately supervising them.

Professional liability insurance will not cover an instructor for copyright infringement claims or offer protection in suits involving libel, slander, invasion of privacy, or defamation of character. These sorts of actions may be considered intentional torts and are not typically covered.

Instructors seeking affordable liability policies should check with professional groups, such as IDEA, ACSM, NCSA, and AFAA, or discuss their needs with insurance agents who may suggest liability coverage be added on the instructor's residence insurance as a "business pursuits rider."

Liability insurance is a must for exercise instructors. They should not begin a class anywhere without knowing what the insurance coverage is and what is excluded. The key thing for instructors to do if they are not given adequate insurance information by a club supervisor is to ask specific questions related to a club's liability insurance policy.

Americans with Disabilities Act

Fitness professionals can be affected by legislative mandates beyond insurance regulations. One of the more recent laws that affect the profession is the **Americans with Disabilities Act**, which became law in 1992. Modeled after the Civil Rights Act, it prohibits discrimination on the basis of disability. The law provides for equal treatment and equal access to programs for disabled Americans. (Previous legislation — Section 504 of the Rehabilitation Act of 1973 — required barrier-free access to all publicly funded facilities.)

The new act extends the same provisions to all areas of public accommodation, including businesses. Therefore, it is essential that fitness professionals make sure that their buildings, equipment, and programs are available to persons with disabilities. Employers must also provide reasonable accommodations for employees with disabilities, including adjusted work stations and equipment as necessary. Therefore, whether a disabled person is an employee or a client, steps must be taken to ensure that the professional and business environment is one that respects the dignity, skills, and contributions of those individuals.

Scope of Practice in the Profession

Group fitness instructors are generally in the business of providing exercise leadership and exercise-related advice. They are not normally physicians, physical therapists, or dietitians (although some may be certified or licensed in these areas).

The primary area in which the **scope of practice** comes into question is generally the health-history or wellness-history form. As described earlier, this form is used as a general screening document prior to the client's entry into a fitness program. Fitness law expert David Herbert says that "wellness-assessment documents should be utilized for...determination of an individual's level of fitness...*never* for the purpose of providing or recommending *treatment* of any condition." Use of such a form in recommending treatment could constitute the practice of medicine without a license.

Another area of interaction between fitness professionals and clients that can cause issues related to the scope of certain professional practices is in dietary and nutritional counseling. According to the American Dietetic Association, most states have statutes that regulate or license nutritionists. In the other states, anyone is able to profess to be a nutritionist. Laws in each state should be examined to ensure that healthcare practice statutes are not violated by fitness professionals who may be surpassing their training and expertise. If a client has complex dietary questions, referral should be made to a registered dietitian (R.D.) or other qualified healthcare professional.

Similarly, group fitness instructors are not psychologists, marriage counselors, or physical therapists and therefore should not provide advice or counseling on issues related to a client's emotional and/or psychological status. Clients should always be referred to licensed practitioners in these and other related areas.

Summary

No program, regardless of how well it is run, can completely avoid all injuries. In an attempt to reduce both injuries to participants and the accompanying legal complications, a group fitness instructor would be wise to adhere to the following guidelines:

1. Obtain professional education, guided practical training under a qualified exercise professional, and current certification from an established professional organization.

2. Design and conduct programs that reflect current professional standards.
3. Formulate and enforce policies and guidelines for the conduct of the program in accordance with professional recommendations.
4. Establish and implement adequate and proper procedures for supervision in all phases of the program.
5. Establish and implement adequate and proper methods of instruction in all phases of the program.
6. Post safety regulations in the facility and ensure that they are rigidly enforced by supervisory personnel.
7. Keep the facility free from hazards and maintain adequate free space for each activity to be performed.
8. Establish and document inspection and repair schedules for all equipment and facilities.
9. Formulate policies and guidelines for emergency situations, rehearse the procedures, and require all instructors to have current first-aid training and CPR certification.

By applying the recommendations presented above, fitness professionals can help reduce the probability of injury to participants. Should legal action result from an injury, the facts of the case would be examined to determine whether negligence was the cause. A properly trained, competent, and certified instructor conducting a program that was in accordance with current professional standards would probably prevail.

References

American College of Sports Medicine. (1997). *ACSM's Health Fitness Facility Standards and Guidelines*. Champagne, Ill.: Human Kinetics.

Herbert, D.L. (1989). Appropriate Use of Wellness Appraisals, *Fitness Management*, September, p.23.

Wong, G. (1994). *Essentials of Amateur Sports Law.* West Port, Conn.: Praeger.

Suggested Reading

Arnold, D.E. (1983). *Legal Considerations in the Administration of Public School Physical Education and Athletic Program.* Springfield, Ill.: Charles C. Thomas.

Gerson, R.F. (1989). *Marketing Health and Fitness Services.* Champaign, Ill.: Human Kinetics Publishers.

Herbert, D.L. & Herbert, W.G. (1989). *Legal Aspects of Preventative and Rehabilitative Exercise Programs,* 2nd ed. Canton, Ohio: Professional and Executive Reports and Publications.

Koeberle, B.E. (1990). *Legal Aspects of Personal Training.* Canton, Ohio: Professional and Executive Reports and Publications.

Nygaard, G. & Boone, T.H. (1989). *Law for Physical Educators and Coaches.* Columbus, Ohio: Publishing Horizons.

Appendix A

Code of
Ethics

The American Council on Exercise (ACE) is a not-for-profit organization committed to the promotion of safe and effective exercise. ACE accomplishes its mission by setting certification and education standards for fitness instructors and through public education and research. Since 1985, ACE has certified more than 85,000 group fitness instructors, personal trainers, lifestyle & weight management consultants, and clinical exercise specialists in 77 countries, making it the largest not-for-profit fitness certifying organization in the world. ACE sets forth this code of ethics to communicate the quality instruction and service the public can expect to receive from ACE-certified fitness instructors.

AMERICAN COUNCIL ON EXERCISE CODE OF ETHICS

As an ACE-certified Professional, I am guided by the American Council on Exercise's principles of professional conduct whether I am working with clients, the public, or other health and fitness professionals. I promise to:

- ✔ Provide safe and effective instruction.
- ✔ Provide equal and fair treatment to all clients.
- ✔ Stay up-to-date on the latest health and physical activity research and understand its practical application.
- ✔ Maintain current CPR certification and knowledge of first-aid services.
- ✔ Comply with all applicable business, employment, and copyright laws.
- ✔ Protect and enhance the public's image of the health and fitness industry.
- ✔ Maintain the confidentiality of all client information.
- ✔ Refer clients to more qualified fitness, medical, or health professionals when appropriate.

Appendix B

Group Fitness Instructor Certification
Exam Content Outline

The purpose of this exam content outline is to set forth the tasks, knowledge, and skills necessary for group fitness instructors to perform their job responsibilities at a minimum professional level. This includes, but is not limited to, teaching the components of fitness to apparently healthy individuals in a group exercise setting. Please note, not all knowledge statements listed here in the exam content outline will be addressed on each exam administered.

It is the position of the American Council on Exercise that the recommendations outlined here are not exhaustive to the qualifications of a group fitness instructor but represent the minimum level of proficiency and theoretical knowledge essential for an aero-bics instructor to: screen and evaluate prospective clients; design a safe and effective exercise program; instruct clients in correct exercise technique to avoid injury; and respond to the typical questions and problems that arise in a group exercise setting.

These recommendations apply only to group fitness instructors training healthy individuals who have no apparent physical limitations or special medical needs. It is not ACE's intent to provide recommendations for instructors delivering specialized programs for highly trained athletes, pre- and postnatal women, older clients, individuals with physical handicaps, the morbidly obese, or individuals known to have coronary heart disease.

American Council on Exercise Exam Contents

Exercise Science	Basic physiology; cardiorespiratory, musculoskeletal, neuromuscular, metabolic, and environmental
	Basic anatomy
	Basic kinesiology
	Correct training techniques
	Basic fitness test terminology and procedures
	Physiological and anatomical considerations of special populations
	Basic psychological issues affecting exercise adherence
	Basic nutrition and weight management

Exercise Programming	Components of a class given the class objective
	Modifications or adaptations
	Selection, modification, and adaptation for special populations
	Establishment of a safe exercise environment
Instructional Techniques	Techniques to monitor exercise intensity
	Teaching strategies to modify incorrect movements
	Modification of group and individual performance
	Correct cueing
	Teaching methodologies
	Injury prevention
	Emergency procedures: first aid, cardiopulmonary resuscitation (CPR), and evacuation plans
Professional Responsibility	Current legal principles and issues
	American Council on Exercise Code of Ethics
	Accepted business standards and practices
	Emergency procedures: first aid, cardiopulmonary resuscitation (CPR), and evacuation plans
	Insurance needs related to group exercise instruction

Domain I: Exercise Science

Task 1:

To demonstrate knowledge of basic cardiorespiratory physiology by applying correct cardiorespiratory physiological principles in order to develop and instruct safe and effective exercise.
Knowledge of:

1. Normal and abnormal static and dynamic exercise, including heart rate, blood pressure, and oxygen consumption.
2. Cardiorespiratory physiology terms as they apply to endurance training (e.g., cardiac output, stroke volume, oxygen consumption, ventilation, respiration, and aerobic capacity).
3. The principles of training as they apply to cardiorespiratory endurance (e.g., overload, specificity, reversibility, progression, frequency, training effect, and adaptation).
4. The benefits of endurance training (e.g., improvement in aerobic capacity, weight control, and reduced stress levels, body fat, and risk of heart disease).
5. The risk factors for coronary artery disease and their impact on normal cardiorespiratory function.
6. The relationship among heart rate, exercise intensity, and oxygen requirement.

Task 2:

To demonstrate knowledge of basic musculoskeletal physiology by applying correct musculoskeletal physiological principles in order to develop and instruct safe and effective exercise.

Knowledge of:

1. The major components of muscular fitness (e.g., muscular strength, endurance, and flexibility).
2. Training principles for improving muscular strength, endurance, and flexibility.
3. The following terms pertaining to muscular fitness: training effect, resistance, overload, specificity, repetitions, sets, frequency, rest periods, progression, and muscle atrophy and hypertrophy.
4. The potential benefits of muscular strength and endurance training (e.g., injury prevention, optimal leisure, and work performance).
5. The various methods of using resistance during muscular fitness training: body weight, gravity, bands, hand weights, and leverage.
6. The risks associated with performing the Valsalva maneuver during resistance training.
7. Static and dynamic stretches and the risks and benefits of each method.
8. Hypermobility, flexibility, and tightness and their relationship to joint mobility.
9. The relationship between joint mobility and muscular flexibility.
10. The risks associated with muscular strength training: improper body mechanics and lifting techniques that may result in acute and chronic overuse injuries.
11. The different muscle fiber types and their individual characteristics.
12. How osteoporosis and osteoarthritis affect the skeletal system.

Task 3:

To demonstrate knowledge of basic neuromuscular physiology by applying correct neuromuscular physiological principles in order to develop and instruct safe and effective exercise.

Knowledge of:

1. Key terms in neuromuscular physiology: motor neurons, motor unit, and neuromuscular junction.
2. The roles of Golgi tendon organs and muscle spindles in the regulation of muscle contraction (e.g., reflex, contraction, and stretch reflex).
3. Motor skills with respect to agility, balance, and coordination.

Task 4:

To demonstrate knowledge of metabolic physiology by applying correct metabolic physiological principles in order to develop safe and effective exercise.

Knowledge of:

1. The fundamentals of metabolic physiology, including anaerobic metabolism (ATP-CP system and glycolysis), oxidative metabolism, and fatty acid oxidation.
2. Aerobic and anaerobic metabolism and the roles of each during various physical activities.
3. The roles of carbohydrates, fats, and proteins as fuel for aerobic and anaerobic exercise.
4. The following definitions: kilocalorie, caloric expenditure, caloric deficit, caloric intake, and energy balance.

Task 5:

To demonstrate knowledge of cardiorespiratory anatomy by identifying correct anatomical structures in order

to develop and instruct safe and effective exercise.

Knowledge of:

1. The basic components of the cardiorespiratory system (e.g., heart, vessels, lungs).
2. The general anatomy of the heart, cardiovascular system, and the cardiorespiratory system.
3. The chambers of the heart.
4. The circulatory pathway through the cardiorespiratory system.
5. The major components of the musculoskeletal system (e.g., bone, muscle, ligaments, tendons).
6. Function of the different joints of the body.
7. The major muscle groups and bones.

Task 6:

To demonstrate competence in the area of basic kinesiology by applying correct kinesiological principles in order to develop and instruct safe and effective exercise.

Knowledge of:

1. The following anatomical and directional terms: anterior, posterior, medial, lateral, dorsal, ventral, plantar, superior, inferior, prone, and supine.
2. The anatomical planes: sagittal, frontal, and transverse.
3. The fundamental movements from the anatomical position (e.g., abduction, adduction, elevation, depression, flexion, dorsiflexion, plantar flexion, and rotation).
4. The types of muscular contractions: isokinetic, isometric, and isotonic (eccentric and concentric).
5. Normal (good) postural alignment and the normal curvature of the back: kyphosis and lordosis.

6. Abnormal curvatures of the back: excessive kyphosis, excessive lordosis, and scoliosis.
7. Differences between agonist, antagonist, and synergist and their opposing muscles.
8. The principle of muscle balance.
9. Healthy back exercises: back range of motion (flexion, extension, and rotation), abdominal strength, pelvic stability, and scapular retraction.
10. The actions and applications of the major muscles: biceps, triceps, deltoids, rectus abdominus, internal and external obliques, transversus, erector spinae, gluteus maximus, gluteus medius, quadriceps, hamstrings, gastrocnemius, soleus, anterior tibialis, posterior tibialis, hip adductors, hip abductors, and iliopsoas.
11. The potential risks associated with certain exercises (e.g., double leg raises, full squats, full neck circles, hurdler's stretch, knee hyperflexion while bearing weight, the plough exercise, and back extension).
12. Factors that affect movement: neurological, proprioceptive, biomechanical, and kinesthetic awareness.

Skill in:

1. Identifying joint type, action, and normal degree of range of motion.
2. Identifying common muscle imbalances and their causes that contribute to abnormal postural alignment.
3. Developing exercises to promote pelvic and scapular stability.
4. Educating participants on proper body mechanics.
5. Designing safe exercises for all major muscle groups.

Task 7:

To demonstrate an understanding of the principles of exercise programming by applying correct training techniques

**in order to develop and instruct safe
and effective exercise.**

Knowledge of:

1. The various components of a conditioning program (e.g., warm-up, cardiorespiratory conditioning, muscular conditioning, and cool-down).
2. The components of an exercise program, including frequency, intensity, duration, mode of activity, and progression.
3. The various methods of determining and monitoring exercise intensity, including target heart rate (THR), Borg's rating of perceived exertion (RPE), and the talk test.
4. The major components of physical fitness, including cardiovascular endurance, muscular endurance, muscular strength, flexibility, and body composition.
5. The current American College of Sports Medicine (ACSM) guidelines for improving and maintaining cardiorespiratory endurance, muscular fitness and flexibility with reference to mode of activity, intensity, duration, and frequency for various levels of fitness.

Task 8:

To demonstrate an understanding of fitness test terminology and results by identifying correct modifications and recommendations in order to develop and instruct safe and effective exercise based upon fitness results.

Knowledge of:

1. The various methods of fitness assessments, including submaximal and maximal aerobic capacity tests, muscular strength and endurance tests, and body composition tests.
2. The rationale for the determination of aerobic capacity, muscular strength and endurance, flexibility, and body composition.

3. How to interpret results from basic field tests: cardiorespiratory endurance, body composition, muscular strength, muscular endurance, and flexibility.
4. The purpose and methods for administering fitness assessments in a group exercise setting.

Task 9:

To demonstrate an understanding of the various physiological and anatomical considerations of special populations by identifying correct modifications and recommendations in order to develop safe and effective exercise.

Knowledge of:

Special Populations: General

1. The benefits of regular exercise for specific conditions such as coronary artery disease, hypertension, diabetes mellitus, musculoskeletal disorders (including rheumatoid arthritis, lower-back problems, and osteoporosis), obesity, and asthma.
2. Modifications necessary for a participant with a medical condition that has been cleared by a physician or appropriate medical personnel.

Special Populations: Older Adults

3. Physiological processes and exercise implications for older adults, including the musculoskeletal, cardiorespiratory, metabolic, and psychosocial systems.
4. Musculoskeletal, cardiovascular, respiratory, and metabolic health concerns common to older adults, including suitable exercise programs.
5. Appropriate motivational reinforcement techniques of older adults.

***Special Populations: Pregnant
and Postpartum Women***

6. The American College of Obstetricians and Gynecologists (ACOG) recommendations

for exercise during pregnancy and the postpartum period, as well as contraindications and warning signs to cease exercise.

7. The risks associated with exercise and pregnancy due to the following: hypoxia, hypothermia, hypoglycemia, and dehydration.

8. Musculoskeletal adaptations due to pregnancy: weight gain, hormonal changes, and postural changes.

Special Populations: Children

9. The special concerns of working with children, including thermoregulation, anaerobic capacity, intensity monitoring, and safety.

10. Musculoskeletal, cardiovascular, respiratory, and metabolic concerns of children involved in exercise programs.

11. Youth fitness testing methods.

12. The importance of program design, including: (1) gradual increase in exercise intensity, (2) improvement in adequate muscular strength and flexibility, (3) proper body mechanics, (4) appropriate clothing and equipment, and (5) short-term intermittent activity.

Skill in:

Special Populations: General

1. Identifying health problems or risk factors that interfere with a participant's ability to exercise safely in class and that may warrant physician referral, such as a recent injury, diabetes, obesity, pregnancy, musculoskeletal problems (including arthritis), hypertension, asthma, and previous difficulty with exercise (including exercise-related chest discomfort, dizzy spells, and extreme breathlessness).

Special Populations: Older Adults

2. Modifying the exercise program in terms of intensity, duration, frequency, and mode.

3. Identifying aging characteristics and exercise implications for the older adult.

4. Designing appropriate exercise programs regarding the aging process and health concerns.

5. Designing effective exercise activities and motivational reinforcement for older adults.

Special Populations: Pregnant and Postpartum Women

6. Designing exercises to accommodate postural changes associated with pregnancy (e.g., lordosis, pelvic widening).

7. Adjusting frequency, duration, intensity, and mode of activity for pregnant women.

8. Monitoring exercise levels during pregnancy using heart rate, RPE, and respiration rate.

9. Modifying muscular training programs with respect to pregnancy-induced musculoskeletal adaptations.

10. Making appropriate modifications necessary to pregnant and postpartum participants accepted in a regular group exercise class.

Task 10:

To demonstrate a basic understanding of various psychological issues by correctly relating them to group exercise program design in order to optimize exercise adherence and the well-being of the participant.

Knowledge of:

1. Motivational techniques used to optimize exercise adherence and other healthy lifestyle behaviors.

2. The issues related to body image.

3. The issues related to self-efficacy and obsessive/compulsive behavior in a group exercise setting.

4. The principles of the learning theory with respect to effective teaching in a group exercise setting.

Task 11:

To demonstrate an understanding of basic nutrition by applying correct nutritional recommendations in order to provide appropriate information to apparently healthy individuals.

Knowledge of:

1. The six categories of nutrients, their functions, and current dietary guidelines according to the U.S. RDA.
2. Special nutritional needs as they apply to osteoporosis and anemia.
3. Nutritional misinformation and misconceptions (e.g., salt tablets and protein powders).
4. Cholesterol, lipoproteins, and triglycerides.
5. Supplements and ergogenic aids (e.g., bee pollen and caffeine).
6. The toxic effects of over-supplementation of vitamins.
7. Hydration with water versus sports drinks.
8. Special dietary needs with respect to referral to a registered dietician.
9. The signs and symptoms of atypical eating behaviors (e.g., anorexia, bulimia, and compulsive overeating).

Skill in:

1. Identifying special dietary needs for the purpose of referral to a registered dietician.

Task 12:

To demonstrate knowledge of environmental physiology by applying correct physiological principles in order to develop safe and effective exercise.

Knowledge of:

1. Concepts from environmental physiology that may affect exercise performance, including heat, humidity, altitude, cold, and pollution.
2. The physiological responses to variations in environmental conditions (e.g., changes in temperature, heart rate, and blood pressure).
3. The physiological adaptations that result from acclimatization.
4. Recommendations and precautions for exercising in heat, humidity, cold, altitude, and pollution.

Task 13:

To demonstrate knowledge of weight management by applying sound nutritional and exercise principles in order to provide appropriate information to apparently healthy individuals.

Knowledge of:

1. Safe and effective weight-loss methods.
2. The number of pounds per week recommended for unsupervised, safe, and effective weight loss.
3. The definition of kilocalories as applied to caloric intake and expenditure.
4. Different protocols of fat weight loss and/or body composition change (e.g., diet and exercise combined, diet alone, etc.).
5. The concepts of energy balance, energy imbalance, and set point theory.
6. Different methods of determining ideal body weight (e.g., height/weight, charts, scale, and body composition).
7. Extreme approaches to weight loss (e.g., fasting, spot reducing, diet pills, and drugs).

Domain II:
Exercise Programming

Task 1:

To determine the content of each class component in order to plan safe and effective group exercise sessions with respect to the objective for the class by adhering to accepted standards of practice.

Knowledge of:

1. The components involved in a group exercise class: warm-up, pre/post-cardiorespiratory conditioning, cardiorespiratory conditioning, cool-down, muscle conditioning, and flexibility exercises/final cool-down.
2. The components of a circuit training class: warm-up, pre/post-cardiorespiratory conditioning, cardiorespiratory/strength training, flexibility exercises, and final cool-down.
3. The components of an aerobic interval training class: warm-up, pre/post-cardiorespiratory conditioning, interval cardiorespiratory/muscular conditioning, cool-down, flexibility exercises, and final cool-down.
4. The major components of a resistance class: warm-up, muscle conditioning, and flexibility/final cool-down.
5. The major components of a stretch class: warm-up and flexibility/final cool-down.

Skill in:

1. Determining the content, combination, and sequence of various types of general group exercise classes.

Task 2:

To demonstrate competence in the design of an exercise class by planning appropriate modifications or adaptations to activities in order to provide safe and effective exercise.

Knowledge of:

1. The physiological effects and appropriate precautions to take with respect to the following substances: beta blockers, diuretics, anti-hypertensives, antihistamines, tranquilizers, alcohol, diet pills, cold medications, caffeine, and nicotine.

2. Modifications and adaptations for participants with medical conditions who have been cleared for exercise by a physician or appropriate medical personnel.
3. Modifications and adaptations for special populations: pregnant and postpartum women, children, and senior citizens.
4. Modifications and adaptations for participants desiring increased exercise intensity.

Skill in:

1. Selecting modifiable exercises for participants with medical conditions who have been cleared for exercise by a physician or appropriate medical personnel.
2. Selecting modifiable exercises for special populations: pregnant and postpartum women, children, and older adults.
3. Selecting modifiable exercises for participants desiring increased exercise intensity.

Task 3:

To accommodate the particular needs of special populations by selecting, modifying, and adapting activities in order to plan a safe and effective exercise class.

Knowledge of:

1. The American College of Obstetricians and Gynecologists (ACOG) guidelines for pregnant and postpartum exercisers.
2. The common musculoskeletal conditions typically associated with older adults.
3. The appropriate modifications for special populations and individuals with medical conditions who have been cleared for exercise by a physician or appropriate medical personnel.

Skill in:

1. The integration of safe and effective exercises for participants with medical conditions and for special populations who have been cleared for exercise by physicians or appropriate medical personnel.

Task 4 :

To establish a safe exercise setting by assessing and appropriately modifying the exercise environment in order to promote comfort and safety for all participants.

Knowledge of:

1. Specific environmental factors as they relate to the safety of the participants in a group exercise class (e.g., air temperature, humidity, exercise surface and area, sound, and altitude).

Skill in:

1. Selecting and/or adapting a safe and effective environment in order to maximize safety for class participants.

Domain III:
Instructional Technique

Task 1:

To demonstrate various methods for monitoring exercise intensity by applying appropriate techniques in class in order to ensure safe and effective participation in exercise.

1. The methods, precautions, and limitations for monitoring exercise intensity: heart rate, talk test, Borg's rating of perceived exertion (RPE), dyspnea scale, and metabolic equivalents (METS).

2. The techniques, precautions, and limitations for monitoring heart rate of the radial, carotid, temporal, and apical sites.

3. The applications, precautions, and limitations in the calculations of target heart range: percent of maximum heart rate method, age-predicted maximum heart rate, measured maximum heart rate.

4. Heart rate responses to exercise: adequate warm-up, aerobic exercise phase,

recovery, abnormal responses, and the effects of medications.

Skill in:

1. Palpating heart rate at the radial, carotid, temporal, and apical sites.

2. Demonstrating correct technique for palpating heart rate at the radial, carotid, temporal, and apical sites.

3. Explaining the talk test, RPE, and dyspnea scale as methods for monitoring exercise intensity.

4. Evaluating intensity monitoring methods and making appropriate adaptations.

5. Modifying group or individual exercise intensity.

6. Identifying signs and symptoms of excessive effort and in making appropriate modifications.

7. Selecting an appropriate intensity monitoring method in order to accommodate the effects of medications on heart rate response.

Task 2:

To demonstrate competence in the modification of incorrect movements by applying appropriate teaching strategies in order to ensure safe and effective exercise.

Knowledge of:

1. The three types of statements used when giving knowledge of results (KR): corrective, value, and neutral.

2. The appropriate uses of the three statements used when giving KR: corrective, value, and neutral.

3. Basic exercise science principles as related to movement: cadence, muscular strength conditioning principles, body mechanics, postural assessment, and intensity precautions.

4. Psychological factors related to feedback and KR.

5. Psychological factors affecting participants with respect to feedback and KR.

Skill in:

1. Recognizing incorrect posture and improper execution.
2. Identifying and using KR and feedback statements.
3. Applying basic kinesiology to the correction of movement.
4. Applying appropriate feedback and KR with respect to the participant.
5. Assessing the effects of muscular imbalances when correcting individual execution.
6. Analyzing posture when correcting individual execution.
7. Analyzing body mechanics when correcting individual execution.
8. Recognizing improper execution.
9. Applying effective instructional techniques for error corrections.
10. Understanding the psychological implications in communicating correction and applying appropriate response.

Task 3:

To select appropriate techniques for modifying and adapting group and individual performance by the application of correct principles of exercise science in order to ensure safe and effective participation.

Knowledge of:

1. The contraindications and resulting adaptations to exercise with respect to musculoskeletal, cardiorespiratory, and metabolic factors affecting exercise for participants who have been cleared by a physician or appropriate medical personnel.
2. The implications and modifications of exercise for older adults, pre- and post-natal women, and children.

3. The risk factors for coronary artery disease.
4. The methods used to accommodate various fitness levels and populations within a class.

Skill in:

1. Incorporating appropriate adaptations for musculoskeletal conditions associated with arthritis, back problems, and osteoporosis.
2. Incorporating adaptations for cardiovascular conditions, including high-risk participants, with respect to isometric muscle contractions, arm positions, resistance training, and exercise intensity and duration.
3. Incorporating adaptations for respiratory conditions associated with chronic obstructive pulmonary disease (COPD), including asthma, bronchitis, and emphysema.
4. Incorporating appropriate adaptations for metabolic concerns associated with hypoglycemia, diabetes, and obesity.
5. Modifying exercises for older adults, children, and pregnant and postpartum participants.
6. Adapting an exercise class to accommodate various fitness levels and populations.
7. Incorporating various fitness levels and populations in the same class.
8. Identifying and assigning intensity modifications for older adults, pregnant and postpartum women, children, and people with medical concerns.

Task 4:

To demonstrate competence in instructional techniques by using correct cueing in order to ensure safe and effective exercise participation.

Knowledge of:

1. The various type and appropriate uses of cues.

2. Voice projection and vocal control.

3. The principles of vocal projection and control necessary for safe and effective verbal cueing.

4. Appropriate volume levels needed to ensure safe and effective cueing.

Skill in:

1. Projecting the voice safely and effectively.

2. Applying basic principles of nonverbal cueing for hearing-impaired participants or participants who do not speak the language of the instructor.

3. Using the voice safely and effectively when cueing.

Task 5:

To demonstrate competence in instructional techniques by applying appropriate teaching methodologies in order to ensure safe and effective exercise participation.

Knowledge of:

1. The principles of exercise instruction.

2. The principles of evaluating performance.

3. The styles of instruction appropriate to the group exercise setting.

4. The nature of the learning process.

5. The domains of learning.

6. The stages of motor learning.

7. The strategies for teaching movement.

8. The strategies for motivating participants.

9. The factors affecting exercise adherence.

Skill in:

1. Designing an exercise class (e.g., goal setting and lesson planning).

2. Selecting appropriate instructional techniques in evaluating performance in the group exercise setting.

3. Using different styles of instruction, such as command, practice, reciprocal, and self-check.

4. Selecting instructional strategies that use the cognitive, affective, and psychomotor domains of learning.

5. Selecting instructional strategies appropriate to the learning level of the participant.

6. Selecting the appropriate instructional strategy for teaching particular exercises.

7. Selecting appropriate instructional strategies to motivate participants to excel.

8. Selecting motivational strategies that affect exercise adherence.

Task 6:

To demonstrate competence in injury prevention by applying the principles of exercise science in order to ensure safe and effective exercise participation.

Knowledge of:

1. Common chronic and acute exercise injuries.

2. The exercise science principles affecting safe and effective exercise.

3. Appropriate exercise selection affecting safe and effective exercise.

4. High-risk exercises.

5. Health concerns that may affect safe exercise performance.

6. Teaching techniques and their effects on safe exercise.

7. Modifications indicated as necessary based on health history and/or fitness assessments.

8. Music volume control as indicated by a decibel meter.

Skill in:

1. Applying exercise science principles for safe and effective exercise (e.g., anatomy, applied kinesiology, body mechanics, effects of muscular imbalances, muscle physiology, and neuromuscular conditioning).

2. Selecting alternatives to contraindicated exercises.

3. Selecting appropriate exercises for safe and effective exercise.

4. Effectively modifying or substituting exercises for participants with health concerns.

5. Applying teaching techniques and their effects on safe exercise (e.g., monitoring exercise intensity, corrective techniques, modifying and adapting, cueing, music considerations, and teaching methodologies).

6. Applying modifications based on health history and/or fitness assessments.

7. Determining appropriate music volume levels in order to avoid hearing damage.

Task 7:

To demonstrate competence in emergency procedures by correct implementation of first aid, cardiopulmonary resuscitation (CPR), and evacuation plans in order to ensure a safe and effective exercise environment.

Knowledge of:

1. When to perform CPR.

2. How and when to activate the EMS system.

3. The signs and symptoms of heat stress syndromes (e.g., heat cramps, heat exhaustion, and heatstroke).

4. Emergency procedures and protocol.

Skill in:

1. Initiating the appropriate first-aid procedures.

Domain IV: Professional Responsibility

Task 1:

To demonstrate an understanding of the various legal issues by applying current legal principles in order to avoid litigation and ensure safe and effective exercise.

Knowledge of:

1. The assumption of risk, including waiver, warning, and informed consent.

2. Liability, including facilities, equipment, supervision, instruction, exercise recommendations, and health screening.

3. Negligence, both contributory and comparative.

4. Copyright law as it applies to music, print media, and film.

5. Scope of practice.

6. Standard of care.

7. Relevant legal terminology.

8. The difference between an independent contractor and an employee.

Skill in:

1. Completing an accident/incident report.

Task 2:

To consistently apply the American Council on Exercise Code of Ethics by exhibiting behavior that is in accordance with this code in order to uphold professional standards.

Knowledge of:

1. The American Council on Exercise Code of Ethics.

2. The American Council on Exercise Professional Practices and Disciplinary Procedures.

3. Appropriate sources for acquiring continuing education offered by individuals, conferences, colleges, universities, seminars, workshops, etc.

4. How to stay current on health and physical activity research.

Task 3:

To demonstrate competence in business issues by application of accepted business standards and practices in

order to maintain or promote the role
of a group exercise instructor.

Knowledge of:

1. Employment practices.
2. Accurate record keeping and incident/accident reporting.
3. Personal and professional objectives.

Task 4:

To demonstrate competence in emergency procedures by implementing first
aid, cardiopulmonary resuscitation, and
evacuation procedures in order to ensure the safety of participants and minimize complications in the event of an
emergency.

Knowledge of:

1. CPR procedures.
2. EMS system activation.

3. The rest, ice, compression, and elevation
(RICE) principle.
4. Contraindications to exercise.
5. The components of a health-screening
instrument.

Task 5:

To demonstrate an understanding of
insurance as it relates to group exercise
instruction by identifying insurance
needs in order to minimize financial risk.

Knowledge of:

1. Professional liability insurance.
2. General liability insurance.
3. Worker's compensation insurance.
4. Health and disability insurance.
5. Business interruption insurance.
6. Property insurance.

Appendix C

Effects of Medications on Heart-rate (HR) Response

Medications	Resting HR	Exercise HR	Maximal Exercising HR	Comments
Beta-adrenergic blocking agents	▼	▼	▼	Dose-related response
Diuretics	↕	↕	↕	
Antihypertensives	▲, ↕ or ▼	▲, ↕ or ▼	usually ↕	Many antihypertensive medications are used. Some may decrease, a few may increase, and others do not affect heart rates. Some exhibit a dose-related response.
Calcium channel blockers	▲, ↕ or ▼	▲, ↕ or ▼	▼ or ↕	Variable & dose-related responses
Antihistamines	↕	↕	↕	
Cold medications: without sympathomimetic activity (SA)	↕	↕	↕	
with sympathomimetic activity (SA)	↕ or ▲	↕ or ▲	↕	
Tranquilizers	↕, or if anxiety-reducing may ▼	↕	↕	
Antidepressants and some antipsychotic medication	↕ or ▲	↕	↕	
Alcohol	↕ or ▲	↕ or ▲	↕	Exercise prohibited while under the influence; effects of alcohol on coordination increase possibility of injuries
Diet pills:				Discourage as a poor approach to weight loss; acceptable only with physician's written approval
with SA	▲ or ↕	▲ or ↕	↕	
containing amphetamines	▲	▲	↕	
without SA or amphetamines	↕	↕	↕	
Caffeine	↕ or ▲	↕ or ▲	↕	
Nicotine	↕ or ▲	↕ or ▲	↕	Discourage smoking; suggest lower target heart rate & exercise intensity for smokers

▲ = increase   ↕ = no significant change   ▼ = decrease

Note: Many medications are prescribed for conditions that do not require clearance. Do not forget other indicators of exercise intensity, e.g., participant's appearance, rating of perceived exertion.

Glossary

Abduction Movement away from the mid-line of the body.

Accent Emphasis on a given beat.

Actin One of the contractile protein filaments in muscles.

Acute injury An injury having a sudden onset, characterized by specific pain and swelling and the inability to use the injured area normally.

Addiction The devotion or surrendering of oneself to something habitually or obsessively.

Adduction Movement toward the midline of the body.

Adenosine diphosphate (ADP) One of the chemical by-products of the breakdown of ATP during muscle contraction.

Adenosine triphosphate (ATP) The immediately usable form of chemical energy needed for all cellular function, including muscular contractions.

Adherence The amount of programmed exercise someone engages in during a specified time period compared to the amount of exercise recommended for that time period.

Adipose tissue *See* Body fat.

Adult-onset diabetes *See* Diabetes mellitus *and* Type 2 diabetes.

Aerobic In the presence of oxygen.

Aerobic fitness *See* Cardiovascular endurance.

Aerobic glycolysis A metabolic pathway that requires oxygen to facilitate the use of glycogen for energy (ATP).

Aerobic power *See* Cardiovascular endurance.

Affective domain One of the three domains of learning; involves the learning of emotional behaviors.

Agonist The muscle directly responsible for observed movement; also called the prime mover.

Alveoli The small membranous air sacs located at the terminal ends of bronchioles where oxygen and carbon dioxide are exchanged between the blood and air in the lungs.

Amenorrhea The condition of having two or fewer menstrual periods per year.

American Society of Composers, Authors, and Publishers One of two performing rights societies in the United States that represent music publishers in negotiating and collecting fees for the non-dramatic performance of music.

Americans with Disabilities Act Civil rights legislation designed to improve access to jobs, work places, and commercial spaces for people with disabilities.

Amino acid The simplest component of dietary protein.

Anaerobic Without the presence of oxygen.

Anaerobic glycolysis A metabolic pathway that does not require oxygen, the purpose of which is to transfer the bond energy contained in glucose (or glycogen) to the formation of ATP.

Anatomical position Standing erect with the feet and palms facing forward.

Anemia A disorder caused by a low hemoglobin content in the blood, which reduces the amount of oxygen available to the body's tissues; symptoms include fatigue, breathlessness after exercise, giddiness, and loss of appetite.

Anaerobic threshold (AT) The point at which exercise intensity can no longer meet the metabolic demands of the muscles aerobically and the muscles have to rely on anaerobic metabolism for ATP.

Anorexia nervosa An eating disorder characterized by self-starvation, distorted body image, and an intense fear of becoming obese.

Antagonist The muscle that acts in opposition to the action of the agonist muscle.

Anthropometric assessment The measurement of the human body and its parts most commonly measured using skinfolds, girth measurements, and body weight.

Antioxidants Chemicals that protect membranes, lipid rich organelles, and lipoproteins (like LDL cholesterol) from being attacked by destructive agents knows as free radicals; include vitamins C and E, betacarotene, and selenium.

Aorta The main artery exiting the left ventricle of the heart.

Apical pulse A pulse point located at the apex of the heart.

Apparently healthy A term to describe participants who have no known diseases, no disease symptoms, and two or fewer cardiovascular disease risk factors.

Applied force An external force acting on a system (body or body segment).

Arrythmias Abnormal heart rhythms.

Arteries Blood vessels that carry oxygenated blood away from the heart to vital organs and the extremities.

Arterioles Smaller divisions of arteries.
Arthritis Inflammatory condition involving a joint. See also Osteoarthritis and Rheumatoid arthritis.

Articulation The point of contact or connection between bones or between bones and cartilage; also called a joint.

Associative stage of learning The second stage of learning a motor skill when performers have mastered the fundamentals and can concentrate on skill refinement.

Assumption of risk A defense used to show that a person has voluntarily accepted known dangers by participating in a specific activity.

Asthma An obstructive pulmonary disease caused by constriction of the breathing passages.

Atria The two upper chambers of the heart (right and left atrium).

Atrophy A reduction in muscle size (muscle wasting) due to inactivity or immobilization.

Autonomous stage of learning The third stage of learning a motor skill when the skill has become habitual or automatic for the performer.

Axial skeleton The bones of the head, neck, and trunk.

Ballistic stretching Dynamic stretching characterized by rhythmic bobbing or bouncing motions representing relatively high-force, short-duration movements.

Basal metabolic rate (BMR) The energy required to complete the sum total of life-sustaining processes, including ion transport (40% BMR), protein synthesis (20% BMR), and daily functioning such as breathing, circulation, and nutrient processing (40% BMR).

Beats Regular pulsations that have an even rhythm and occur in a continuous pattern of strong and weak pulsations.

Beta adrenergic agent Medications used for cardiovascular and other medical conditions that block or limit sympathetic nervous system stimulation; commonly called "beta blockers."

Beta oxidation *See* Fatty acid oxidation.

Binge eating disorder Characterized by frequent binge eating (without purging) and feelings of being out of control when eating.

Bioelectrical impedance A non-invasive body-composition assessment method measuring electrical current flow through the body.

Biomechanical balance Balancing the musculoskeletal stress of various movements.

Blanket license A certificate or document granting permission that varies and applies to a number of situations.

Blood pressure The driving force that pushes blood through the circulator system; the pressure exerted by the blood on the walls of the arteries, measured in millimeters of mercury.

Body composition The makeup of the body considered as a two-component model: lean body mass and fat mass.

Body fat A component of the body, the primary role of which is to store energy for later use.

Body mass index (BMI) A relative measure of body height to body weight to determine degree of obesity.

Broad ligament The ligament that extends from the lateral side of the uterus to the pelvic wall; keeps the uterus centrally placed while providing stability within the pelvic cavity.

Broadcast Music, Inc. One of two performing rights societies in the U.S. that represent music publishers in negotiating and collecting fees for the non-dramatic performance of music.

Bronchial tree Name given to describe the continuous branching of the trachea into the bronchi and bronchioles of the lungs.

Bronchioles The smallest tubes that supply air to the alveoli in the lungs.

Bronchitis An obstructive pulmonary disease caused by inflammation of the mucus membranes and bronchial tubes in the lungs.

Bulimia nervosa An eating disorder characterized by binge eating followed by self-induced vomiting, fasting, or the use of diuretics or laxatives.

Burnout A state of emotional exhaustion caused by stress from work or responsibilities.

Caffeine A relatively harmless and naturally occurring central nervous system stimulant that can be found in about 63 different species of plants (notably coffee and cocoa beans, cola nuts, and tea leaves) and any products made from those plants.

Calcium The most abundant mineral in the body; involved in the conduction of nerve impulses, heart function, muscle contraction, and the operation of certain enzymes; an inadequate supply of calcium contributes to osteoporosis.

Calorie (note capital C) *See* Kilocalorie.

calorie (note lowercase c) The amount of heat necessary to raise the temperature of 1 gram of water 1 degree Celsius; often used incorrectly in place of kilocalorie. (1 kilocalorie = 1000 calories).

Cancer Uncontrolled multiplication of certain cells of the body, which can lead to death in the host.

Capacity The total amount of energy produced.

Capillaries The smallest divisions from arterioles and leading to venuoles; site of exchange of nutrients and metabolic waste products.

Carbohydrate A primary foodstuff used for energy; dietary sources include sugars (simple) and grains, rice, potatoes, and beans (complex). Carbohydrate is stored as glycogen in the muscles and liver and is transported in the blood as glucose.

Cardiac output The amount (quantity) of blood pumped from the heart per minute.

Cardiorespiratory endurance *See* Cardiovascular endurance.

Cardiorespiratory fitness (CRF) The ability to perform large muscle movement over a sustained period; related to the capacity of the heart-lung system to deliver oxygen for sustained energy production. Also called cardiorespiratory endurance or aerobic fitness.

Cardiorespiratory segment The portion of a group exercise class designed for improving cardiorespiratory endurance and body composition and keeping the heart rate elevated for a sustained time period.

Cardiovascular disease (CVD) General term for any disease of the heart.

Cardiovascular endurance The capacity of the heart, blood vessels, and lungs to deliver oxygen and nutrients to the working muscles and tissues during sustained exercise and to remove metabolic waste products that would result in fatigue.

Carotid pulse A pulse point located on the carotid artery in the neck about 1 inch below the jaw line, next to the esophagus.

Cartilage A smooth, semi-opaque material that absorbs shock and reduces friction between the bones of a joint.

Central nervous system (CNS) The brain and spinal cord.

Cerebral palsy An injury to the brain before, during, or after birth, resulting in spasticity (tight muscles) making smooth, fluid movement difficult.

Cervical vertebrae The seven vertebral bones of the neck.

Cholesterol A fatty substance found in blood and body tissues and in certain foods (it is absorbed relatively intact in the diet). In the body it is produced by the liver and is a basic unit for many cells and hormones in the body.

Chondromalacia A gradual softening and degeneration of the articular cartilage, usually involving the back surface of the patella (kneecap). This condition may produce pain and swelling or a grinding sound or sensation when the knee is flexed and extended.

Chronic bronchitis Characterized by increased mucus secretion and a productive cough lasting several months to several years.

Chronic obstructive pulmonary diseases (COPD) Term for a spectrum of airway disorders including asthma, bronchitis, and emphysema.

Circumduction A biplanar movement involving the sequential combination of flexion, abduction, extension, and adduction.

Class objectives Specific objectives for each class meeting, clarifying what the instructor expects the participants to accomplish during each exercise session; objectives help instructors focus on the purpose of each selected exercise and activity.

Coccyx The four small vertebral bones making up the "tailbone."

Cognitive domain One of the three domains of learning; describes intellectual activities and involves the learning of knowledge.

Cognitive stage of learning The first stage of learning a motor skill when performers make many gross errors and have extremely variable performances.

Collagen The main constituent of connective tissue, such as ligaments, tendons, and muscles.

Combinations Two or more movement patterns combined and repeated in sequence several times in a row.

Command style of teaching A teaching style in which the instructor makes all decisions about rhythm, posture, and duration while participants follow the instructor's directions and movements.

Compilations Original, copyrightable sequences or a program of dance steps or exercise routines that may or may not be copyrightable in themselves.

Complex carbohydrates Starch and dietary fibers made up of longer chains of carbohydrate molecules.

Concentric A type of isotonic muscle contraction where the muscle develops tension and shortens when stimulated.

Congenital Born with (i.e., a condition).

Connective tissue The tissue that binds together and supports various structures of the body. Ligaments and tendons are connective tissues.

Contract An agreement or promise between two or more parties that creates a legal obligation to do or not to do something.

Contractile proteins The protein myofilaments that are essential for muscle contraction.

Contraindication Any condition that renders some particular movement, activity, or treatment improper or undesirable.

Copyright The exclusive right, for a certain number of years, to perform, make, and distribute copies and otherwise use an artistic, musical, or literary work.

Creatine phosphate (CP) A high-energy phosphate compound found within muscle cells, used to resynthesize ATP for immediate muscle contraction.

Cueing Visual or verbal techniques, using hand signals or minimal words, to inform participants of upcoming movements.

Defendant The party in a lawsuit who is being sued or accused.

Dehydration The condition resulting from excessive loss of body fluids.

Delayed onset muscle soreness (DOMS) Soreness that occurs 24 to 48 hours after strenuous exercise, the exact cause of which is unknown.

Dependence The condition of being influenced or controlled by something else.

Depression The action of lowering a muscle or bone.

Diabetes mellitus A metabolic disorder where the body cannot control blood glucose level by either a total or partial lack of the hormone insulin resulting in an inability to metabolize carbohydrates.

Diaphragmatic breathing A deep, relaxing breathing technique that helps COPD patients improve their breathing capacity.

Diaphysis The shaft of a long bone.

Diastasis recti The separation of the recti abdominal muscles along the midline of the body.

Diastolic blood pressure The pressure in the arteries during the relaxation phase (diastole) of the cardiac cycle.

Dietary Fiber *See* Fiber.

Dietary-induced thermogenesis The thermic (heat producing) effect of food; energy spent on digesting and absorbing food, approximately 10% of all energy expenditure.

Disability insurance Insurance that provides income protection in the event of an injury to the instructor.

Disaccharides Double sugar units called sucrose, lactose, and maltose.

Distal Farthest from the midline of the body, or from the point of attachment of a body part.

DNA adducts A cancer-promoting condition that occurs when a molecule bonds to DNA, which can cause a cellular mutation.

Dorsiflexion Movement of the foot up toward the shin.

Dowager's hump An exaggerated outward curve of the thoracic spine, often associated with vertebral fractures and osteoporosis.

Downbeat The regular strong pulsation in music occurring in a continuous pattern at an even rhythm.

Duration The length of time of an exercise session.

Dynamic stretching *See* Ballistic stretching.

Dyspnea Difficult or labored breathing.

Eating disorders Disturbed eating behavior that jeopardizes a person's physical or psychological health.

Eccentric A type of isotonic muscle contraction where the muscle lengthens against a resistance when it is stimulated; sometimes called "negative work."

Echocardiography A sensitive test to identify heart defects.

Electrocardiogram (EKG or ECG) A recording of the electrical activity of the heart.

Elevation The action of raising a muscle or bone.

Emphysema An obstructive pulmonary disease characterized by the gradual destruction of lung alveoli and the surrounding connective tissue, in addition to airway inflammation, leading to reduced ability to inhale and exhale.

Endomysium The thin layer of connective tissue covering each individual muscle fiber in skeletal muscle.

Endosteum A soft tissue lining the internal surface of the diaphysis on a long bone.

Energy The potential to perform work or activity.

Energy deficit Burning more calories than one is consuming, which promotes weight loss.

Epimysium The layer of connective tissue that entirely surrounds skeletal muscles, which thickens into tendons at either end of the muscle.

Epiphyses The ends of a long bone, usually wider than the shaft (singular: Epiphysis).

Ergogenic aid An energy-enhancing substance thought to improve athletic performance.

Essential body fat Fat thought to be necessary for maintenance of life and reproductive function.

Essential fatty acids Fat that cannot be produced by the body and must be supplied by the diet. Linoleic acid is the only essential fatty acid.

Estrogen Hormones produced by the ovary.

Eversion Rotation of the foot to direct the plantar surface outward.

Excess post exercise oxygen consumption (EPOC) *See* Oxygen debt.

Exercise evaluation A process of evaluating an exercise based on its effectiveness and safety.

Exercise-induced asthma (EIA) Over 80% of all asthmatics experience asthma during exercise. EIA is probably caused by the cooling and then drying of the respiratory tract that accompanies the inspiration of large volumes of dry air during exercise.

Exercise intensity The specific level of physical activity at which a person exercises that can be quantified (e.g., heart rate, work, RPE); usually reflected as a percentage of one's maximal capacity to do work.

Exercise physiology The study of how the body functions during physical activity and exercise.

Exercise specificity *See* Specificity.

Extension An increase in the angle between the anterior surfaces of articulating bones.

External rotation Outward turning about the vertical axis of bone.

Fast twitch (FT) fiber A muscle fiber type specialized for anaerobic metabolism, recruited for rapid, powerful movements such as jumping, throwing, and sprinting.

Fat-soluble vitamins Vitamins which, when consumed, are stored in the body (particularly the liver and fat tissues); includes vitamins A, D, E, and K.

Fatty acid The simplest component of dietary fat, important for the production of energy during low-intensity exercise.

Fatty acid oxidation A metabolic pathway involving the breakdown of fatty acids (digested dietary fat) for the production of ATP.

Feedback An internal response within a learner; during information processing, it is the correctness or incorrectness of a response that is stored in memory to be used for future reference.

Fetus The developed embryo and growing human in the uterus, from usually three months after conception to birth.

Fiber Carbohydrate chains the body cannot break down for use and which pass through the body undigested.

Field tests Fitness tests that can be used in mass testing situations.

Flexibility The ability to move joints through their normal full range of motion.

Flexion A decrease in the angle between the anterior surfaces of articulating bones.

Food Guide Pyramid A guide to assist the public with daily food choices that will accomplish dietary goals. Published in 1992 by the U.S. Department of Agriculture and the U.S. Department of Health & Human Services.

Force A push or a pull, which causes or tends to cause a change in a body's motion or shape.

Fracture Any break in the continuity of a bone, ranging from a simple crack to a severe shatter of the bone with multiple fracture fragments.

Freestyle choreography A way of designing the cardiovascular segment of a class that uses movements randomly chosen by the instructor.

Frequency The number of exercise sessions per week resulting in a training effect.

Frontal plane A plane that divides the body into front (anterior) and back (posterior) halves.

Functional capacity The maximum physical performance represented by maximal oxygen consumption.

General liability insurance Insurance for bodily injury or property damage resulting from general negligence such as wet flooring, an icy sidewalk, or poorly maintained equipment.

Glucometer A devise used by diabetics to check blood sugar.

Glucose A simple sugar; the simplest form of carbohydrate used by the body to produce energy (ATP).

Glycemic index A measurement of the impact on blood glucose levels after ingestion of carbohydrates.

Glycogen The storage form of glucose found in the liver and muscles.

Glycolysis Breakdown of glucose, or its storage form glycogen.

Golgi tendon organ (GTO) A sensory organ within a tendon that, when stimulated, causes an inhibition of the entire muscle group to protect against too much force.

Graded exercise test A physician-supervised diagnostic examination to assess a participant's physiological response to exercise in a controlled environment.

Health screening A vital process that identifies individuals at high risk for exercise-induced heart problems that need to be referred to appropriate medical care as needed.

Heart rate (HR) The number of heart beats per minute.

Heart rate reserve The result of subtracting the resting heart rate from the maximal heart rate; represents the working heart-rate range between rest and maximal heart rate within which all activity occurs.

Heat index Guidelines regarding when exercise can be safely undertaken or when it should be avoided based on measures of heat and humidity.

Hemoconcentration An increase in the number of red blood cells as a result of a decrease in the volume of plasma.

Hemoglobin (Hb) A protein molecule in red blood cells specifically adapted to carry oxygen molecules.

Hemorrhagic stroke Disruption of blood flow to the brain caused by the presence of a blood clot or hematoma.

Heterocyclic amines Compounds that increase cancer risk, created by charbroiling and grilling foods.

High density lipoprotein (HDL cholesterol) Cholesterol that helps move body lipids from places of storage to places of use; referred to as "good" cholesterol.

Homocysteine A normal by-product of metabolism that can promote development of heart disease.

Hydration The chemical combination of a substance with water.

Hydrogenation A process by which liquid fats are turned into solids.

Hydrostatic weighing An underwater test that measures the percentage of lean body weight and body fat, based on the principle that fat floats and muscle and bone sink; considered the gold standard of body composition assessment due to its accuracy.

Hyperextension Extension of an articulation beyond anatomical position.

Hyperglycemia An abnormally high content of sugar in the blood.

Hypertension High blood pressure.

Hyperthermia A life threatening increase in core body temperature.

Hypertrophic cardiomyopathy A congenital heart defect involving a thickening of the heart muscle.

Hypertrophy An increase in the size of individual muscle cells.

Hypoglycemia A blood sugar deficiency caused by too little glucose, too much insulin, or too much exercise in the insulin dependent diabetic.

Hypoxia Decrease in the amount of oxygen in inspired air that usually occurs at high altitudes.

Inclusion style of teaching A teaching style that enables multiple levels of performance to be taught within the same activity.

Incontinence The loss of sphincter control that results in the inability to retain urine, semen, or feces.

Independent contractors People who conduct business on their own on a contract basis and are not employees of an organization.

Individual medical insurance Insurance that provides hospitalization and major medical coverage.

Inferior Located below.

Informed consent A written statement signed by a client prior to testing that informs them of testing purposes, processes, and all potential risks and discomforts.

Inguinal ligament The ligament that extends from the anterior, superior, iliac spine to the pubic tubercle.

Insoluble fiber Fiber that does not bind with water, fluids, or cholesterol, accelerating the passage of foods through the body while slowing the digestive processes (includes cellulose, hemicellulose, and lignins found in wheat bran, vegetables, and whole-grain breads/cereals).

Insulin A hormone secreted into the bloodstream by the pancreas that regulates carbohydrate metabolism.

Insulin reaction The result of hypoglycemia, not enough sugar in the blood, in which diabetics experience symptoms such as anxiety, confusion, and irritability; if unchecked may lead to insulin shock.

Insulin shock The condition produced when there is excessive insulin present in the bloodstream, causing rapid pulse, dizziness or headache, disorientation, and fainting with possible unconsciousness.

Intensity Physiological stress on the body during exercise; indicates how hard the body should work to achieve a training effect.

Internal fat Fat stored deep inside the body.

Internal rotation Inward turning about the vertical axis of bone.

Interval training Exercising at high-intensity levels for brief periods (10 seconds to 5 minutes) with intervening rest or relief periods at a lower intensity to allow heart rate to decline.

Inversion Rotation of the foot to direct the plantar surface inward.

Iron deficiency anemia A nutritional deficiency characterized by a lack of hemoglobin or poorly formed red blood cells.

Ischemia Lack of blood flow to the heart muscle.

Ischemic stroke A sudden disruption of cerebral circulation in which blood supply to the brain is either interrupted or diminished.

Isokinetic A type of muscular contraction where tension developed within the muscle changes throughout the range of motion; performed with the use of special equipment; also referred to as "variable resistance" exercise.

Isometric A type of muscular contraction where the muscle is stimulated to generate tension but no joint movement occurs.

Isotonic A type of muscular contraction where the muscle is stimulated to develop tension and joint movement occurs.

kcal *See* Kilocarie.

Kegel exercises Controlled isometric contraction and relaxation of the muscles surrounding the vagina to tone and gain control of the pelvic floor muscles.

Kilocalorie (kcal) The term to express energy intake and expenditure in nutrition and exercise. A calorie is a unit of energy, specifically the amount of heat needed to increase the temperature of 1kg of water 1°C; one kcal equals 1,000 calories.

Kinesiology The study of the principles of mechanics and anatomy in relation to human movement.

Kinesthetic awareness (Kinethesis) The perception of body position and movement in space.

Kyphosis Excessive posterior curvature of the spine, typically seen in the thoracic region.

Lactic acid (LA) A byproduct of anaerobic glycolysis thought to cause localized muscle fatigue associated with very high-intensity exercise.

Lateral Away from the midline of the body, or the outside.

Lateral flexion Bending of the vertebral column to the side.

Law of acceleration Newton's second law of motion stating that the force acting on a body in a given direction is equal to the body's mass times its acceleration in that direction.

Law of inertia Newton's first law of motion stating that a body at rest will stay at rest and a body in motion will stay in motion unless acted upon by an external force.

Law of reaction Newton's third law of motion stating that for every applied force there is an equal and opposite reactive force.

Lean body mass The components of the body including muscles, bones, nervous tissue, skin, blood, and organs.

Lecithin A type of fat called phospholipid manufactured by the body and having both a water-soluble and fat-soluble portion.

Lever A rigid bar that rotates around a fixed support (fulcrum) in response to an applied force.

Liability Legal responsibility.

Ligament Strong, fibrous tissue that connects one bone to another.

Linear progression Consists of one movement that transitions into another without cycling sequences.

Linoleic acid The only essential fatty acid; *See also* Essential fatty acids.

Lipids The name for fats used in the body and blood stream.

Lipoproteins A complex of lipid and protein molecules, which transport cholesterol and other lipids throughout the body.

Lordosis Excessive anterior curvature of the spine that typically occurs at the low back (may also occur at the neck).

Low back pain (LBP) A general term to describe a multitude of back conditions, including muscular and ligament strains, sprains, and injuries. The cause of LBP is often elusive; most LBP is probably caused by muscle weakness and imbalances.

Low-density lipoprotein (LDL cholesterol) Cholesterol involved in the artery-blocking process; referred to as the "bad" cholesterol.

Lumbar vertebrae The five vertebrae in the low back, just below the thoracic vertebrae and just above the sacrum.

Macronutrients The main contributors to energy intake in the diet; carbohydrate, protein, and fat.

Maximal heart rate The highest heart rate a person can attain.

Maximal heart rate formula A formula for determining target heart rate based on a percentage of the maximal heart rate.

Maximal oxygen uptake ($\dot{V}O_2$ max) The point at which the body's ability to take in oxygen from the atmosphere via the pulmonary system, transport it via the cardiovascular system, and utilize it via the muscular system reaches a point of little or no change with an additional workload; a direct measure of cardiorespiratory endurance.

Measure One group of beats in a musical composition marked by the regular occurrence of the heavy accent.

Medial Toward the midline of the body, or the inside.

Megadoses Large levels of intake of vitamins and minerals, possibly dangerous to health.

Meter The organization of beats into musical patterns or measures.

Micronutrients Special chemicals needed in minute amounts; found widely in foods; vitamins and minerals.

Minerals Inorganic (non carbon-containing) compounds the body requires that must be provided in the diet.

Mitochondria A highly specialized structure within cells where aerobic glycolysis takes place for energy production; sometimes called the "powerhouse" of the cell.

Mobility The degree to which an articulation is allowed to move before being restricted by surrounding tissues.

Monosaccharides Single sugar units called glucose, fructose and galactose.

Monounsaturated fat A type of unsaturated fat (liquid at room temperature) that has one spot on the fatty acid for the addition of a hydrogen atom (e.g., oleic acid in olive oil).

Motor domain One of the three domains of learning; involves the learning of motor skills.

Motor end plate The location of the synapse of a motor neuron and muscle cell; also called the neuromuscular junction.

Motor neurons Nerve cells that conduct impulses from the CNS to the periphery signaling muscles to contract or relax, regulating muscular movement.

Motor skill The degree to which movements using agility, balance, and coordination are executed.

Motor unit A motor nerve and all the muscle fibers it stimulate.

Multiple sclerosis A common neuromuscular disorder involving the progressive degeneration of muscle function, including increased muscle spasticity.

Muscle spindle The sensory organ within a muscle that is sensitive to stretch and thus protects the muscle against too much stretch.

Muscular endurance The ability of a muscle or muscle group to exert force against a resistance over a sustained period of time.

Muscular strength The maximal force a muscle or muscle group can exert during contraction.

Myofibrils Thread-like protein strands composing individual muscle cells.

Myofilaments Collective term for the contractile proteins of a muscle fiber, actin and myosin.

Myosin Contractile protein in a myofibril.

Near-infrared (NIR) light interactance A body-composition assessment technique that analyzes the amount of near-infrared light reflected from the biceps based on the principle that body fat absorbs light while lean body mass reflects light.

Negligence Failure of a person to perform as a reasonable and prudent professional would perform under similar circumstances.

Neuron The basic anatomical unit of the nervous system; the nerve cell.

Neuropathy A chronic disease linked to diabetes involving diminished sensations in distal extremities (peripheral neuropathy) or altered heart rate (autonomic neuropathy).

Neutral spine position The balance of vertebrae in the three naturally occurring curves: two slight anterior curves at the neck and low back and one slight posterior curve in the thoracic region.

Nitrates/Nitrites Preservatives used in certain foods (hot dogs, lunch meats) that are converted to carcinogenic nitrosamines, which may increase risk for stomach cancers.

Nitrosamines Carcinogenic compounds converted from nitrate/nitrite preservatives in the stomach.

Nutrients Components of food needed by the body. There are six classes of nutrients: water, minerals, vitamins, protein, carbohydrates, and fats.

Nutrition The study of nutrients in foods and of their digestion, absorption, metabolism, interaction, storage, and excretion.

Obesity Excessive storage of body fat, defined as at least 20% above ideal weight; typically more than 30% body fat for women and more than 23% body fat for men.

Omega-3 fatty acids Fats (found in cold water fish) that can lower blood cholesterol, help prevent blood clots, and may lower high blood pressure.

Osteoarthritis A degenerative bone disease involving a wearing away of joint cartilage.

Osteoporosis A condition in which bones weaken and soften due to progressive loss of calcium.

Overload The principle that a physiological system subjected to above-normal stress will respond by increasing in strength or function accordingly.

Overweight A term to describe an excessive amount of weight for a given height, using height-to-weight ratios.

Oxidative enzymes Enzymes that initiate fat metabolism by breaking down free fatty acids into Aceytl CoA.

Oxidative glycolysis *See* Aerobic glycolysis.

Oxygen consumption ($\dot{V}O_2$) The process by which oxygen is used to produce energy for cellular work; also called oxygen uptake.

Oxygen debt The temporary elevation of oxygen consumption levels upon cessation of exercise to "pay back" the oxygen deficit created at exercise onset.

Oxygen deficit A situation created at exercise onset when actual oxygen consumption does not immediately meet the physiological requirement for oxygen.

Oxygen uptake *See* Oxygen consumption.

Oxylates Substances that bind and decrease calcium absorption in the body.

Part-to-whole teaching strategy A teaching strategy involving breaking a skill down into its component parts and practicing each skill in its simplest form before placing several skills in a sequence.

Partial pressure The pressure of each gas in a multiple gas system, such as air, which is composed of nitrogen, oxygen, and CO_2.

Peak flow meter A device used to measure the flow of air through the lungs; useful for COPD patients to aid in activity selection.

Pelvic floor The muscles and tissues that act as a support or reinforcement to the lower border of the pelvis.

Performing rights society An organization to which the copyright or publisher assigns the non-dramatic performing rights in a musical composition.

Perineal The fibromuscular tissue located between the lower part of the vagina and the anal canal.

Periosteum A connective tissue sheath surrounding the outer surface of the diaphysis of a long bone.

Phosphocreatine *See* Creatine phosphate.

Phosphagens Adenosine triphosphate (ATP) and creatine phosphate (CP), two high-energy phosphate molecules that can be broken down for immediate use by the cells.

Phospholipid A fatty substance that has a fat-soluble end and a water-soluble end; an essential part of cell membranes that does not supply calories.

Photosynthesis Process by which plants turn radiant energy (sunlight) into chemical energy.

Phrase Two or more measures of music.

Physical activity Daily movement through either planned activity (exercise) or daily living activities; the most variable component of total energy expenditure at 10% – 30%.

Physical Activity Readiness Questionnaire (PAR-Q) A brief, self-administered medical questionnaire recognized as a safe pre-exercise screening measure for low-to-moderate (but not vigorous) exercise training.

Physical fitness The physical components of well-being that enable a person to function at an optimal level.

Physiological balance The balance of movement intensity (when sequencing moves) combined with movement selection based on the duration of the class.

Phytate A non-nutrient component of plant seeds that binds with minerals, forming insoluble complexes that the body excretes unused.

Phytochemicals Biologically active compounds in plants thought to have anti-cancer and anti-heart disease properties when consumed as part of a healthy diet.

Placenta The vascular organ in mammals that unites the fetus to the maternal uterus and mediates its metabolic exchanges.

Plaintiff A party who brings a suit against another party in a court of law.

Plantar fasciitis Inflammation of the plantar fascia, a broad band of connective tissue running along the sole of the foot; caused by stretching or tearing the tissue, usually near the attachment at the heel.

Plantar flexion Distal movement of the plantar surface of the foot; opposite of dorsiflexion.

Plasma The liquid portion of the blood.

Plyometrics High-intensity movements, such as jumping, involving high-force loading of body weight on the landing phase of the movement.

Polycyclic aromatic hydrocarbons Compounds that increase cancer risk, created by char-broiling and grilling foods.

Polyunsaturated fat A type of unsaturated fat (liquid at room temperature) that has two or more spots on the fatty acid available for hydrogen (e.g., corn, safflower, soybean oils).

Posterior Toward the back or dorsal side.

Postpartum The period of time after childbirth.

Practice style of teaching A teaching style that provides opportunities for individualization and includes practice time and individualized instructor feedback.

Pre-class preparation Methods or principles for successful group exercise instruction, including professional attributes such as knowing participants' health histories, being available to orient new participants before class, and having music/equipment cued and ready to go before class begins.

Preparticipation (pre-exercise) screening The process of determining someone's health and fitness status before beginning an exercise program.

Primary bronchi The two main branches of the trachea or windpipe.

Prime mover A muscle responsible for a specific movement.

Professional liability insurance Insurance to protect an instructor against professional negligence or failure to perform as a competent and prudent professional would under similar circumstances.

Progesterone Hormone produced by the corpus luteum, adrenal cortex, and placenta, the function of which is to facilitate growth of the embryo.

Prognosis Assessment of progress toward recovery from an accident or condition.

Program goals Goals established by the instructor to aid participants in developing personal fitness goals, reflecting what the instructor expects students to gain from participation in the group exercise program.

Pronation Internal rotation of the forearm causing the radius to cross diagonally over the ulna and the palm to face posteriorly.

Proprioception The reception of stimuli produced within the body.

Proprioceptive neuromuscular facilitation (PNF) A stretching technique involving statically stretching a muscle immediately after maximally contracting it against resistance.

Proprioceptors Somatic sensory receptors in muscles, tendons, ligaments, joint capsules, and skin that gather information about body position and the direction and velocity of movement.

Protein Compound composed of amino acids that is the major structural component of all body tissue; complete protein is protein containing all nine amino acids essential to health.

Proximal Nearest to the midline of the body or point of attachment of a body part.

Psychological balance Balancing movement complexity with simplicity to avoid compromising form, technique, and safety, and to limit participant frustration.

Public performance Playing a recording of a copyrighted musical composition at a place where a substantial number of persons outside of a normal circle of a family and its social acquaintances are gathered.

Publisher The entity to which the owner of a copyrighted artistic, musical, or literary work assigns such copyright for licensing and income collection purposes.

Pulse rate The wave of pressure in the arteries that occurs each time the heart beats.

Radial Pulse A pulse point located on the thumb side of the wrist.

Range of motion (ROM) The number of degrees that an articulation will allow one of its segments to move.

Rating of perceived exertion (RPE) A scale that correlates the participants' perceptions of exercise effort with actual intensity level.

Receptor Nerve tissue that is sensitive to changes in its environment.

Reciprocal style of teaching Teaching style that involves using an observer or partner to provide feedback to the performer.

Recommended daily allowances (RDA) The amounts of selected nutrients that adequately meet the known nutrient needs of most healthy Americans.

Recovery heart rate The number of heartbeats per minute following the cessation of vigorous physical activity. As cardiorespiratory fitness improves, the heart rate returns to resting levels more quickly.

Relaxin A hormone of pregnancy that softens connective tissue.

Repetition reduction teaching strategy Teaching strategy involving reducing the number of repetitions that make up a movement sequence.

Repetitions The number of successive contractions performed during each weight-training exercise.

Respiration The exchange of oxygen and carbon dioxide between the cells and the atmosphere.

Respiratory ventilation The movement of air into and out of the lungs.

Resting heart rate The number of heartbeats per minute when the body is at complete rest; usually counted first thing in the morning before any physical activity.

Reversibility principle The training principle explaining that training adaptations will gradually decline if not reinforced by a "maintenance" program.

Rheumatoid arthritis A chronic disease caused by an immune response leading to inflammation of the joint membrane.

Rhythm A regular pattern of movement of sound that can be felt, heard, or seen.

RICE An immediate treatment for injury: rest, ice, compression, and elevation.

Risk factor A characteristic, inherited trait or behavior related to the presence or development of condition or disease.

Risk management Minimizing the risks of potential legal liability.

Risk stratification The classification of participants into risk strata to identify the need for referral to a healthcare provider, to ensure safety of exercise testing and participation, and to determine the appropriate type of exercise test or program.

Rotation Movement in the transverse plane about a longitudinal axis; can be "internal" or "external."

Round ligament Ligaments found on the side of the uterus near the fallopian tube insertion to help the broad ligament keep the uterus in place.

Sagittal plane A plane that divides the body into right and left halves.

Sarcomere The basic functional unit of the myofibril containing the contractile proteins that generate skeletal muscle movements.

Saturated fats Fatty acids carrying the maximum number of hydrogen atoms; these fats are solid at room temperature and are usually of animal origin.

Scapulohumeral rhythm Combined action of scapular and humeral movement.

Scapulothoracic articulation The articulation of the scapula with the thorax beneath it.

Sciatica Severe pain in the leg running from the back of the thigh down the inside of the leg as a result of the compression of, or trauma to, the sciatic nerve.

Scoliosis Excessive lateral curvature of the spine.

Scope of practice The range and limit of responsibilities normally associated with a specific job or position.

Self-check style of teaching A teaching style that relies on individual performers to provide their own feedback.

Sensory neurons Nerve cells that convey electrical impulses from sensory organs in the periphery (such as the skin) to the spinal cord and brain (CNS).

Serum lipids Lipids found circulating in the blood.

Shin splints A general term for any pain or discomfort on the front or side of the lower leg in the region of the shin bone (tibia); a common, chronic aerobics injury with several causes.

Shoulder joint complex The three segments of the shoulder: the scapula, clavicle, and humerus.

Simple carbohydrates Single sugars (monosaccharides) and double sugars (disaccharides).

Simple-to-complex teaching strategy Advanced teaching strategy that treats a sequence of movement patterns as a whole, teaching small changes (adding small amounts of complexity) to progressively challenge the exercise participant.

Sliding filament theory Explanation for how muscle contraction occurs via the interaction of action and myosin myofilament proteins and ATP.

Slow-to-fast teaching strategy Teaching strategy used to allow participants to learn complex movement at a slower pace, emphasizing proper placement or configuration of a movement pattern (e.g., teaching a movement at half-tempo).

Slow twitch (ST) fiber A muscle fiber type designed for use of aerobic glycolysis and fatty acid oxidation, recruited for low-intensity, longer-duration activities such as walking and swimming.

Soluble fiber Fiber that binds fluid to delay stomach emptying and glucose absorption, lower blood cholesterol, and aid against constipation.

Spatial teaching strategy Teaching strategy used when introducing participants to a new body position, involving describing the position of different portions of the body.

Specificity Exercise training principle explaining that specific exercise demands made on the body produce specific responses by the body; also called exercise specificity.

Sphincter A circular muscle whose function is constricting an opening.

Spinal bifida A defect in the arch of the vertebra that results in a failure to fuse; usually occurs at the base of the back or the lower spine.

Spinal cord injury A traumatic injury that damages or severs the spinal cord, causing paraplegia or quadriplegia, paralysis, or weakness in limbs.

Sprain Overstretching or tearing of a ligament and/or joint capsule, resulting in discoloration, swelling, and pain.

Standard of care Appropriateness of an exercise professional's actions in light of current professional standards and based on the age, condition, and knowledge of the participant.

Static stretching Holding a nonmoving (static) position to immobilize a joint in a position that places the desired muscles and connective tissues passively at their greatest possible length.

Statute of limitations A formal regulation limiting the period within which a specific legal action may be taken.

Steady state The term that describes the point at which the energy needs of the body during exercise are being met aerobically.

Step test (submaximal) A test for cardiovascular fitness that requires the subject to step up and down from a bench at a prescribed rate for a given period.

Strain Overstretching or tearing of a muscle or tendon.

Stress fracture An incomplete fracture caused by excessive stress (overuse) to a bone. Most common in the foot (metatarsal bones) and lower leg (tibia).

Stretch reflex An involuntary motor response that, when stimulated, causes a suddenly stretched muscle to respond with a corresponding contraction.

Stroke volume (SV) The amount (quantity) of blood pumped per heart beat.

Structured choreography A way of designing the cardiovascular segment of a class that uses formally arranged step patterns repeated in a predetermined order.

Subcutaneous fat Fatty deposits or fat pads of storage fat found under the skin.

Superior Located above.

Supination External rotation of the forearm (radioulnar joint) that causes the palm to face anteriorly.

Supine Face up.

Supine hypotension An abnormal reduction in blood pressure related to position (lying on the back).

Symphysis pubis The fibrocartilaginous joint between the pelvic bones in the midline of the body.

Syncopation A rhythmic device that temporarily shifts the normal pattern of stresses to unstressed beats or parts of beats.

Synergist A muscle that aids another muscle in its action.

Systolic blood pressure The force generated by the heart during its ventricular contractile phase (systole).

Tachycardia Elevated heart rate over 100 bpm.

Talk test A method for measuring exercise intensity using observation of respiration effort and the ability to talk while exercising.

Target heart rate (THR) Number of heartbeats per minute that indicate appropriate exercise intensity levels for each individual; also called training heart rate.

Target heart-rate range Exercise intensity that represents the minimum and maximum intensity for safe and effective exercise; also referred to as training zone.

Tempo The rate of speed of music, usually expressed in beats per minute.

Temporal pulse Pulse point located on either temple.

Tendinitis Inflammatory response to microtrauma from overuse of a tendon.

Tendon Thickened connective tissue at the ends of skeletal muscle that connects muscle to bone.

Tennis elbow Pain on the outside of the elbow at the attachment of the forearm muscles.

Teratogenic Non-genetic factors that can cause birth defects in the fetus.

Thermoregulation Regulation of the body's temperature.

Thoracic vertebrae The 12 vertebrae to which the ribs are attached.

Tibial stress syndrome *See* Shin splints.

Tidal volume Depth of breathing.

Total energy expenditure Amount of energy expended in a 24-hour period, which includes basal metabolism, physical activity, and dietary-induced thermogenesis.

Trace minerals Minerals required in very minute amounts for health.

Trans fatty acids Fatty acids created during hydrogenation that provoke heart disease.

Transient osteoporosis The temporary increase in the porosity of the bone as a result of dietary calcium deficiency.

Transverse plane Plane that divides the body into upper (superior) and lower (inferior) parts.

Triglycerides The form of 95% of diet fats and stored fats in adipose tissue, consisting of a glycerol backbone and three fatty acids.

Type 1 diabetes Type of diabetes mellitus caused by the non-functioning (destroyed) insulin producing beta cells in the pancreas; these diabetics produce little or no insulin and require daily insulin injections.

Type 2 diabetes The most common form of diabetes mellitus, resulting from an inability to use insulin produced by the pancreas because of the target cells' reduced sensitivity to insulin; may require insulin injections, oral medications, or simply diet modifications.

Unsaturated fats Fatty acids that contain double bonds between carbon atoms and thus are capable of absorbing more hydrogen; liquid at room temperature and usually of vegetable origin.

Upbeat The regular, weak pulsation in music occurring in a continuous pattern at an even rhythm.

Valsalva maneuver Holding the breath when a great deal of force is exerted (such as when lifting a very heavy weight), increasing thoracic pressure and possibly impeding venous blood return.

Value statement Feedback that projects a feeling about a performance, using words such as "good," "well done," or "poor job."

Vascular disturbances A disruption of circulation.

Vascularity An increase in the number and size of blood vessels enhancing blood supply and oxygen delivery to muscle cells.

Vasoconstriction Narrowing of the opening of blood vessels (notably the smaller arterioles) caused by contraction of the smooth muscle lining the vessels.

Vasodilation Widening of the openings of blood vessels caused by relaxation of the smooth muscle lining the vessels.

Veins Blood vessels that carry deoxygenated blood toward the heart from vital organs and the extremities.

Ventilation Rate and depth of breathing.

Ventricles The two lower chambers of the heart (right and left ventricles).

Venuoles Smaller divisions of veins.

Vertebrae Bones that form the spinal column.

Vital signs Measurable bodily functions, including pulse rate, respiratory rate, blood pressure, skin color, and temperature.

Vitamins Organic (carbon-containing) compounds required for optimal health that the body cannot manufacture on its own and must therefore be consumed.

VO$_2$ max *See* Maximal oxygen uptake.

Waiver Voluntary abandonment of a right to file suit.

Water The most important nutrient in the body responsible for all energy production, temperature control (especially during vigorous exercise), transportation of all nutrients and waste products in and out of the body, and lubrication of joints and other structures.

Water-soluble vitamins Vitamins that must be supplied daily, as the body excretes excess amounts (rather than storing them); includes vitamin C and the B complex vitamins.

Wolff's Law Principle stating that bone is capable of adjusting its strength in proportion to the amount of stress placed on it.

Index

A

inguinal, 259, 260, 267, 269, 270, 273
    joint, 13
    round, 259-60, 273
    talofibular, 287
lignins, 110
linea alba, 258, 259, 260, 267
linear momentum, 69
linear progression, 194-95
linoleic acid, 106
lipids, 104, 113
"little lat," 93
locomotion, 54, 76
log sheets, 216, 217, 221
long bones, 41, 42-43
    gross anatomy, 44
longissimus, 60, 83
lordosis, 71, 79, 80, 295
low back exercises,
    for pregnant women, 267
low back pain, 81, 229, 295-96
low-density lipoprotein (LDL)
    cholesterol, 113
lower extremity, movements and range of
    motion, 70
lower trapezius, 88
low-impact class, 152
low variability exercises, 236
lumbar lordosis, 262, 267
    in pregnancy, 271
lumbar plexus, 39
lumbar spine, 71, 151
    alignment, 78-79
lateral flexion, 78
    range of motion, 78
lumbar vertebrae, 45, 58
lumbosacral angle, 262
lunges, 76, 288
lungs, 37
lycopene, 111

M

MacLellan, M. A., 199
macronutrients, 101
Magill, R. A., 180
magnesium, 108, 109
mainstreaming, 182
maintenance, of strength, 13
manganese, 108, 109
marrow, 41
Martin, J. E., 220
maternal blood glucose, 255
maximal oxygen consumption ($\dot{V}O_2$ max),
    19, 20, 22, 164
    norms for men and women, 146, 147
measure, 192
mechanical energy, 99
medial compartment, of the thigh, 56, 57,
    59, 60
medial hip muscles, 74-75

mediastinum, 37
medical history, 128, 303
medical information release form, 135
medical insurance, 309
medical/physical examination, 133-36, 138
mediolateral axis, 49
medullary cavity, 42
megadoses, of micro-nutrients, 109
meniscus, 47, 291
menopause, 43, 44-45
metabolic equivalent (METs) system, 146-
    47
metabolism, 99
    and muscles, 6-8
metacarpals, 42
metatarsals, 42
meter, 192
micronutrients, 106-9
microphone, 199
middle deltoid, 91-92
middle trapezius, 88, 89, 90, 91
military press, 290
    seated, 92
mind-body classes, 273
minerals, 102, 103, 106, 107-9
mineral salts, 44
mirroring techniques, 197
mirrors, 143, 185
Missett, Judi Sheppard, 194
mitochondria, 6, 7, 17
modifications, 159, 160, 166, 284, 294
    of exercise intensity, 200
    for participants with injury limita-
        tions, 298
    for pregnant women, 273
molybdenum, 108
monosaccharides (single sugars), 101, 102
monoterpenes (polyphenols), 111
monounsaturated fats, 104-5, 114-15
Mosston, M., 188
motivation. *See* exercise adherence
motor domain, 181
motor end plate, 9
motor neurons, 8, 40
motor skill, 2
motor unit, 9, 13
movement
    biomechanical principals of, 68-70
    neurological factors affecting, 40-41
movement cues, 197
movement execution, 284, 298
movement pattern, 32-count, 193
mucilages, 110
mucous membrane, 37
multifidus muscles, 60
multilevel classes, 201
multiple sclerosis, 242-43
muscle balance, 78, 80-81, 167
    in pregnancy, 256-57
muscle cramps, in pregnancy, 264

muscle fiber distribution, 6-8
muscle groups, varying, 162
muscle "pull," 286
muscles, 46
    of the lower extremity, 54-61
    and metabolism, 6-8
    orientation, 73
    that act at the ankle and foot, 54-55,
        56
    that act at the elbow, 63, 65
    that act at the hip joint, 58-59, 59
    that act at the knee joint, 55-57, 58
    that act at the scapulothoracic artic-
        ulation, 67, 68
    that act at the shoulder joint, 63-66
    that act at the trunk, 59-61, 61
    that act at the wrist, 62-63, 64
    that need strengthening, 168
    that need stretching, 168
    of the upper extremity, 61-67
muscle spindle, 14, 15, 41
muscle tension, 10, 11
muscular contraction, types of, 10
muscular strength and endurance, 2, 11-
    13, 13
    program, 153, 167-70
    tests, 147
muscular system, 52-67
    basic organization of, 9-10
musculoskeletal injuries, 298
    factors associated with, 283-85
    general, 285-87
    specific, 287-95
    symptoms of, 282
    types of, 282-83
musculoskeletal system
    imbalances and dysfunctions during
        pregnancy, 256-64
    response to pregnancy, 253-54
music, 155
    beat, 192, 193
    in cardiorespiratory segments, 162-
        63
    and copyright law, 313
    in muscular strength and endurance
        segment, 170
    pitch control, 186
    selection of, 183, 192-94
    volume, 186
    in warm-up, 158-59
musical phrases, 192-93
myofibrils, 9, 12
myofilaments, 9
myosin, 9, 10, 12
myotatic stretch reflex, 171

N

nasal cavities, 37
National Academy of Science, 109

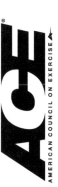

AMERICAN COUNCIL ON EXERCISE

YES, I would like to receive information on the following ACE certifications:

❏ Lifestyle & Weight Management Consultant   ❏ Personal Trainer
❏ Group Fitness Instructor   ❏ Clinical Exercise Specialist

Name _____

Address _____

City _____ State _____ ZIP _____

Home Phone (___) _____

Work Phone (___) _____

E-mail _____

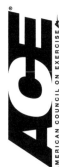

AMERICAN COUNCIL ON EXERCISE

YES, I would like to receive information on the following ACE certifications:

❏ Lifestyle & Weight Management Consultant   ❏ Personal Trainer
❏ Group Fitness Instructor   ❏ Clinical Exercise Specialist

Name _____

Address _____

City _____ State _____ ZIP _____

Home Phone (___) _____

Work Phone (___) _____

E-mail _____

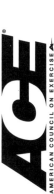

AMERICAN COUNCIL ON EXERCISE

YES, I would like to receive information on the following ACE certifications:

❏ Lifestyle & Weight Management Consultant   ❏ Personal Trainer
❏ Group Fitness Instructor   ❏ Clinical Exercise Specialist

Name _____

Address _____

City _____ State _____ ZIP _____

Home Phone (___) _____

Work Phone (___) _____

E-mail _____

AMERICAN COUNCIL ON EXERCISE

YES, I would like to receive information on the following ACE certifications:

❏ Lifestyle & Weight Management Consultant   ❏ Personal Trainer
❏ Group Fitness Instructor   ❏ Clinical Exercise Specialist

Name _____

Address _____

City _____ State _____ ZIP _____

Home Phone (___) _____

Work Phone (___) _____

E-mail _____

BUSINESS REPLY MAIL

FIRST-CLASS MAIL   PERMIT NO. 202113   SAN DIEGO CA

POSTAGE WILL BE PAID BY ADDRESSEE

AMERICAN COUNCIL ON EXERCISE®
PO BOX 910449
SAN DIEGO CA 92191-9961

NO POSTAGE
NECESSARY
IF MAILED
IN THE
UNITED STATES

BUSINESS REPLY MAIL

FIRST-CLASS MAIL   PERMIT NO. 202113   SAN DIEGO CA

POSTAGE WILL BE PAID BY ADDRESSEE

AMERICAN COUNCIL ON EXERCISE®
PO BOX 910449
SAN DIEGO CA 92191-9961

NO POSTAGE
NECESSARY
IF MAILED
IN THE
UNITED STATES

BUSINESS REPLY MAIL

FIRST-CLASS MAIL   PERMIT NO. 202113   SAN DIEGO CA

POSTAGE WILL BE PAID BY ADDRESSEE

AMERICAN COUNCIL ON EXERCISE®
PO BOX 910449
SAN DIEGO CA 92191-9961

NO POSTAGE
NECESSARY
IF MAILED
IN THE
UNITED STATES

BUSINESS REPLY MAIL

FIRST-CLASS MAIL   PERMIT NO. 202113   SAN DIEGO CA

POSTAGE WILL BE PAID BY ADDRESSEE

AMERICAN COUNCIL ON EXERCISE®
PO BOX 910449
SAN DIEGO CA 92191-9961

NO POSTAGE
NECESSARY
IF MAILED
IN THE
UNITED STATES